THE CHILD WITH DELAYED SPEECH

Clinics in Developmental Medicine No. 43

The Child with Delayed Speech

Edited by

MICHAEL RUTTER and J. A. M. MARTIN

1972

Spastics International Medical Publications

LONDON: William Heinemann Medical Books Ltd.

PHILADELPHIA: J. B. Lippincott Co.

ISBN O 433 20334 X

Reprinted 1977

Printed in England at THE LAVENHAM PRESS LTD., Lavenham, Suffolk.

Contents

Introduction

Inspired by the late Dr. Simon Yudkin, and generously financed by the Spastics Society in the United Kingdom, a group of interested physicians and others* have regularly met together over the past four or five years to discuss problems of children with speech and language disorders. We have met in various different centres and have benefited greatly from the actual practical experience of seeing cases with our colleagues and discussing their ways of handling these problems. Two years ago we ran a meeting for some eighty people in York when papers covering many aspects of the field were presented. This conference had been structured to illustrate some of the most important clinical issues, but the working party thought that a simple publication of the Conference proceedings would not be adequate. Instead we were asked to prepare a comprehensive introductory text suitable for the family doctor, paediatrician, child psychiatrist, ENT specialist and others struggling with the clinical problems presented by children with delayed speech development.

Our colleagues on the working party gave us an entirely free hand to proceed as we wished, and although about half of the papers presented here are based on those given at the original York Meeting, many of them have been freshly commissioned and written for this book. We believe that a clinician reading the book will get a useful introduction to this field, and some indications of where he might profitably extend his reading.

There is one particular subject which we have not covered, namely the place of education and the rôle of teachers in helping these children. It is clear that they bear the brunt of the work and all of us who are concerned with speech and language disorders should be acquainted with the techniques and methods that an experienced teacher will use to try and help the child to communicate and to learn in spite of his handicaps. To attempt to summarise these in a single chapter seemed impossible, so we decided to omit the field of education as a main topic for consideration. Nevertheless, we want to emphasise the need for all professionals involved in the care of children with speech and language disorders to know and to understand what teachers can do to help such children.

It is difficult to obtain a precise figure for the numbers of children with speech and language disorders. However, it is evident from the estimates given in chapter 4 that the problem is an important and large one. Far more attention needs to be paid to the early recognition of the problems and the treatment of these children. Although it is clear that the majority of children with speech delay do learn to talk and to communicate reasonably well, it is also clear that in some cases emotional, social and educational sequelae may remain if adequate treatment is not forthcoming. Delayed speech and language development may be of great significance to the whole future of the child. It is with this thought that we present this volume to the reader.

*See list of working party members overleaf.

Michael Rutter and J. A. M. Martin

CHAPTER 1

The Normal Development of Speech and Language

MICHAEL RUTTER and MARTIN BAX

In this chapter we give a rather didactic description of the normal development of speech and language which forms a basis from which to assess children who show deviation or retardation of development.*

Development is described longitudinally without a clear separation of the different aspects of language (phonetic, semantic, syntactic, etc.) This is because in the normal child these skills tend to develop in close conjunction with each other (Herriot 1970) and because they are not functionally independent. However, syntactical and semantic skills are not the same (Suci 1969) and particularly in cases of abnormal development they may progress at different rates. Because of this it is essential for each aspect of language to be assessed separately when a child is seen for suspected speech delay (see chapter 3).

Brain Development

The emergence of speech and language is dependent on a certain level of biological maturation, so that it is appropriate to start with a consideration of the relevant aspects of brain growth (Marshall 1968). At birth, the human brain is about a quarter of its adult weight but by the third birthday the brain is some four-fifths of adult weight. It is not only increase in weight that occurs after birth; neural structures grow considerably, there is more myelination, and the net of intercommunicating nerve fibres extends and becomes more complex. These microscopic changes are parallelled by alterations in the chemical composition of the brain.

It is important that different parts of the brain mature at different rates. Thus, the motor area advances more quickly than the sensory areas and the auditory association areas lag somewhat behind the visual. Whereas the study of brain structure indicates whether the brain *might* be functional, it cannot indicate whether the brain is in fact functioning. Nevertheless, these findings suggest that the infant's understanding of what he hears takes longer to develop than his appreciation of what he sees.

If the normal disparity in rates of development between different parts of the cortex were greater in some children than others, this might offer some clue as to why some children are so much behind in one aspect of development (such as speech) in spite of a normal rate of development in others. In addition, the neonatal brain is more susceptible to injury by virtue of its immaturity and rapid rate of growth, so that neurological sequelae following encephalitis are most common in the first months of life. However, so far as language is concerned, this vulnerability is to a great extent

---

*While the account is didactic it is based on extensive research evidence. As this has been considered in more detail in several lengthy reviews we have usually referred to the appropriate review rather than overload the chapter with references to the original research reports.

compensated for by the great plasticity of the immature brain. Accordingly, the effects of unilateral lesions in early childhood tend to be transient because the brain can transfer functions from one side to the other. This means that a persisting language impairment very rarely follows unilateral lesions (such as caused by a cerebral abscess) in the first few years of life. This is markedly different from the situation in adult life (Lenneberg 1967, Rutter *et al.* 1970).

Neonatal Period

Even *in utero* the fetus may kick or move in response to a loud noise and it has long been observed that neonates can respond to different sounds (Kessen *et al.* 1970). This is evident from observations that most newborn babies will blink to the sound of a tuning fork, turn their eyes or *condition* to sounds, and startle or still in response to whistles. Auditory evoked responses have also demonstrated neonatal auditory sensitivity. Experimental studies under laboratory conditions (Friedlander 1970) have shown not only that neonates can hear, but also that they can discriminate between different types of sounds (although this skill is crude compared with what they can do a few months later). However, these observations are difficult and time-consuming to make and ordinarily the clinician seeing a baby for a short time will be fortunate if he is able to positively identify responses to sound at this age. Both the differences in responsiveness due to the baby's state of arousal or wakefulness and the complexity of most natural stimuli make this differentiation problematic. A mother's voice may seem to sooth a baby when he is disturbed, but if this involves him being picked up, other sensations of smell, touch, temperature and kinaesthetic sense may all play a part in helping him to settle.

In the neonatal period, crying constitutes the main type of sounds produced by babies. The ability to cry actually precedes birth as shown by the presence of intrauterine crying. Recent studies by Wolff (1969) and by Wasz-Höckert and his colleagues (1968) have shown that there are several distinct types of cry (such as those reflecting pain, hunger or pleasure) with definable accoustic characteristics. Another interesting feature of the newborn's cry is the fact that the mother is able to identify her baby's cry when the baby is still at a very early age.

Abnormal cries have also been described and these occur when parts of the brain are damaged or stressed. The most easily distinguishable is that associated with the rare 'cri du chat' syndrome, and other examples are the short shrill cry of the brain-damaged infant and the low-pitched cry of the infant with Down's syndrome.

The First Year

During the first few months of life there is a marked development in the baby's ability to make fine auditory discriminations (Friedlander 1970). At 20 weeks babies can discriminate between phonemes as similar as 'p' and 't', 'b' and 'g', or 'i' and 'a'. By their first birthday, before they can speak, babies will not only discriminate but will respond to language differences which concern who is speaking, the intonation used, vocabulary and amount of repetitiveness in what is said. This has been shown, for example, by the 'Playtest' equipment, in which the baby can operate switches controlling a loudspeaker and a stereotape player with a pre-programmed selection of

2

two channel tapes. By the baby's differential playing (electrically recorded) of the two tapes it can be shown that he responds to differences, such as between flat and bright intonation and between conversations of high and low redundancy. Of course, it is not possible in studies of very young babies to be sure how much the infant *understands* (as distinct from differentiates) in what is said to him. However, it is clear that toddlers and young children will often understand words or phrases said to them well before they can produce the words themselves. Language comprehension normally precedes language production (Fraser *et al.* 1963, Lovell and Dixon 1967) and the process of developing an understanding of language begins in infancy well before speech emerges.

Babies show an extraordinary interest in language even when this consists of a disembodied voice coming out of a loudspeaker with no surplus stimulus cues such as facial expression or physical contact. The amount babies vocalise, too, is much affected by what they hear (see chapter 5), and parental interaction with children during these early months is most important.

The successful development of speech requires that the child's ability to hear and to listen has developed normally during the first year of life. A child's turning response to his mother's voice is the best confirmation of the integrity of the auditory apparatus during the first year. By 5 or 6 months, babies will clearly turn to soft sounds made some 18 to 24 inches from their right or left ear. The efficient localisation of sound may develop in one side before the other.

Features of the child's response to sound at 6 months often show how sounds become linked to other aspects of personal interaction. The child may fail to respond to a quiet 'th' or 'sss' made behind his line of vision. If the examiner then comes back in front of the baby he can quickly condition a response. He smiles at the baby and makes the requisite noise; the baby smiles in return. The examiner then retreats behind the baby and makes the same noise; the baby turns smiling towards him. The baby has associated the friendly face with the sound and displays not only a simple hearing response but also a social response to the human face.

At about 7 months there is much variation in infants' responses to a sound made at an angle of 45° to the head. Frequently there is a horizontal turning of the head followed by a vertical movement to locate the source of sound. The eyes, too, play a part here, but at around 10 to 12 months direct localisation to the sound will often be noted. Even so, the variation in the rate at which children develop is large and some 5-year-olds still have difficulty immediately locating sounds made directly above their heads.

Vocalisations develop greatly during the first year (McCarthy 1954, Murphy 1964, Ervin-Tripp 1966, Rebelsky *et al.* 1967). In the initial weeks, respiration and feeding activities are mixed with other vocalisations such as the cry, yawn, sneeze, gurgle, belch and cough. During the early months crying gradually decreases in frequency and cooing increases with the production of vowel sounds from the front of the mouth, such as 'oo', and then middle vowels like 'ugh' or 'agh'. Back vowels take longer to develop. The back consonants ('g', 'k' and 'r') appear quite early in connection with swallowing and belching, but their emergence is mainly a transient phase and during the first 3 months vowel sounds predominate. By 4 to 6 months, lip and tongue consonants are developing with the production of sounds like 'ébé', 'pth', and 'élé', but there is often still much 'singing' with 'àaa', 'aàa', 'aaà' like vowel sounds.

The young child's understanding of gesture is developing at the same time and frequently he can respond to and wave 'bye-bye' before he can say it. The normal child often uses gestures to communicate for a brief period before he can communicate in words. This tendency is much more marked in twins and triplets or when speech is retarded, but will not occur if the neural structures underlying the relevant linguistic and cognitive functions are not intact.

The first meaningful words normally appear at about 12 months of age, but there is considerable variation so that in some 5 per cent of children this occurs by 8 months, and in another 5 per cent it does not occur until after 18 months (Morley 1965). At the same time as the first words are being spoken the child is also likely to be using long 'sentence' patterns of sounds with complex inflections and intonations. Murphy (1964) noted how children may string words together with a litanical quality; for example, saying over and over 'dinkie', 'wee-wee', 'potty', in a way that gradually rises to a crescendo. At this age (around the first birthday) the child often does not seem to know to whom he is talking or whether he is being listened to. He just talks for himself in what Piaget (1926) termed 'egocentric' speech. Words may be used to attract attention, to play with sounds or to accompany action, as well as to communicate. The way language develops is dependent not only on language competence but also on the child's general level of cognition and social maturity.

The Second Year
At the beginning of the second year, after a gap of a month or so following the first meaningful word, there is a gradual increase in vocabulary which markedly accelerates from about 18 months so that by 2 years of age the average child will understand several hundred words and regularly use some 200. However, as with nearly all aspects of speech development, there is very wide individual variations and a few normal children may use only a dozen or so words by their second birthday. Data are lacking, but it is likely that the variation in *understanding* of words is less than the variation in production. The great majority of the first words learned are nouns and the main speech activity is naming objects and, a bit later, pictures in a book. At first, words may have a very restricted meaning so that 'doggie' is used only to refer to one particular pet; gradually its use is extended to other living dogs, and then to miniature toy dogs and finally to semi-impressionistic artists' drawings in his picture books. However, just as often the converse applies so that a word may start with a very general meaning before it becomes specific. Thus, 'dog' may be applied to all animals to begin with and only after the word 'cat' is appreciated is it restricted to canines.

A child's first words are little more than reflex responses to an object but particularly during the latter half of the second year he develops a flexibility in the use of words that indicates the beginnings of true language. This may be apparent in several different ways. The child may learn to use familiar words for objects never seen before. Having learned 'dog' with respect to his family's tiny short-haired toy terrier, he will also use 'dog' when he first encounters a strange large long-haired Afghan hound. Or

4

he may start using words to ask for some object which he wants and which is not present. Lewis (1951) gives the example of a child who was in the habit of naming each item on the table as he sat down to breakfast. One morning after his usual recital he noted that his favourite honey was missing. In a few moments he pointed to the closed cupboard in which honey was kept and called 'Ha-a'—his word for honey. This first progression from reflex labelling to symbolic naming was the beginning of language.

Even during this early stage of single word utterances, words are used in different ways to convey a variety of meanings (Lenneberg 1967). Thus, 'Daddy' may be said with distinctive intonation patterns to mean 'Daddy, I want this', 'Daddy, come here', 'Daddy, what is that?' or 'Look, there's Daddy'. This observation has led some workers to regard single word utterances as primitive syntactic units—in a sense the beginning of early sentence formation.

After words have first appeared, but before phrases are used, there is an intermediate stage when words may be linked in a fixed way such as 'go-now' or 'get-down' as if they were single words and without the child realising that he is using a combination of words. The child begins to use word combinations about the time of his second birthday. To begin with these may consist merely of phrases he has heard from his parents but soon he is using new phrases in a new way that he has never heard before. Having learned what 'bye-bye' means he may apply it in novel ways such as 'bye-bye car' to indicate that the car has gone, or 'bye-bye milk' to show that he has finished his drink. Braine (1963) has divided words into two classes, 'pivot' and 'open'. Pivots are descriptive words (such as 'bye-bye' in the above examples) that can be linked with a wide range of other words in the open class (such as 'car' and 'milk' in the same examples). Typically, a child has many words in the open class but only a few in the pivot class. While this distinction is an over-simplification (Huxley 1969), it is useful in showing how children learn *language* (which they can use in an infinite variety of ways) rather than just a fixed number of phrases copied from others (McNeill 1970). This is evident from the rapid rise in word combinations (from 14 to over 2,500 over a period of 6 months in one child studied), by the fact that children use word combinations that they could never have heard, and from the observation that the combinations follow certain rules. Thus, it appears that pivot words almost never occur in combination with one another. Unfortunately, it is hard to back-up this last statement as it is not always easy to recognise the pivot of the two-word utterance and we cannot always be sure how to characterise the sentence grammatically (Lenneberg 1967).

Following the use of nouns, verbs increase in frequency, as do adjectives and adverbs. By the second birthday, the proportion of nouns used is falling as a function of the greater use of other parts of speech. Pronouns generally appear just before 2 years and prepositions just after. Conjunctions are rare before 30 months (McCarthy 1930).

During the second year, children's understanding of language markedly increases so that they are able not only to respond to single words, but are able to understand and follow simple instructions to perform common actions, to get up or sit down, or to fetch something which is in sight. The child is all the time listening to the speech around him, understanding more and more of adult conversation, as well as gaining information and following straightforward instructions. He is taught nursery rhymes and his enjoyment of their rhythm and simple language helps to reinforce basic speech patterns. Oft-repeated stories, too, add their share to the building-up of language skills.

Those aspects of play which reflect language also develop in striking fashion (Sheridan 1969). Early in the second year infants begin to use common objects (such as a hairbrush or a cup and saucer) in a way that indicates an understanding of their use and function. Some months later the child will extend functional play to involve dolls and large toys and, by his second birthday, he may be expected to use miniature toys in similar fashions. This may be readily observed in the doctor's office by giving the child the appropriate play material and seeing what he does with it. For example, placing a miniature baby doll in a cot from a set of dolls' house furniture, 'bathing' a doll in the toy bath, pushing a toy car, 'talking' into a toy telephone, or pouring an imaginary cup of tea using a toy tea set would all indicate appreciation of functions and the beginnings of imaginative play. The development of play reflects the growth of 'inner language' which constitutes an essential element in the emergence of spoken language.

The first half of the second year is also the time when imitative gestural games such as 'peek-a-boo', 'bye-bye' and 'pat-a-cake' are prominent features of the child's activities. The linguistic function of gestural imitation is unclear but these activities have a communicative purpose and are usually impaired in cases of severe global language retardation.

Two to Five Years

During the pre-school years following the child's second birthday there is a tremendous upsurge in the child's competence in all aspects of speech and language. Vocabulary increases from some 200 words to several thousand and the length of the average utterance rises by about one word per year, from just less than 2 words at 2 years to just less than 5 words at 5 years (McCarthy 1954). The average age of first using two word phrases is 18 months and by two years of age nearly 90 per cent are using at least simple word sequences (Morley 1965). The way words are used also changes. Exclamatory remarks decrease and questions increase. At 2 years most questions are of the 'What?' variety, by 3 years 'Where?' and 'Who?' queries are becoming more prominent, and 4 is the age of asking 'Why?' (Watts 1947). While questions are frequently used to seek information, it is obvious that many times questions are asked to which the child already knows the answers. It seems that he is mainly concerned to hear how the adult formulates a reply; perhaps he is seeking information about language rather than about any object or event. In the same way toddlers spend a lot of time talking to themselves—partly as an accompaniment of games but sometimes as little more than a play with words, practising different word combinations and different ways of saying things. This is well illustrated in Weir's study (1962) of the pre-sleep monologues of a 30-month-old child.

At the same time as vocabulary and utterance length are increasing, sentences are becoming more often functionally and structurally complete, and more often complex or compound (about 6-7 per cent by the time of starting school). Adverbial clauses are heard but are never common. Prepositions first start being used about the age of 2 and increase in frequency over the next couple of years; conjunctions first appear after about 30 months and the definite and indefinite articles ('the' and 'a') are increasingly used. To begin with children tend to refer to themselves by name, but soon personal pronouns are accurately used.

A child's first sentences are telegrammatic, containing only the key words and none of the connecting words. He may say 'go shops' to mean 'Can we go to the shops?' or 'I am going to the shops'. Connecting words are introduced during the second year but the use of different tenses takes longer. The present tense is used first, the future tense becomes common after the third birthday, and the past tense follows shortly after.

When children are first learning to speak they frequently go through a stage when they often echo the last few words of whatever is said to them (Fay 1967). Sometimes the exact words are repeated, but sometimes the words are slightly altered or added to. For example, in response to the question 'What did my dog do?' the child might reply 'your dog do', indicating some measure of understanding. Pure echolalia (and, to a lesser extent, mitigated echolalia) is a function of poor understanding of language (Fay and Butler 1968). In children with *language* retardation, echolalia is much more persistent than in normal children, but there is no association between echolalia and speech articulation. In normal children, echolalia generally does not persist beyond 30 months.

As children grow older, speech becomes more specific. As vocabulary increases, the word 'it' is used less, being replaced by common or proper nouns. Quantitative expressions such as 'some', 'any' or 'several' are used more and children become both more precise and more detailed in their response to questions.

Exactly how words are learned is not known, but it is evident that the process involves meaning and understanding rather than mere reflex associative learning (Morton 1971). The ease with which a word is recognised when it is flashed on a screen for a very brief period is a function of how often the word occurs in the language. Accordingly, common words like 'table' and 'car' are more easily recognised than the less frequent 'cable' and 'tar', although phonetically they are similar. The importance of what words mean is well shown by two experimental findings. First, the recall of adverbs derived from adjectives (*e.g.* 'quickly') is a function of the frequency of usage of the adjectives from which the words were derived, and not the words themselves. Second, the recognition (when flashed briefly on a screen) of words such as 'bark' with two distinct meanings (of the tree and of the dog) is a function of how often each *meaning* occurs in the language, and not the frequency of the word itself. In other words, 'bark' is recognised at a threshold appropriate for its use for *one* meaning, a threshold only half that appropriate for the frequency with which the word itself occurs in the language. Phonetically, 'bark' is one word, but linguistically it is two, and learning involves linguistic rather than phonetic units.

At the same time as children are learning new words their articulation of these words is steadily improving. Some two thirds of children are easily intelligible from the beginnings of speech, but one third go through a phase when they cannot be under-

7

stood. In the Newcastle study, 69 per cent were intelligible to strangers by two years of age and 84 per cent by three years of age (Morley 1965). However, 4 per cent were still unintelligible on entry to school at five years. The assessment of phonological maturation is best done by examining children's pronunciation of consonants in view of the marked regional variations with respect to vowels (Anthony *et al.* 1971). Some consonants appear correctly much earlier than others (the timing also depends on whether the consonant is at the beginning, middle or end of a word). These phonetic studies indicate that the sounds 'd', 'p', 't', 'h', 'l', 'm', 'k', 'n', hard 'g' and 'ing' are usually correctly articulated by 3 or $3\frac{1}{2}$ years; 'br', 'mm', 'fl', 'r', soft 'g', 'pl', 'v' and 'y' are generally right by 5 or $5\frac{1}{2}$ years, but 'sh', 'cl', 'ds', 's', 'ch', 'sm', 'sp', 'str', 'sk' are often incorrect until well after the child starts school, and 'th' sounds take longest of all to develop.* To the untrained observer, approximations to these sounds are often heard early.

Usually children can perceive linguistically significant contrasts and distinctions before they can produce them correctly (de Hirsch 1970). However, there is a complex relationship between perception and articulation and discrimination errors may sometimes be the result rather than the cause of misarticulation.

It is said that the essence of language lies in the development of grammar and certainly syntactical development has been the chief preoccupation of psycholinguists in recent years. Between 2 and 4 years the child learns most of the principal grammatical rules. It is important to note that children do learn *rules*, not just specific grammatical constructions (Brown and Bellugi 1964). This can be shown by their ability to apply rules to nonsense words (Berko 1958, Blake and Williams 1968). For example, a child may be shown a picture of a bird-like object and then a picture of two of them. He is told 'This is a *wug*. Now there is another one. There are two of them. There are two ....'. Children will reply 'wugs' although they have never heard the word before. Their ability to transform verbs into the past tense can be assessed by showing them a picture of a man performing some odd action and saying 'This is a man who knows how to *bip*. He is *bipping*. He did the same thing yesterday. What did he do yesterday? Yesterday he ....'.

Children's possession of grammatical rules is also shown by their production of phrases and constructions that they are most unlikely to have heard—such as those involving grammatical rules wrongly generalised (*e.g.* 'I digged a hole' or 'I breaked a cup'). Their use of indefinite articles often involves similar effects. Thus, they learn that you must put 'a' before a noun, and so use phrases like 'a Jimmy' or 'fix a Lassie' (which neglect the exception that the indefinite article is not used for proper nouns) or 'a your ear' or 'a my pencil' (neglecting the further exceptions that the indefinite article is not placed before possessive pronouns), or 'a hands' or 'a shoes' (neglecting the exception that the indefinite article is not put before plurals). What is important in these examples is not that the child used incorrect grammar but rather that he had learned syntactical principles which he was applying to new words. The process to be

---

*Of course, there is no one-to-one connection between these letters and the sounds they are meant to represent; amongst other things their pronunciation depends on the position within the word. However, as most readers will not be familiar with the international phonetic alphabet this representation is thought more appropriate.

explained is the acquisition of rules (exactly what the rules are is still uncertain) rather than the learning of particular items of speech in rote fashion.

The traditional grammar of nouns, verbs and adjectival clauses is of very little help in understanding linguistic development and psycholinguists have developed new ways of studying grammar (Huxley 1969). Chomsky has emphasised the need to study what children know of language (their competence) rather than merely what they say and he has suggested that grammar is best considered in terms of its *deep* structure (see Herriot 1970 for a clear exposition of Chomsky's views). For example, 'John is eager to please' and 'John is easy to please' have a similar surface structure but in the former 'John' is the subject of the sentence in the deep structure and in the latter the object of the verb. This deep structure grammar is based on phrase structure rules and transformational rules. Transformational rules reveal the relations between different sentences expressing the same idea. For example, 'The window was broken by the brush', 'Did the brush break the window?' and 'Wasn't the window broken by the brush?' are all transformations of 'The brush broke the window'. The first is a passive transformation, the second a question transformation and so forth. The essence of Chomsky's theories is that grammar should describe not just the sentences that have occurred, but all sentences that could occur in a language. This notion remains valid, and his suggestions on what sort of rules might underlie the development of grammar have stimulated much research and put new life into the study of language. Unfortunately, the specifics of his views have not survived the test of experiment. It no longer seems likely that the number of transformations is a valid index of the difficulty of processing sentences and it appears that grammar cannot be regarded as totally independent of meaning (Herriot 1970, Morton 1971) as Chomsky claimed. Even the notion of deep structure has come under criticism (Olson 1970).

Nevertheless, the distinction between childrens' understanding of language (competence) and their speech (performance) remains valid. It is also true that what has to be explained is the acquisition of grammatical *rules*. But it has to be accepted that we still do not know what are the rules that are learned and even less about how they are learned. Parents seem to pay little attention to correcting children's grammar (more attention is paid to the truth of what is said and correct pronunciation), and it appears that somehow children must extract these rules by paying attention to what they hear. The capacity to do this is a distinctively human characteristic although it is possible that primitive rudiments of grammar may be learned by chimpanzees (Gardner and Gardner 1969, Premack 1971).

Five Years Onwards

Whereas most of the main principles of grammar have been learned by age 5 years, considerable linguistic development continues to take place after the child starts school (Chomsky 1969, Kessel 1970). A child's understanding of the complexities of language increases in relation to his ability to make abstractions. This emphasises that language cannot be considered as independent of general cognitive development (see chapter 15). The development of language during the school years has largely been studied by examining children's responses to structural ambiguities (as for example in the sentences 'They fed her dog biscuits', where the meaning is

9

dependent on whether the pause comes before or after 'dog', or 'He told her baby stories' when the same applies with respect to 'baby'). The distinction between 'tell' and 'ask' has also been used as an indicator of language competence. For example, children may be given a set of 4 pictures which show various types of interaction between a boy and a girl. The child has to decide which correctly represents the sentence 'The boy asks the girl what toothpaste to use' (in which case the boy should be cleaning his teeth), or 'The boy tells the girl what toothpaste to use' (in which case the girl should be doing so). At the present time, knowledge on these later stages of language development is too fragmentary to allow any succinct conclusions, but it is evident that after 5 years, children's ability to use language continues to develop and, in particular, the involvement of language in cognition and thought processes becomes more secure.

Sex Differences

Numerous studies have shown that girls are slightly more advanced than boys in language development (McCarthy 1954, Rebelsky *et al.* 1967), a difference that parallels the greater maturity of girls in all aspects of physical development (Rutter 1970). However, the sex difference in rate of language development is quite small and largely confined to the later stages of development. Indeed, what is striking is that the sex difference is so small within the normal range in view of the fact that marked *delays* in development are so much commoner in boys than girls (Ingram 1959, 1969).

Probably, the difference in rate of development is less important than the evidence pointing to possible sex differences in the *pattern* of language development. In girls, pre-speech babbling and attention to sounds at 6 months is of some value in predicting speech development, whereas it is much less so in boys. Similarly, girls' use and understanding of words at 18 months gives a fair prediction of their verbal skills at 8 years, whereas this long-term prediction is not possible in boys (Moore 1967). The sex difference applies also in the relation between early speech and later intelligence. Why this should be so is not known. It may relate to sex differences in early interest patterns, to differences in cultural expectations, to biological differences in sensitivities to auditory and visual stimuli or to the much wider variation in rate of development in boys than in girls. It may also be a function of sex differences in response to environmental stresses and deprivations. Boys appear more vulnerable to psychological stress than are girls and certainly they are more susceptible to biologic hazards (Tanner 1962, Rutter 1970). How far these apply to environmental influences in language development is uncertain, but the issue requires more attention than it has generally received in the past.

Conclusions

For the sake of simplicity, in this chapter language development has been described in isolation from other aspects of the developmental process. Language is a cognitive skill with affective components which performs a communicative function in a social context. Accordingly, delay or distortion in these other features of a child's development is likely to influence the emergence of language and, conversely, retardation of language will affect other aspects of psychological development (see chapter

15). While language development proceeds on the basis of biological maturation, it is inevitably much influenced by the child's life experiences (see chapter 5). While it is helpful to try and break down function to analyse individual components, this isolation is artificial, and 'real life' development is more complex and involves simultaneous development along all the integrated parameters.

REFERENCES

Anthony, N., Bogle, D., Ingram, T. T. S., McIsaac, M. W. (1971) *The Edinburgh Articulation Test.* Edinburgh: Churchill-Livingstone.

Berko, J. (1958) 'The child's learning of English morphology.' *Word*, **14**, 150.

Blake, K. A., Williams, C. L. (1968) *Use of English Morphemes by Retarded, Normal and Superior Children Equated for CA.* Athens, Georgia: University of Georgia Press.

Braine, M. D. S. (1963) 'The ontogeny of phrase structure: the first phrase.' *Language*, **39**, 1.

Brown, R., Bellugi, U. (1964) 'Three processes in the child's acquisition of syntax.' *Harvard Educ. Rev.*, **34**, 133.

Chomsky, C. (1969) 'The acquisition of syntax in children from 5 to 10'. *in Aspects of the Theory of Syntax.* Cambridge, Mass.: M.I.T. Press.

Ervin-Tripp, S. (1966) 'Language development.' *in* Hoffman, L. W., Hoffman, M. L. (Eds.) *Review of Child Development Research*, Vol. 2. New York: Russell Sage Foundation. p. 55.

Fay, W. H. (1967) 'Childhood echolalia: a group study of late abatement.' *Folia phoniat.* (*Basel*), **19**, 297.

—— Butler, B. V. (1968) 'Echolalia, IQ and the developmental dichotomy of speech and language systems.' *J. speech Res.*, **11**, 365.

Fraser, C., Bellugi, U., Brown, R. (1963) 'Control of grammar in imitation, comprehension and production.' *J. verbal Learning.* **2**, 121.

Friedlander, B. Z. (1970) 'Receptive language development in infancy: issues and problems.' *Merrill -Palmer Quart.*, **16**, 7.

Gardner, R. A., Gardner, B. T. (1969) 'Teaching sign language to a chimpanzee.' *Science*, **165**, 664.

Herriott, P. (1970) *An Introduction to the Psychology of Language.* London: Methuen.

de Hirsch, K. (1970) 'A review of early language development.' *Develop. Med. Child Neurol.* **12**, 87.

Huxley, R. (1969) 'Research in language development.' *in* Wolff, P. H., Mac Keith, R. (Eds.) *Planning for Better Learning.* Clinics in Developmental Medicine, No. 33. London: S.I.M.P. with Heinemann. p. 77.

Ingram, T. T. S. (1959) 'Specific developmental disorders of speech in childhood.' *Brain*, **82**, 450.

—— (1969) 'Developmental disorders of speech.' *in* Vincken, P. J., Bruyn, G. W. (Eds.) *Handbook of Clinical Neurology*, Vol. 4. Amsterdam: North Holland. p.407

Kessel, F. S. (1970) 'The role of syntax in children's comprehension from ages six to twelve.' *Monogr. Soc. Res. Child. Develop*, **35**, (6).

Kessen, W., Haith, M. M., Salapatek, P. H. (1970) 'Infancy.' *in* Mussen, P. H. (Ed.) *Carmichael's Manual of Child Psychology*, Vol.1, 3rd edn. New York: Wiley, p. 447.

Lenneberg, E. H. (1967) *Biological Foundations of Language.* New York: Wiley.

Lewis, M. M. (1951) *Infant Speech.* London: Harrap.

Lovell, K., Dixon, E. M. (1967) 'The growth of the control of grammar in imitation, comprehension and production.' *J. Child. Psychol. Psychiat.*, **8**, 31.

McCarthy, D. (1930) *The Language Development of the Preschool Child.* Institute of Child Welfare Monograph Series, No.4. Minneapolis: University of Minnesota Press.

—— (1954) 'Language development in children.' *in* Carmichael, L. (Ed.) *Manual of Child Psychology.* 2nd edn. London: Chapman & Hall. p. 492.

McNeill, D. (1970) 'The development of language.' *in* Mussen, P. H. (Ed.) *Carmichael's Manual of Child Psychology*, 3rd edn., Vol. 1. New York: Wiley, p. 1061.

Marshall. W. A. (1968) *Development of the Brain.* Edinburgh: Oliver & Boyd.

Moore, T. (1967) 'Language and intelligence: a longitudial study of the first eight years Part 1. Patterns of development in boys and girls.' *Hum. Develop.*, **10**, 88.

Morley, M. E. (1965) *The Development and Disorders of Speech in Childhood.* 2nd edn. Edinburgh: E. & S. Livingstone.

Morton, J. (1971) 'Psycholinguistics.' *Brit. med. Bull.*, **27**, 195.

Murphy, K. (1964) 'Development of normal vocalisation and speech'. *in* Renfrew, C., Murphy, K. (Eds.) *The Child who does not Talk.* Clinics in Developmental Medicine, No. 13. London: S.I.M.P. with Heinemann, p. 11.

Olson, D. R. (1970) 'Language and thought: aspects of a cognitive theory of semantics.' *Psychol. Rev.* **77**, 257.

Piaget, J. (1926) *The Language and Thought of the Child.* New York: Harcourt, Brace.

11

Premack, D. (1971) 'Language in chimpanzee?' *Science*. **172**, 808.

Rebelsky, F., Starr, R. H., Zella, L. (1967) 'Language development: the first four years.' *in* Brackbill, Y. (Ed.) *Infancy and Early Childhood*. London: Collier-Macmillan. p. 289.

Rutter, M. (1970) 'Sex differences in children's responses to family stress.' *in* Anthony, E. J., Koupernick, C. (Eds.) *The Child and his Family*. New York: Wiley, p. 165.

—— Graham, P., Yule, W. (1970) *A Neuropsychiatric Study in Childhood*. Clinics in Developmental Medicine, Nos. 35/36. London: S.I.M.P. with Heinemann.

Sheridan, M. (1969) 'Playthings in the development of language.' *Hlth. Trends* **1**, 7.

Suci, G. J. (1969) 'Relations between syntactic and syntactic factors in the structuring of language.' *Lang. Speech*, **12**, 69.

Tanner, J. (1962) *Growth at Adolescence*. 2nd edn. Oxford: Blackwell.

Wasz-Höckert, O., Lind, J., Vuorenkoski, V., Partanen, T., Valanne, E. (1968) *The Infant Cry: A Spectrographic and Auditory Analysis*. Clinics in Developmental Medicine, No. 29. London: S.I.M.P. with Heinemann.

Watts, A. F. (1947) *Language and Mental Development of Children*. London: Harrap.

Weir, R. H. (1962) *Language in the Crib*. The Hague: Mouton.

Wolff, P. H. (1969) 'The natural history of crying and other vocalisations in early infancy.' *in* Foss, B. M. (Ed.) *Determinants of Infant Behaviour*, Vol. 4. London: Methuen. p. 81.

CHAPTER 2

The Classification of Speech and Language Disorders in Young Children

T. T. S. INGRAM

Disorders of speech in childhood should be classified according to linguistic and phonetic criteria. A number of useful and appropriate quantitative and qualitative tests of articulation are now available. Close study of the results of these may reveal patterns of sound substitutions which may be very idiosyncratic but which are consistent in an individual child.

Linguistic studies of the developing speech of the young child are much less complete than those of articulatory development, and a satisfactory theoretical framework on which to base a classification of language disorders in childhood has yet to be devised. Nevertheless, there are encouraging signs that linguists are becoming increasingly interested in children with language disorders (Huxley 1969). In the future it is to be hoped that classification will primarily be on the basis of linguistic and phonetic criteria, but at present this is impossible. In these circumstances, a classification based on the major function of speech which is disordered and associated clinical findings is justifiable for practical purposes, and this has been in use in Edinburgh since 1956 (Ingram 1959a, Table I).

TABLE I

Clinical classification of speech disorders in childhood

(1)   Disorders of voicing (dysphonia)
(2)   Disorders of respiratory co-ordination (dysrhythmia)
(3)   Disorders of speech sound production with demonstrable dysfunction
      or structural abnormalities of tongue, lips, teeth or palate (dysarthria)
      (a) Due to neurological abnormalities
               upper motor neurone lesions
               nuclear agenesis
               lower motor neurone lesions
               abnormal movement patterns
      (b) Due to local abnormalities
               jaws and teeth
               tongue
               lips
               palate
               pharynx
               mixed
(4)   Disorders of speech sound production not attributable to dysfunction or
      structural abnormality of tongue, lips, teeth or palate, but associated
      with other disease or adverse environmental factors (secondary speech
      disorders)
      (a) Associated with mental defect
      (b) Associated with hearing defect
      (c) Associated with true dysphasia
      (d) Associated with psychiatric disorders
      (e) Associated with adverse environmental factors
               (combinations of the above)
(5)   The developmental speech disorder syndrome
      (specific developmental speech disorders)
(6)   Mixed speech disorders comprising two or more of the above categories

Inevitably, since this is clinically orientated, it is more likely to appeal to paediatricians and other clinicians than to phoneticians and linguists.

The disorders of speech will be considered in turn. It will be noted that the first category 'Dysphonia' deals with disorders of the voice. The second category 'Speech Dysrhythmia' deals with disorders of the co-ordination of respiratory movements and speech and the third category 'Dysarthria' with disorders of articulation. The fourth category 'Secondary Speech Disorders' consists of an assortment of disorders of articulation and language which are secondary to disease not directly affecting the structure or function of the lips, tongue and palate, and the fifth category consists of what I have called 'Developmental Speech Disorder Syndrome' (Ingram 1959b). The sixth category consists of 'Mixed Speech Disorders' in which more than one type of speech disorder is present. For example, a child with cleft palate may also suffer from the effects of hearing loss and mental retardation which cause secondary speech disorders, in addition to dysarthria attributable to his cleft palate.

Dysphonia

Dysphonia implies loss of voice and is characterised by hoarseness. It affects girls more often than boys and in most hospital speech clinics accounts for 3 to 4 per cent of children referred. Characteristically, the voice is more normal when the child tries to shout than when he tries to talk at a normal volume (Greene 1964).

The commonest cause of dysphonia in childhood is chronic or recurrent laryngitis which often dates from infancy. Associated with this is often a history that the child has always had a marked tendency to shout rather than to speak in a normal voice. This history seems to be particularly common in dysphonic children who come from large families. It is sometimes very difficult to know whether their shouting is a result of the dysphonia or a cause of it. Since the prevalence of shouting, large families and upper respiratory tract infections in early life are all more common in social classes 4 and 5 than in the upper social classes, it is hardly surprising that dysphonia tends to occur more frequently in the lower social classes.

Parents commonly report that the dysphonic voice of their child varies in quality and loudness from day to day and even from hour to hour. Usually the voice is more normal first thing in the morning and deteriorates as the end of the day is reached.

On examination, low grade inflammatory changes are frequently found, often with nodules on the vocal cords.

Treatment is difficult, especially in young children, for rest of the voice is required and, if there is evidence of infection, antibiotics should be given for a prolonged period. Rest of the voice may be necessary for as long as six to eight weeks and it is virtually impossible to achieve this, even in hospital conditions, until the child is 7 or 8 years of age. Removal of nodules from the cords does not appear to be of great therapeutic value. Papillomata are multiple tumours within the larynx which may cause dysphonia. These tumours very rarely become malignant, but their removal may be followed by a considerable improvement in the voice and, in view of this, all children with dysphonia lasting more than a week or two, and not directly related to acute upper respiratory tract infection, should be subjected to laryngoscopy (Birrell 1954).

Speech Dysrhythmia in Childhood

Speech dysrhythmia implies that there is an inco-ordination between respiratory and articulatory function. This disturbance may cause prolongation of word sounds, arrest or 'blocking' of speech, most often at the beginning of sentences, or repetitive stammer or stutter.

It has been pointed out by a number of authors that some degree of speech dysrhythmia is physiological. If one listens to the speech of apparently normal adults, a high proportion of their utterances consist of hesitations, repetitions, and various other 'non-fluencies' (Johnson 1955, van Riper 1957). It has been suggested that the differences between patients who stammer and normal adults is more to do with the patient's awareness of the characteristics of his speech than the actual characteristics themselves (Travis 1957).

Physiological speech dysrhythmia is likely to be particularly marked in children aged between $2\frac{1}{2}$ and 4 years, when they are at a stage of acquiring vocabulary and new grammatical structures at a rapid rate. A proportion of their utterances at this stage may be 'non-fluent', and it has been suggested that if parents begin to attract the attention of the child to his 'non-fluencies' at this time, the child is likely to become sensitive about them and his consequent anxiety will be likely to perpetuate them (Johnson 1959). Speech dysrhythmia at this age is commonly referred to as 'clutter', but there seems to be no very marked symptomatic distinction between 'clutter' and later pathological speech dysrhythmia. When hesitations, prolongations and repetitions persist or disappear for a period and then recur, most often in the early school years, the patient is considered to suffer from a pathological speech dysrhythmia or 'to have a stammer', or 'to have a stutter'.

The study of patients with 'stutter' in Newcastle, carried out by Andrews and Harris (1964), suggested that 3 to 4 per cent of children of school-age stammered for a period. Most often this was only for a matter of weeks or months, and the stammer cleared up after this time, usually without treatment. In about 1 per cent of children, however, speech dysrhythmia, 'stammer or stutter', was more persistent and lasted until the age of 15 years or even into adult life. In the majority of patients with 'persistent speech dysrhythmia', symptoms appeared between the ages of 2 and 8 years.

The Causes of Stammer

It is not proposed to review the very large number of causes of stammering which have been suggested. A relatively high proportion of children who stammer have a family history of a similar speech disturbance. This has been regarded as suggesting a genetic pre-disposition by some authors, but Johnson (1959) suggests that the positive family history is important in alerting parents to the possibility that their offspring may have a speech disorder and therefore in attracting their attention to physiological clutter. Andrews and Harris (1964) thought that 'stuttering may be transmitted as a single dominant gene, the penetrance being modified by other genetic and environmental factors'.

Stammer or stutter and various other manifestations of speech dysrhythmia have also been regarded as anxiety symptoms, but Andrews and Harris (1964) found no real excess of psychiatric symptoms in the children they studied who stammered. It has been suggested that stammer may be caused by environmental stress, but these workers were unable to establish this as a single cause in any high proportion of their patients, though they stated 'stuttering can be regarded as a product of certain adverse environmental factors, acting upon a genetic matrix'. This statement would be accepted by the majority of clinicians and speech therapists who work with stammering children.

The Development of Speech Dysrhythmia

As already noted, in about 1 per cent of the child population speech dysrhythmia tends to be persistent and the symptoms become progressively severe as the child grows older (Bloodstein 1960a and b, 1961). This author defines four stages in the development of speech dysrhythmia.

In the first stage there is repetition of speech sounds and sometimes of two or more syllables. Repetition tends to occur most often at the beginning of sentences or phrases, particularly when the child is excited. The severity of the speech disorder varies greatly from hour to hour and day to day.

In the second stage, prolongation, hesitation and complete arrest of utterance (blocking) occurrs in addition to repetitions which tend to become more frequent than in the first stage. In many cases, a child in this stage shows involuntary movements accompanying his hesitations. There might be grimacing or unwanted movements of the limbs. Inevitably during this stage, a high proportion of children become more and more aware of their speech difficulties.

In the third stage, hesitation and blocking become more important than repetitive stammer. Affected children tend to 'get stuck' much more frequently than in stage 2, especially when they are excited or anxious. By this stage, patients are usually very aware of their speech difficulties and begin to avoid making spontaneous remarks whenever possible. They may avoid sounds which they believe precipitate 'blockings' and circumlocutions appear.

In the fourth stage, 'blockings' and arrests of the flow of speech are so severe that the child's power of communicating, using spoken language, is severely restricted. By this time, the patient spends much of his life avoiding situations in which spontaneous utterance is required, and tends whenever possible to use monosyllables rather than to indulge in conversation. In severely affected patients it is not uncommon to find that avoiding 'speaking situations' has become a major preoccupation in their lives.

Other authors have defined the different stages in the development of speech dysrhythmia in different terms, but those described by Bloodstein would be accepted by most clinicians as representing a recognisable description of the stages of the development of speech dysrhythmia as they see them in speech clinics. Nevertheless, it must be admitted that not all patients pass through the stages in a regular fashion. It is not too uncommon, for example, to find that after a sudden severe episode of emotional trauma, a child aged 6 or 7 years is found to be in what Bloodstein would call 'stage 3', without apparently having passed through the two preceding stages.

16

The Management of Speech Dysrhythmia

Management in young children below the age of 7 or 8 years consists of indirect treatment—largely in attempting to modify the environment to minimise the effects of his speech disorder. It is important to make sure that parents understand that drawing the child's attention to his speech defects is likely to exacerbate them and that they should not continually attract his attention to his 'non-fluencies' by attempting to correct them.

After the age of 7 or 8 years, the child is increasingly able to co-operate in direct speech therapy. A huge number of different types of speech therapy for stammering have been described (Moore 1946, van Riper 1954).

One of the most promising of these is training in so-called 'syllabic speech'. Patients using this technique are told to speak syllable by syllable with a regular unaltering rhythm. This results in diminished intonational variation and a certain monotony of speech. Children are taught that speech pulses should be evenly spaced.

It takes considerable time for them to learn the technique of so called 'syllable-timed speech' and the co-operation of the patient and his family is essential. Usually a period of intensive therapy is given in a group situation together with other children suffering from speech dysrhythmia. This may last from two to three weeks. Following this initial period of intensive therapy, it is important that there should be continual 'reinforcement' of what has been learned so that he is motivated to continue using syllable-timed speech. In spite of this, a great many children tend to neglect using syllable-timed speech, except on special occasions, and resort to stammering. Nevertheless, at the end of treatment, they have at their command a method of avoiding the worst effects of stammer or hesitation. This represents a considerable gain in many cases.

Dysarthria

Dysarthria is a term used to denote defective articulation which is attributable to disorders of function or of structure of the articulatory organs; namely, the tongue, lips and palate, and related structures including the teeth, larynx and nose. From the point of view of classification it is useful to distinguish between (1) conditions which are isolated structural defects of teeth, lips, tongue, palate or related parts; (2) disease of related structures; (3) the disproportion between different parts of the articulatory apparatus; and (4) neurological disease which impairs the control of voluntary movement of the articulatory organs during speech.

A variety of local structural abnormalities may prevent normal articulation.

Structural Defects of the Tongue

Agenesis is a relatively rare condition and usually there is not complete absence of the tongue but hypoplasia of the organ, which is tied down to the floor of the mouth by bands of fibrous tissue so that it lacks mobility as well as size. Speech is often remarkably unimpaired and can be improved if the mobility of the tongue can be increased by section of the fibrous bands (Ardran *et al.* 1964). Macroglossia occasionally occurs, for example in Hurler's syndrome and in Down's syndrome, but rarely as an isolated malformation. Since there are so many other factors affecting speech in the majority of patients who show macroglossia, it is difficult to assess its significance in causing articulatory difficulties.

Tongue-tie

Tongue-tie is the common name given to the condition found when the frenum of the tongue is so short that it impedes tongue movement and particularly tongue protrusion. It is in fact exceedingly uncommon to find children who suffer from this condition to such an extent that articulation of speech is impaired. In patients with speech difficulties attributable to tongue-tie, it is almost invariably found that there is a history of feeding difficulties in infancy attributable to inadequate tongue movement.

The management of children thought to be tongue-tied is always difficult, for most parents cannot be convinced that speech difficulty is unrelated to the anatomical deformity. In these circumstances it is often helpful to cut both the frenum and the argument before embarking on any other form of speech therapy.

Hare-lip and Cleft Palate

Hare-lip is by far the commonest of the abnormalities of the lips encountered in childhood. It is interesting to note that the incidence of cleft lip (without associated cleft palate) varies very greatly in different communities, *e.g.* the incidence is much higher in Newcastle-upon-Tyne than it is in Edinburgh (Drillien *et al.* 1966). Very few patients who suffer from cleft lip alone show articulatory abnormalities once they have cut their permanent teeth—whether their lips have been repaired or not.

Multiple factors contribute to the speech handicaps of children who suffer from cleft palate. In the majority of cases, the severity of the articulatory abnormalities is proportional to the degree of nasal escape. The degree of nasal escape is determined not only by the extent of the initial palatal defect but also upon the expertise of the surgeon who closed the cleft, whether or not infection was present when he did so, and to some extent upon the ability of the child to compensate for his palatal incompetence—which is probably related to some degree to his intelligence.

It is worth emphasising that the problem of defective speech in children who suffer from cleft palate is not one to be explained purely on anatomical principles. A high proportion of patients suffer from hearing impairment as a result of middle-ear infection, others are mentally defective or of below average intelligence, and still others have associated primary or secondary abnormalities of the jaws which contribute to articulatory difficulties. For example, it has been shown that the tongue movements of a high proportion of patients with cleft palate are abnormal (Berry 1949, Nylen 1961).

In addition to dysarthria, many patients who suffer from cleft palate show secondary speech disorders attributable to hearing impairment, commonly the result of otitis media, or to associated mental retardation (Drillien *et al.* 1966).

Diseases of Related Structures

Diseases of structures related to the lips, tongue and palate, may produce articulatory abnormalities.

Undoubtedly the commonest single abnormality of this type is due to a pathological enlargement of the adenoids which causes impairment of the nasal airway and hyporhinophonia. Children with chronically large adenoids speak as if they had a continual 'cold in the nose'. The nasal sounds *n*, *m* and *ng* are defective and articulation of other consonants is also faulty.

Recurrent or chronic tonsillitis is often associated with adenoiditis. If there is much peritonsillar infection, there is a marked tendency for the child to move the body of the tongue and the soft palate as little as possible and to produce speech sounds more forward in the mouth than is usual. The articulatory pattern is highly characteristic and can be recognised almost immediately by any experienced speech therapist or doctor interested in speech disorders. Sometimes the articulatory abnormalities are accompanied by visible tongue thrust with the tip of the tongue protruding between the teeth during speech. The tendency to tongue thrust may persist even when infected tonsils and adenoids have been removed.

A rare cause of hyporhinophonia is choanal atresia, in which condition, the normal canalisation of the nasal passages which should take place in fetal life has failed to occur.

Disproportion

Malocclusion of the jaws is a relatively common condition inconstantly associated with dysarthric speech disorders. Relative retrusion of the lower jaw (Fig. 1) is referred to by orthodontists as the 'skeletal two malformation', to be contrasted with the 'skeletal three malformation' in which there is relative protrusion of the mandible or prognathous. In the latter condition, the upper front incisors may be opposed in the same vertical plane to the lower front incisors or may be anterior to the upper incisors when the jaws are shut.

In the 'skeletal two malformation' there is commonly underdevelopment of the lower jaw which usually tends to correct itself as the child grows older. For a time however, the lower jaw seems to be too small to contain the mass of the tongue and this is protruded during speech so that tongue thrust results with inter-dental sigmatism. When hypomandibulosis is associated with cleft palate it is known as the Pierre Robin syndrome. In this condition, the tongue is very liable to fall back into the cleft of the palate in early infancy and to cause respiratory obstruction in the new born period and feeding difficulties are likely to be severe.

In 'skeletal three malformation', the central upper and lower incisors are opposed in the same vertical plane or the lower incisors may be anterior to the upper incisors and there tends to be lateralisation of 's' and 's' combination sounds which produces a characteristic articulatory pattern. Other patients with 'skeletal three malformation' oppose their lateral incisors but have a gap between their central incisors through which there is an escape of air and often tongue intrusion. Again, the articulatory pattern tends to be characteristic (Hopkin and McEwan 1955, Hopkin 1962).

Another form of disproportion which may cause dysarthria is when the nasopharyngeal aperture is unduly large, so that, though the palate is of normal size and has a full range of movement, it is inadequate to close off the nasopharynx completely during speech. This means that all vowel sounds and some consonants are

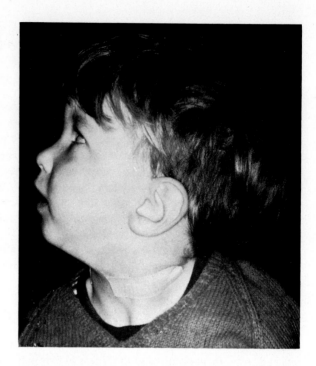

Fig. 1. Hypomandibulosis.

distorted and there is a characteristic articulatory pattern associated with hyper-rhinophonia. This so-called 'palatal disproportion' syndrome is often first manifest in feeding difficulties in early infancy, milk continually coming down the nose during feeding. In other cases, however, adequate occlusion of the nasopharyngeal orifice is achieved by the posterior margin of the soft palate coming into contact with the adenoid pad. It is only when the adenoids are removed that nasal escape becomes apparent.

Patients who suffer from the palatal disproportion syndrome may often be recognised at sight because of their typical facies with an excessively long and often broad maxilla—a trait which is commonly familial. The speech of these patients is characteristic. There is excessive nasal escape during speech and this impairs the articulation of all vowel sounds and consonants except *n*, *m* and *ng*.

The speech has been termed 'cleft palate speech without a cleft palate' and this is a fair description. The degree of nasal escape can be estimated in a rough way by asking the child to utter an 'e' or an 'a' sound and holding a finger or a mirror beneath his nose as he does so. If the palate is fully efficient, no air should escape from the nose when these sounds are produced. If there is nasal escape, the warmth of the air coming from the nose can be appreciated by the finger or by the clouding on a mirror. More accurate methods of assessing the adequacy of nasopharyngeal closure may be obtained by using flowmeters and by x-ray palatography, in which the position of the soft palate at rest, and when the child is producing the vowel and consonant sounds, can be observed.

A number of operations are available to lessen the effects of nasal disproportion. In some of these, posterior pharyngeal wall is pushed forwards so that the posterior margin of the soft palate can contact it. In pharyngoplasty, a flap of mucous membrane is raised from the posterior pharyngeal wall and attached to the palate so that the nasopharyngeal orifice is reduced in area. Pharyngoplasty has proved its worth over the years. In the hands of an experienced plastic surgeon the results are good. Recently attempts have been made to slide posteriorly the whole of the soft palate so that occlusion between it and the posterior pharyngeal wall is improved.

Malocclusion of the jaws and the palatal disproportion syndrome both tend to be familial, and it is not too uncommon to find parents with marked hyperrhinophonia who are quite unaware of their speech defect.

Neurological Causes of Dysarthria

Dysarthria may be caused by lesions in the brain, the cerebral hemisphere, the basal ganglia, the cerebellum or the cranial nerves, or the function of the nerve endings may be affected, as in myasthenia gravis, or by disease of the muscles of the lips, tongue and palate themselves.

Approximately 50 per cent of children who suffer from cerebral palsy have speech defects which are sufficient to impair their ability to communicate significantly (Hansen 1960, Ingram 1964a).

Dysarthria is uncommon in patients with unilateral cortical abnormalities, although it occurs more frequently than the literature on the subject would indicate (Luria 1966). Dysarthria however occurs in a high proportion of patients with bilateral cerebral lesions. Thus the majority of patients who suffer from diplegia with involvement of the upper limbs, and virtually all patients who suffer from bilateral hemiplegia and dyskinesia, show dysarthric speech defects. In diplegia in which there is paresis of voluntary movement of the affected organs associated with spasticity, speech tends to be slow and sounds are produced with obvious effort. In particular, there is difficulty in producing complex consonant clusters and words in which large movements of the tongue have to be co-ordinated with movements of the lips and palate. Often there is associated hyperrhinophonia, hyporhinophonia or rhinolalia mixta (in which there is sometimes hyperrhinophonia and at other times hyporhinophonia). Many affected patients have defects of involuntary swallowing, so that there is drooling of saliva from the mouth. Frequently there is tongue thrust and feeding difficulties which persist into later childhood.

In children who suffer from severe bilateral cerebral palsy, it is often very difficult to assess the relative significance of dysarthria and secondary speech disorders in the causation of speech difficulties. It is not too uncommon, for example, to find that in severely affected diplegic patients there is paresis of the lips, tongue and palate, hearing defect, and mental deficiency (Fig. 2).

In dyskinetic (choreo-athetoid) cerebral palsy, the main cause of dysarthria is involuntary movement of the lips, tongue and palate. This occurs in the majority of patients, though it is commonly associated with secondary speech disorders attributable to mental retardation and/or hearing loss, and dysrhythmia attributable to the lack of co-ordination between respiratory and articulatory muscles during efforts to

21

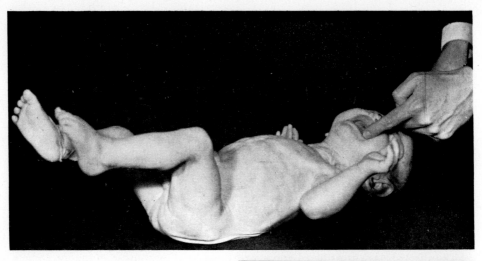

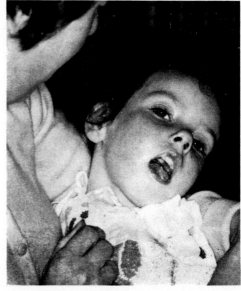

Fig. 2. Marked rooting and lip reflexes in diplegic baby aged 11 months. Note mouth opening.

Fig. 3. Reflex mouth opening and tongue protrusion in severe dyskinesia.

make speech. As a result, articulation on inspiration may occur, and involuntary movements and arrests of movement of the lips, tongue and palate are frequently found, accompanied by bizarre mispronunciations with inconstant nasal escape and the inconstant substitution or omission of consonant and vowel sounds. Often there is considerable drooling and it is not uncommon to find that feeding patterns are infantile in type and that the children have never learned to chew and still show marked routine sucking and swallowing reflexes (Fig. 3).

In ataxic cerebral palsy there is weakness and inco-ordination of the movements of the lips, tongue and palate. Speech tends to be slow and monotonous and even in children there is the same characteristic scanning intonation that is found in adults with disease of the cerebellum or cerebellar connections, *e.g.* in multiple sclerosis.

In ataxic diplegia, the type of cerebral palsy characteristically associated with hydrocephalus, the lips, tongue and palate tend to be paretic and inco-ordinate. In such patients, however, there seem to be no inhibitions so far as speech is concerned. They are garrulous to a degree and tend to parrot what they have heard, even if they can only do this inaccurately.

Nuclear agenesis, or Moebius' syndrome, is commoner than is generally realised. In this condition, nuclei of the cranial nerves have failed to develop or the connections between the hemispheres and cranial nerve nuclei are missing. The cranial nerves themselves may be defective and the muscles that they innovate may be hypoplastic in some cases but not in all. The clinical manifestations of nuclear agenesis vary considerably. In some patients the eyes alone are affected. In others, the eyes and face are affected but the tongue and palate are spared, and in yet others, the tongue and palate are paretic so that there is feeding difficulty, often with nasal escape of milk and sometimes with aspiration complicated by respiratory infection. Drooling from the mouth is almost constant. In patients in whom the lips, tongue and/or palate are involved, there tends to be rather slow speech development, gross dysarthria and hyperrhinophonia or rhinolalia mixta. Pharyngoplasty may be effective in reducing the amount of nasal escape in some patients, and orthodontic appliances may encourage more normal swallowing patterns and reduce drooling. A high proportion of children with nuclear agenesis, however, are severely affected and it is important not to subject them to unrealistic speech therapy.

Persistent palatal paresis, the result of poliomyelitis, is seen very uncommonly today, but occasionally viral or toxic encephalopathy is complicated by paresis of the lips, tongue and/or palate.

Lesions of the peripheral nerves causing dysarthria are uncommon, but occasionally, as a result of tonsillectomy or other trauma to the pharynx, the palatal nerves are damaged and lower motor neurone type of palatal paresis results.

A variety of other neurological conditions may present for the first time as dysarthric speech disorders. In the last two years, cases of progressive muscular atrophy, amyotrophic lateral sclerosis, Refsum's syndrome, myasthenia gravis, dystrophia myotonica and facio-scapulo-humeral dystrophy have appeared for the first time in the speech clinic. That they should do so underlines the fact that all children who are sent for speech therapy should be subjected to a medical examination before therapy is begun.

Secondary Speech Disorders

Secondary speech disorders are those abnormalities of speech sound production which are not attributable to dysfunction or structual abnormalities of the tongue, lips or palate but which are associated with other diseases or with adverse environmental factors.

In the majority of patients of this category, the speech disorder consists of retardation of speech development. This may be part of a generalised retardation of behavioural development, as is commonly found in mental retardation, or relatively specific retardation of speech development, as is found in hearing loss.

23

In a proportion of patients, the characteristics of the speech disorder indicate the causal factor. For example, in high-tone hearing loss, the omission of particular high frequency speech sounds is characteristic. In elective mutism, the child's ability to talk normally in certain circumstances and his inability (or refusal) to talk in others is characteristic.

Mental Retardation

Mental defect is the commonest single cause of slow speech development in most clinics. In the Royal Hospital for Sick Children, Edinburgh, more than half of the children referred who had no words by the age of two years were found to be mentally retarded (Ingram 1964*a*). This is to be expected, for, as has been demonstrated in a number of studies, motor milestones in a significant proportion of mentally retarded patients may be within normal limits, whereas milestones of speech adaptive and social behaviour development are invariably achieved late (Illingworth 1966). Even so, it has to be borne in mind that the degree of retardation of speech development is not always proportional to the severity of mental defect in later life (Karlin and Strazzulla 1952). In general, it may be said that idiots rarely use spoken language as a form of communication even in later life. The language of imbeciles is very limited but feeble-minded children use language freely, though they tend to make articulatory errors typically found in normal children at a much younger age.

In a high proportion of mentally defective children with speech defects, contributory causal factors to the speech disorder may be found. Mentally defective children, for example, more frequently come from poor home backgrounds than do those of superior intelligence. There is a greater tendency for them to be environmentally deprived because parents and other social contacts obtain less feed-back from the mentally defective child than from the child of average intelligence. The effects of improving social contacts of severely retarded children have been well described by Renfrew (1964). A higher proportion of mentally retarded children than children of average intelligence suffer from hearing defects. The hearing of mentally retarded children should be studied with the same care as that of children with speech defects who are of average intelligence.

In general, it has been shown that feeble-minded children of school-age make the same articulatory errors as normal children of a much younger age (Bangs 1942).

Hearing Loss

In recent years, screening tests to detect hearing loss in infants have been used increasingly (Fisch 1964). As a result, deafness is suspected or confirmed in an increasing proportion of infants before they have reached the stage of beginning to talk, especially if they are known to be 'at risk' because of a family history of deafness or a history of maternal rubella during pregnancy, or if they were born before term or had known birth injury or hyperbilirubinaemia in the neonatal period. Nevertheless, a significant number of children appear in most speech clinics at the age of 3 or 4 years with limited speech who, on examination, are found to suffer from impaired hearing.

The importance of otitis media in early infancy, especially common in the second six months of life, as a cause of hearing loss is still not fully appreciated. A significant proportion of patients with retarded speech development who are referred to speech clinics have a history of persistent or recurrent otitis media, often with aural discharge which has been treated with 'eardrops'. All too often, perforation of an ear drum in a young child is regarded as a clinical nuisance rather than as a minor clinical disaster (Miller *et al.* 1960). The hearing loss is usually similar throughout the frequencies from 250 to 8,000, though occasionally high tone loss may occur (Maran 1966). Patients who suffer from cleft palate or the palatal disproportion syndrome are especially liable to suffer from middle ear disease and they should be regarded as 'at risk'. Any upper respiratory tract infections that they acquire should be treated energetically with antibiotics in a prophylactic fashion in order to diminish the chances of their speech being affected by the complication of hearing loss.

The management of a young child with hearing impairment depends upon a number of variables, including the severity of the loss, the child's age at the time of diagnosis, the presence or absence of other complicating physical or intellectual handicaps and the facilities which are available locally. Whereas in previous years there was a tendency to place children with hearing loss in schools for the deaf or schools for the hard of hearing, in recent years the policy has been increasingly to try to keep them within the normal community and to avoid segregation (Reed 1964).

Acquired Dysphasia

Much confusion has been caused by the loose use of the term 'dysphasia' (congenital dysphasia, developmental dysphasia, congenital developmental dysphasia, childhood aphasia) applied to children who are slow to develop spoken language (Brain 1965). It is important to recognise that dysphasia implies the loss of acquired language functions. A child affected by birth injury can hardly be described as having 'lost language functions' for he had no language functions to lose at the time he sustained brain damage. The only effect his brain damage may have on his speech is that its subsequent development may be delayed. It is more accurate and more useful to talk about his 'retardation of speech development', and to describe in which way his speech has been affected, than to talk about 'developmental dysphasia'.

After the child has begun to talk, damage to the dominant hemisphere more often causes speech disorders than does damage to the non-dominant hemisphere (Basser 1962). The effects on speech of damage to the dominant hemisphere will depend to some extent on the situation and extent of the lesion in the brain, and to some extent upon the maturity of speech functions at the time the damage was sustained. In a child aged 10 or 11 in whom speech development is virtually complete, the clinical picture is likely to be that found in dysphasia in adults. In the younger child of age two or three years, however, there is likely to be some impairment of the language which has been acquired and, in addition, subsequent slowing of speech development. This is the classical picture of acquired dysphasia in childhood (Guttman 1942).

Alajouanine and L'Hermitte (1965) emphasised the poverty of the spoken language of children who suffer from acquired dysphasia in childhood. They wrote: 'Every child showed peculiar behaviour of psycho-motor inhibition, resulting in a reduction of oral and written language and a reduction of gesture activities. Spon-

25

taneous speech was nearly nil. To get these children to speak it was necessary to multiply incentives and encouragements to repeat questions and orders.' They also noted that the duration of total speech loss after brain injury appeared to be more severe in younger than in older children, and that, even when there was apparent recovery of spoken language, difficulties in reading and spelling often persisted. A high incidence of associated emotional difficulties was found.

Necessarily, speech therapy for acquired dysphasia in the young child has to be indirect. It is often helpful, for example, to place the child in a play group or nursery situation and to encourage him to mix with other children of his own age. In older children, the treatment is much more like that of adult patients. The speech therapist can do a great deal in the early days when the child has lost speech to reassure him that his speech will recover and then to treat him directly, and, in co-operation with his teachers, help him to minimise the affects of his language disorder on education.

Psychiatric Disorders

Inevitably, abnormalities of the child's total behaviour are reflected in disorders of spoken language. For example, the child who has been over-indulged and 'babied' from an early age is likely to show retardation of behaviour development, including retardation of language development. This is especially likely to occur in the youngest child of a large family when his every need is met by parents or older brothers and sisters, without his having to indicate his needs using spoken language.

Retardation of speech development may also be found in the protected child who behaves in a withdrawn manner, shuns the company of other children and is very often, unusually silent.

In elective mutism, children talk in some circumstances but not in all. For example, they may talk freely with their parents and brothers and sisters at home but refuse to utter a single word at school or outside their homes. In a high proportion of cases, there are other manifestations of emotional maladjustment, particularly withdrawal symptoms such as solitariness, inability to make good relationships with children of the same age, and over-dependence on parents and other members of the family (Haskell 1964). Children may remain silent at school for as long as two or three years, yet talk freely at home during this time and show normal speech in these surroundings.

A proportion of children who show elective mutism later manifest psychotic symptoms, but in the majority the condition should be regarded as a neurotic disturbance which can be successfully treated by psychiatrists, though treatment is often protracted and requires in-patient management in the first instance. The eventual prognosis for speech is good in the majority of cases.

The speech defects in infantile autism have attracted much attention in recent years (Wolff and Chess 1964, Rutter 1966). Cunningham (1966) described the characteristics of the speech of one autistic child as follows: 'There was less speech giving information or communicating meaning to others than in normal children with the same mean sentence length. There was more immediate repetition of his own remarks or the experimenters, though delayed repetition was rare. Affirmation was indicated by the repetition of a question. Personal pronouns tended to be reversed so that he might use 'me' instead of 'you'. Sentences were more often grammatically incomplete than with younger children of corresponding sentence length. There appeared to be some difficulty in understanding speech. He scarcely ever asked questions. There was a general shortage of all kinds of pronouns.'

The diagnosis of typical infantile autism is not difficult, but many other children, particularly those with evidence of brain damage, present with slow speech development and abnormal behavioural manifestations of 'autistic type'. In these patients, diagnosis between auditory imperception, true peripheral hearing loss, mental retardation and even temporal lobe epilepsy may be extremely difficult. Some children with hearing loss, for example, behave in a withdrawn fashion, have retarded speech development and show many of the features of autism described by Creak *et al.* (1961) and Wing (1966).

Adverse Environment

The effects of adverse environment on speech development are profound. This has been shown particularly in children who have spent their infancy and early years of childhood in institutions and have been deprived of normal mothering (McCarthy 1954). The effects of institutionalisation are particularly severe if the child is mentally retarded or suffers from hearing defects.

It is not only institutionalised children, however, who suffer from adverse environmental conditions. Studies of immigrant children, particularly in the United States, have shown that a high proportion show retarded maturation of spoken language (Labov 1966, Cazden 1968).

In the United Kingdom, Bernstein (1961, 1962) has for years emphasised the limited language abilities of children of low social class living in poor conditions in which frequently there is little communication using spoken language. He describes a 'restricted code' of language which is adequate for interpersonal contact and an 'elaborated code' which is required if ideas are to be exchanged. The children with only 'a restricted code' are at a considerable disadvantage when they go to school and a high proportion have difficulty in the early stages of learning to read and spell.

It is important always to take account of the fact that secondary speech disorders are very frequently the result of a combination of intrinsic and adverse environmental factors. For example, a deaf child in a poor home is likely to be relatively neglected because his parents find that he doesn't give them verbal 'feedback'. The diagnosis of his condition is likely to be made later than if he came from a more privileged home. Treatment of his hearing loss is liable to be delayed.

The Developmental Speech Disorder Syndrome

This is a descriptive term given to the retardation of speech development which affects apparently healthy children of average or superior intelligence who come from normal home backgrounds.

The definition of 'retarded speech development' is necessarily arbitrary. For present purposes, retarded speech development is considered to be present when the child has no words by the age of 18 months or no phrases by the age of 30 months.

The developmental speech disorder syndrome occurs more commonly in boys

27

than girls. In most speech clinics, two or three times as many boys as girls are affected (Ingram 1959*b*, 1969). In a high proportion of patients there is a positive family history of slow speech development and there is an excess of left-handed and ambidextrous parents, uncles and aunts, brothers and sisters. Often too there is a history of uncles and aunts, parents, or brothers and sisters having difficulties in the early stages of learning to read and write (McCready 1926, Brain 1965).

The developmental speech disorder syndrome is really a misnomer, for it comprises a number of different conditions in which there is retardation of articulatory and/or language development. A high proportion of children are merely retarded in articulatory and language development. For example, they may use spoken language at the age of 4 as a normal child of similar intelligence would at the age of $2\frac{1}{2}$ or 3 years. In other cases, speech development is deviant as well as being retarded; for example, omissions and substitutions of consonants are not those which are typically found in younger children, or there may be a marked discrepancy in the degree of maturation of the verbal comprehension, spoken language and articulation as measured by standard tests.

Nevertheless, with these reservations, it is useful to consider the developmental speech disorder syndrome as comprising a spectrum of speech pathology which varies from the 'mild' to the 'very severe'. Mildly affected children are those whose language development is within normal limits, but whose articulatory development is retarded. Often their mothers say 'He has the words but cannot say them.' On examination it is found that the child is substituting or omitting the later acquired consonants and consonant clusters inconsistently, though his vocabulary and grammatical structures in spoken language may be within normal limits.

Moderately severely affected children are those in whom there is some retardation of language development as well as retardation in the maturation of articulatory patterns. There is no difficulty in the comprehension of spoken language, but the children usually show some limitation of active vocabulary and their grammatical structures are typically those of children younger than their age. Their articulatory abnormalities are more severe than those found in children who are mildly affected and more consonants and consonant clusters are found to be omitted or substituted though vowels are commonly normal. Thus scores on a standardised test of articulatory development tend to be lower than those found in mildly affected patients (Anthony *et al.* 1971).

As well as being late in developing spoken language, moderately severely affected children have a slower rate of progress once language development starts. It may take them, for example, two or three years to make the progress that a child with normal speech development would make in a year or 18 months.

Severely affected patients (Table II) not only have difficulty in expressing themselves using spoken language but are also slow to comprehend spoken language. Parents may note that their offspring was slow to recognise his name and slow to understand simple commands, even though his hearing appeared normal. In such patients, maturation of spoken language is more retarded than in moderately severely affected children and articulatory patterns are still more immature. It is not unusual to find that severely affected children of high intelligence learn to interpret what is said to

TABLE II

Classification of the developmental speech disorder syndrome

Severity	Description	Other Terms
Mild	Retardation of acquisition of word sounds, language normal	dyslalia
Moderate	More severe retardation of word sound acquisition and retarded spoken language development, comprehension normal	developmental expressive dysphasia
Severe	Still more severe retardation of word sound acquisition and spoken language development, impaired comprehension of speech	developmental receptive dysphasia, word deafness, auditory imperception
Very severe	Gross failure of speech development, impaired comprehension of language and significance of other sounds, often apparent deafness	auditory imperception, central deafness

them by lip reading in their toddler years and continue to do so until their ability to comprehend the spoken word develops. This severe form of the developmental speech disorder syndrome has been referred to as 'developmental receptive dysphasia' or 'auditory imperception' (Ingram 1964*b*). A high proportion of children in this category fail to develop verbal fluency even when they are adults and have considerable difficulty in achieving more than elementary reading and spelling.

A small minority of children who suffer from the developmental speech disorder syndrome are very severely affected and appear to have difficulties in discriminating sounds, other than those of speech, in early years. In the first two or three years of life they may, in fact, appear to be deaf. As they grow older they usually show attention to sounds and learn to discriminate between sounds of different types and to localise them, but a significant proportion never learn to discriminate speech sounds accurately and for practical purposes are 'non-communicators'. In the past, a high proportion of such patients have found their way into schools for the deaf. It may be that in some cases this is the appropriate placement for them. For practical purposes they are 'deaf' so far as spoken language is concerned (Murphy 1964).

At all grades of severity, the developmental speech disorder syndrome is a challenge to speech therapists. Mildly affected children rarely require direct speech therapy, but placing them in conditions where the use of spoken language is encouraged is helpful in a high proportion, and many pre-school children benefit enormously from being placed in nurseries where contact and play with other children is supervised by a trained adult, other than the parents. Moderately severely affected children often benefit from the same regime, but clearly these children need the most energetic speech therapy from the time they are diagnosed. Severely affected children with receptive difficulties pose major problems both for the therapist and for the teacher. Often it is better to delay primary education in school for a year or more in order to try to avoid the almost inevitable reading and spelling difficulties which result if they are put into school at the normal age. It is clear that very severely affected children can be helped if they are accurately diagnosed at an early age, but this has only happened in the last twenty years and it is very difficult to know just how successful modern methods of speech therapy are likely to be in any large series of such patients (McGinnis 1963). Training of severely and very severely affected children is a matter for highly trained specialists, for few individual speech therapists, teachers of the deaf, neurologists or paediatricians will see sufficient numbers of these children to work out appropriate programmes for treatment.

The Diagnosis of Speech Disorders in Childhood

In recent years there has been a tendency for paediatricians and other doctors to regard the diagnosis of speech disorders as almost entirely within the province of the speech therapist. This is probably due in large part to the fact that doctors are given inadequate training in the diagnosis of speech disorders. Nevertheless, it must be recognised that a large proportion of children referred to speech therapists, suffer from other disease (Table I). Often the diagnosis in such patients depends upon medical findings rather than phonetic or linguistic criteria.

The speech therapist is entitled to expect that every child referred to her should have had a careful medical assessment. This must include a family history, a history of the birth, a developmental history, an account of the illnesses suffered by the child and a careful physical examination. An indication of the need for this is perhaps that in the last three years such different diseases as nuclear agenesis, Down's syndrome, phenylketonuria, congenital dystrophia, myotonica, myasthenia gravis and facio-scapulo-humeral dystrophy, in addition to 'sub-cultural' mental defect, cerebral palsy, and 'minimal cerebral dysfunction', have been diagnosed amongst patients referred to the speech clinic in the Royal Hospital for Sick Children, Edinburgh.

In many cases, the services of other specialists will be required. These include, ear, nose and throat surgeons, audiologists, plastic surgeons, psychologists, child psychiatrists, and social workers.

It is important, however, that paediatricians, in particular, should become more aware of their responsibilities in helping speech therapists in the diagnosis and management of children who suffer from speech disorders.

REFERENCES

Alajouanine, T., L'Hermitte, F. (1965) 'Acquired aphasia in children.' *Brain*, **88**, 653.
Andrews, G., Harris, M. (1964) *The Syndrome of Stuttering*. Clinics in Developmental Medicine, No. 17. London: Spastics Society with Heinemann.
Anthony, A., Bogle, D., Ingram, T. T. S., McIsaac, M. W. (1971) *The Edinburgh Articulation Test*. Edinburgh: Churchill Livingstone.
Ardran, G. M., Becket, J. M., Kemp, F. H. (1964) 'Aglossia congenita.' *Arch. Dis. Childh.*, **39**, 389.
Bangs, J. L. (1942) 'A clinical analysis of the articulatory defects of the feeble minded.' *J. speech Dis.* **7**, 343.
Basser, L. S. (1962) 'Hemiplegia of early onset and the faculty of speech with special reference to the effects of hemispherectomy.' *Brain*, **85**, 427.
Bernstein, B. (1961) 'Social class and linguistic development: a theory of social learning.' *in* Halsey, A., Floud, J., Anderson, C. A. (Eds.) *Education, Economy and Society*. New York: The Free Press of Glencoe. p. 288.
—— (1962) 'Linguistic codes, hesitation phenomena and intelligence.' *Lang. Speech*, **5**, 31.
Berry, M. (1949) 'Lingual anomalies associated with palatal clefts.' *J. speech Dis.*, **14**, 288.
Birrell, J. F. (1954) 'Hoarseness in childhood.' *Speech*, **18**, 40.

Bloodstein, O. (1960a) 'The development of stuttering. I. Changes in nine basic features.' *J. speech Dis.*, **25**, 219.

—— (1960b) 'The development of stuttering. II. Developmental phase.' *J. speech Dis.*, **25**, 366.

—— (1961) 'The development of stuttering. III. Theoretical and clinical implications.' *J. speech Dis.*, **26**, 67.

Brain, Lord (1965) *Speech Disorders—Aphasia, Apraxia and Agnosia*. 2nd edn. London: Butterworth.

Cazden, C. B. (1968) 'Three sociolinguistic views of the language and speech of lower class children with special attention to the work of Basil Bernstein.' *Develop. Med. Child Neurol.*, **10**, 600.

Creak, M. (Chairman) (1961) 'Schizophrenia syndrome in childhood—progress report of a working party.' *Develop. Med. Child Neurol.*, **3**, 501.

Cunningham, M. A. (1966) 'A five year study of the language of an autistic child.' *J. Child Psychol. Psychiat.*, **7**, 143.

Drillien, C. M., Wilkinson, E. M., Ingram, T. T. S. (1966) *The Causes and Natural History of Cleft Lip and Palate*. Edinburgh: E. & S. Livingstone.

Fisch, L. (1964) 'The contribution of audiology.' *in* Renfrew, C., Murphy, K. (Eds.) *The Child who does not Talk*. Clinics in Developmental Medicine, No. 13. London: S.I.M.P. with Heinemann. p. 55.

Grady, P. A. E., Daniels, J. C. (1964) *A Survey of the Incidence of Speech Defect in Children*. Educational Papers, No. 1. University of Nottingham.

Greene, M. C. L. (1964) *The Voice and its Disorders*. 2nd edn. London: Pitman.

Guttman, E. (1942) 'Aphasia in children.' *Brain*, **65**, 205.

Hansen, E. (1960) 'Cerebral palsy in Denmark.' *Acta psychiat. neurol. scand.*, Suppl. 146.

Haskell, E. (1964) 'Elective mutism.' *in* Renfrew, C., Murphy, K. (Eds.) *The Child who does not Talk*. Clinics in Developmental Medicine, No. 13. London: S.I.M.P. p. 150.

Hopkin, G. B. (1962) Mesiocclusion—A Clinical and Roentgenographic Study. Ph.D. Thesis, University of Edinburgh.

—— McEwen, J. D. (1955) 'Speech defects and malocclusion—a palatographic investigation.' *Dent Pract.*, **6**, 123.

Huxley, R. (1969) 'Our first language.' B.B.C. Radio 3 Talk. (Published, *Listener*, 29th. January, 1970).

Illingworth, R. S. (1966) *The Development of the Infant and Young Child, Normal and Abnormal*. 3rd edn. Edinburgh: E. & S. Livingstone.

Ingram, T. T. S. (1959a) 'A description of classification of common disorders of speech in childhood.' *Arch. Dis. Childh.*, **34**, 444.

—— (1959b) 'Specific developmental disorders of speech in childhood.' *Brain*, **82**, 450.

—— (1964a) *Paediatric Aspects of Cerebral Palsy*. Edinburgh: E. & S. Livingstone.

—— (1964b) 'Auditory imperception and related disorders.' *Proc. roy. Soc. Hlth.*, **40**, 000.

—— (1969) 'Developmental disorders of speech.' *in* Vinken, P. J., Bruin, W. (Eds.) *Handbook of Clinical Neurology*. Vol. 4. Amsterdam: North Holland. p. 407.

Johnson, W. (1955) *Stuttering in Children and Adults*. Minneapolis: University of Minnesota.

—— (1959) *The Onset of Stuttering*. Minneapolis: University of Minnesota Ptess.

Karlin, I. W., Strazzulla, J. (1952) 'Speech and language problems of mentally deficient children.' *J. speech. Dis.*, **17**, 286.

Labov, W. (1966) *The Social Stratification of English in New York City*. Washington: Center of Applied Linguistics.

Luria, A. R. (1966) *Higher Cortical Functions in Man*. London: Tavistock Publications.

McCarthy, D. (1954) 'Language development in children.' *in* Carmichael, L. (Ed.) *Manual of Child Psychology*, 2nd edn. New York: John Wiley, p. 492.

McCready, E. B. (1926) 'Defects in the zone of language (word-deafness and word-blindness) and their influence in education and behavior.' *Amer. J. Psychiat.*, **6**, 267.

McGinnis, M. (1963) *Aphasic Children*. Washington: Volta Bureau.

Maran, A. G. D. (1966) 'The causes of deafness in childhood.' *J. Laryng.*, **80**, 495.

Miller, F. J. W., Court, S. D. M., Walton, W. S., Knox, G. (1960) *Growing up in Newcastle-upon-Tyne*. London: O.U.P.

Moore, W. R. (1946) 'Hypnosis in a system of therapy for stutterers.' *J. speech Dis.*, **11**, 117.

Murphy, K. (1964) 'Language and speech disorders.' *in* Renfrew, C., Murphy, K. (eds.) *The Child who does not Talk*. Clinics in Developmental Medicine, No. 13. London: S.I.M.P. with Heinemann. p. 203.

Nylen, B. O. (1961) 'Cleft palate and speech.' *Acta radiol. (Stockh.)*, Suppl. 203.

Reed, M. (1964) 'Principles of the education of deaf and partially deaf children.' *in* Renfrew, C., Murphy, K. (Eds.) *The Child who does not Talk*. Clinics in Developmental Medicine, No. 13. London: S.I.M.P. with Heinemann. p. 112.

Renfrew, C. (1964) 'Spoken language in intellectually handicapped children.' *in* Renfrew, C., Murphy, K. (Eds.) *The Child who does not Talk*. Clinics in Developmental Medicine, No. 13. London: S.I.M.P. with Heinemann. p. 135.

Rutter, M. (1966) 'Behavioural and cognitive characteristics.' *in* Wing, J. K. (Ed.) *Early Childhood Autism*. London: Pergamon. p. 51.

Travis, L. E. (1957) 'The unspeakable feelings of people with special reference to stuttering.' *in* Travis, L. E. (Ed.) *Handbook of Speech Pathology*. London: Peter Owen. p. 916.

van Riper, C. (1954) *Speech Correction*, 3rd edn. New Jersey: Prentice-Hall.

—— (1957) 'Symptomatic therapy for stuttering.' *in* Travis, L. E. (Ed.) *Handbook of Speech Pathology*. London: Peter Owen. p. 878.

Wing, J. K. (1966) *Early Childhood Autism*. London: Pergamon.

Wolff, S., Chess, S. (1964) 'A behavioural study of schizophrenic children.' *Acta psychiat. scand.* **40,** 438.

CHAPTER 3

Clinical Assessment of Language Disorders in the Young Child

MICHAEL RUTTER

Speech And Language: Definitions

It is ironic that in the field of language, of all places, words have come to have so many contradictory meanings that communication between different workers has often been mis-communication. This difficulty particularly applies to the terms 'speech' and 'language' which, unfortunately and misleadingly, have sometimes been used interchangeably.

In providing definitions, it should first be made clear that in individual children there may well be considerable practical problems in making some of these distinctions. However, if there are clear conceptual distinctions, as there are, then progress can only come by our striving to apply these to the clinical situation.

'Language' is a system of symbols (Lewis 1968)—a symbolic code that allows the generation of novel messages which, by the nature of the system, would be understandable to anyone who knows that system. There are, therefore, at least three key features: (1) it must involve symbols*; (2) the symbols must form part of a system in which each symbol has a systematic relation with each other symbol; and (3) as a consequence of this system, it has a capacity for generating novel messages (Carroll 1964). The essence of language is its productivity (Lenneberg 1967). Given a knowledge of a language it is possible to produce an infinite number of new sentences never used before which would still be understood by anyone else who knew the language.

Obviously, the language with which we are most familiar is spoken language but there are other types of language. For example, there are a variety of gestural and sign languages such as those used by the deaf and by American Indians (Latif 1934), there is Braille which is distinctive in using touch as the medium, and, of course, there is written language. In English the written language bears a one-to-one relationship to spoken language, but this is not so in many Eastern and Far Eastern languages.

The purpose of language is communication, but it is necessary to emphasise that all communication is not language. There are also forms of non-linguistic interpersonal communication as evidenced by smiling, welcoming movements, turning away and so forth (Ekman and Friesen 1969).

The definition of 'speech' poses more problems. In a Spastics Society meeting on language delay, Sheridan (1964) defined 'speech' as 'the use of systematised vocalisations to express verbal symbols or words'. Whereas I think this is both succinct and accurate, the definition does bring out the difficulty that speech refers both to spoken language and to word-sound production, that is the process of vocalisation or articu-

---

*Symbol, i.e. something that stands for something else by convention or code rather than just by similarity or resemblance.

33

lation (Worster-Drought 1968). Accordingly, for most purposes, rather than use the term 'speech', I will specify to which aspect I am referring.

Scheme for Assessment of Speech and Language

The final diagnosis of conditions associated with speech delay must often wait on the results of specialised investigations. On the other hand, much can be learned merely by observing the child's use and understanding of speech and language. The purpose of this chapter is to present a much simplified outline of some of the chief aspects of speech and language which are susceptible to simple clinical observations (see Table I). The scheme represents the basic minimum required in an initial clinical evaluation. Different specialists will each want to extend different aspects. This chapter deals only with the central core which should be common to the assessments of all—paediatricians, otologists, psychiatrists, audiologists, psychologists, neurologists and speech therapists.

TABLE I

Scheme for assessment of speech and language

Imitation
'Inner Language'
Comprehension of Language

a) 'hearing behaviour' (hearing
(listening and attention
(understanding of spoken language

b) understanding of gesture
c) understanding of written language

Vocalisation and Babble
Language Production

a) mode used (spoken language, gesture, etc.)
b) syntactical complexity
c) semantic complexity
d) abnormal qualities to spoken language
e) social situations in which communication occurs
f) amount of communication

Word-Sound Production
Phonation·
Rhythm of Speech
Other Aspects of Development

a) cognition
b) socialisation and interpersonal relationships

Clinical assessment is largely described with respect to the 4-year-old child, as this age is convenient for the description of a wide range of phenomena. It is necessary to stipulate this as many manifestations change with development and with maturation. However, implicit in the description of vocalisation, babble and language comprehension in differential diagnosis, is the assumption that assessment can and should take place in the non-talking child before the age of 2 years. Early assessment is essential.

The order in which an assessment is carried out is of no great moment, but it is necessary to have some kind of overall scheme in mind in order to ensure a comprehensive evaluation of a child's speech and language.

In order to derive most meaning from the assessment the scheme used should be based on the normal developmental process, and defects and deficiencies should be related to this process (Reynell 1969a). It will be obvious that this description of assessment owes much to the work of others, particularly to Sheridan (1964), Ingram (1969a and b), Morley (1965) and Lenneberg (1964a, 1967).

Imitation

The rôle of imitation in the acquisition of language is both complex and ill-understood. The presence of well developed imitative skills is no guarantee of normal language development, as illustrated by the case of mongols (Lenneberg 1967). Nevertheless, serious deficiences in imitation are warning signals that all may not be well with language. The assessment of imitation is, therefore, particularly necessary in children under the age of 2 years who are referred because they are not yet speaking. Parents should be asked if the child readily engages in imitative games such as 'peek-a-boo', 'pat-a-cake' and 'ring-o-roses', and whether he waves 'good-bye' or tries to copy his mother's actions in dusting, hoovering the carpet, and making the beds. In the clinic an attempt should be made to confirm these reports by getting the child to copy actions in the form of a game. There should be concern if a 2-year-old child is not showing any of these imitative actions. Of all the language disorders, autism is most characteristically associated with a defect in this area*. Imitation of sounds may be similarly assessed by determining if the child will copy 'blowing a raspberry' and making sounds such as 'puh', 'mm', 'dada'.

'Inner Language'

The concept of 'inner language' refers to the availability of verbal concepts regardless of whether or not the child talks. Language has a crucial mediating function in cognition and thought (Herriot 1970). But it is important in this connection to make clear once again that by language I do not mean speech. The confusion between speech and language is illustrated by Furth's book (1966) which he called 'Thinking Without Language'. He rightly makes the point that deaf children who cannot speak can sometimes rival normal children in their performance of cognitive tasks. But, of course, as easily demonstrated by their use of gesture and sign language, they are *not* devoid of language. In developmental disorders, too, it can be shown that children who cannot talk can yet have normal understanding of language (Lenneberg 1962).

An accurate measure of a child's availability of verbal concepts or 'inner language' would require psychological investigations well beyond the scope of the initial clinical assessment of a non-speaking child. However, many children's games and toys demand the use of 'inner language' and these may be used as a guide (Sheridan 1969). Two levels may be distinguished: (a) meaningful use of objects and (b) pretend or make-

*Although autistic children often echo semi-automatically what is said to them, they are usually markedly deficient in the ability to imitate to order (either gesture or sound) and they less often spontaneously imitate in a flexible (as distinct from automatic and stereotyped) manner.

believe play. By the age of 18 months or so, children should be able to use real objects such as a hair-brush, spoon or cup, in a way that clearly indicates that they have understood their use. By their second birthday children should be able to do the same thing with miniature toys (Sheridan 1969). The clinician should ask the parent in detail about the way the child plays and what toys he uses. Does he push toy cars in the appropriate fashion or does he just spin the wheels? Does he 'talk' into a toy telephone or does he just take it apart? In the clinic the same functions may be assessed by handing the child objects such as a baby's brush and comb, a doll, a toy car or a toy telephone and observing what he does with them.

During the third and fourth years, the normal child shows a progressive development in his ability to play imaginative games and the clinician should enquire about this type of play. Does the child play at 'tea-parties', at dressing and undressing dolls, at 'mothers and fathers' or 'schools'? Does he use toy cars for races or driving into a garage or does he just push them in a stereotyped fashion? In the clinic the child's capacity for make-believe can be assessed by noting his play with a tea set and with doll's house furniture and family figures. The clinician should attempt to find out whether the child uses toys in a way which implies a story or a sequence of events and ideas. It is important to use toys appropriate to the child's age and interests so that whereas the above objects would be suitable for a 4-year-old, toy soldiers might arouse more interest in a boy of 7 or 8 years.

By 4 years of age the child should be beginning to produce recognisable drawings and the parents should be asked whether he uses crayons, felt-tip pens or paints. Does he draw at all, does he just scribble, or produce patterns, or does he produce figures and shapes which can be seen to represent something? In the clinic the child may be asked to draw a man as a means of assessing this. In this connection it is not the motor control or skill which is of prime interest but rather the extent to which the child puts meaning into his drawings.

The main condition in which there is a serious deficiency in 'inner language' is autism—the most global of all the language disorders. In the rare cases of developmental language disorder involving a severe defect in comprehension, 'inner language' may also be impaired although not usually to the same extent as in the autistic child. The mentally retarded child also may be deficient in imagination and fantasy but usually this deficiency is in keeping with his overall cognitive impairment. In other conditions such as deafness, elective mutism, and developmental disorders not involving receptive problems, 'inner language' is substantially normal.

Comprehension of Language
Evaluation of a child's comprehension of language is of prime importance in differential diagnosis (particularly in the child who does not talk at all). But also it is probably of considerable prognostic importance, at least in relation to autistic children (Rutter *et al.* 1967) and to children with a developmental language disorder (Griffiths 1969). The matter so far has been subject to very little systematic study but clinical experience suggests that in these conditions the degree of impairment in language comprehension gives a fair guide to the likelihood of the child later attaining competence in spoken language (Morley 1964).

The comprehension of spoken language involves several elements which may be grouped under the general term 'hearing behaviour'. Firstly there is *hearing*, that is the reception of sounds by the ear and their transmission to the brain; secondly there is *listening*, the act of paying attention to the sounds received with the object of interpreting their meaning (Sheridan 1964); and thirdly there is *comprehension*, that is the central coding and interpretation of the sound signals reaching the brain.

The ability to make quite complex discriminations between sounds and even between different voices and different intonations is present from early infancy (Hammond 1970), and during the first year of life there is a progressive growth in the child's capacity to understand what is said to him (Friedlander 1970).

To assess whether the child hears, the parents should be questioned closely on the child's response to everyday sounds. Does he look up when an aeroplane flies overhead? Does he ever turn around when the radio is switched on or off when he is not looking? Does he go to the door when the bell rings? In the clinic the child's responses should be carefully observed when interesting and meaningful noises of low intensity are made to one side and out of his sight (not in the midline). The rustling of a sweet paper, the ringing of a bell, the whirr of a friction car may be suitable stimuli (see chapter 7 for a more detailed description). The older child with some language may be asked to repeat whispered numbers. In this assessment it is particularly important that the sounds should be made without giving the child any tactile, visual, or vibratory cues.

Attention and listening should be gauged by noting the manner of the child's response to sounds of an intensity which it has been established he can hear. The clinician should note whether the child looks up when his name is called, whether he looks at the person who is speaking to him, and whether he is alert and attentive when given instructions. The child's responses should be noted both during direct interaction (such as when being spoken to while he and the clinician are playing together) and when the examiner tries to attract his attention when the child is playing on his own. In order to differentiate the autistic child it is also necessary to assess the child's response to any attempt to communicate with him. The deaf child or the child with a receptive developmental language disorder will watch faces and gestures intently trying to get clues from lip movements, facial expression and accompanying hand movements. In contrast, the young autistic child usually fails to hold eye-to-eye gaze and seems to pay no attention to anyone speaking to him.

The comprehension of spoken language needs to be assessed by noting the child's response to instructions spoken (at a volume he can hear) without any visual, contextual or gestural cues. A defect in comprehension can be gauged by the discrepancy between what the child can do spontaneously and what he can do on verbal command; or between the instructions he will follow if they are given with gesture and demonstration and those he will follow if they are just spoken without gesture, indication by looking, or any other non-verbal clues. For example, he may be asked to pick up something from the floor, get something from the desk, take a toy across the room, touch the door, turn around, or put his hands on his head. The instructions may be made more complicated by adding adverbs or qualifying phrases, *e.g.* 'turn around twice' or 'close the door slowly'. More precisely, his ability to understand prepositions may be tested by asking him to put one of the miniature toys in, on, under, or beside another. It is important to differentiate what the child cannot understand and what he just will not do, and sometimes it is helpful to get the mother to ask the child to do things. In any case, the parent should always be asked what things they can ask the child to do at home if no gestures are used. Will he understand being asked to get something from another room or from inside a drawer? It is important to check that the situation is not one which offers non-verbal clues to what is being asked. For this reason, routine requests are usually of no avail in assessing comprehension of spoken language. Thus, the child may put on his coat when asked merely because he sees other people doing the same or because he knows they always go out at that time. Reynell's Developmental Language Scales (1969b) provide a more systematic measurement of language comprehension.

The comprehension of gesture is primarily of value in terms of a comparison between understanding spoken language and understanding gesture, as already mentioned. The understanding of written language is not usually relevant in the pre-school child. However, it is noteworthy that some children with a severe defect in the comprehension of spoken language are appreciably better in their understanding of what is written—an important point in considering how to communicate with the child.

Different disorders are characterised by defects in different elements of 'hearing behaviour'. Thus, the severely deaf child neither hears, understands nor pays attention to sounds, but he *is* likely to watch people's faces closely to get clues on what they are trying to communicate. The mentally retarded child hears normally but may be inattentive to sounds and his comprehension will be limited. The autistic child hears but is markedly inattentive: characteristically, he does *not* watch faces and he comprehends little. The elective mute and the child with an executive developmental language disorder is normal on all counts. The diagnostic features with regard to comprehension are summarised in Table II.

TABLE II

Comprehension in differential diagnosis

	'Inner language'	*Hearing*	*Attention to sounds*	*Watching face*	*Understanding spoken language*	*Understanding gesture*
Severe deafness	+	−	−	+	−	+
Moderate deafness	+	loud only	loud only	+	loud only	+
High frequency loss	+	low freq. only	+	+	limited	+
Mental retardation	limited	+	±	+	limited	±
Autism	−	+	−	no	poor	±
Developmental language disorder (receptive)	variable	±	−	+	poor	+
Developmental language disorder (executive only)	+	+	+	+	+	+
Elective mutism	+	+	+	+	+	+

38

In this Table there is no mention of language retardation due to psychosocial deprivation. This is a condition which is not uncommon—particularly in immigrant children who have experienced very poor child-minding arrangements (see chapter 12). Its omission from the Table merely reflects the lack of adequate studies of language development in these children. My own experience and what is available in the literature suggests that it is unusual in this condition to get any significant impairment in 'inner language' or any aspect of language comprehension (see chapter 12). Thus, language delay due to psychosocial deprivation would be represented by normal or near-normal function in all elements of this Table.

Vocalisation and Babble

The sounds produced by the child in the clinic should be noted and the parents should be asked about the child's vocalisation at home. Many parents have difficulty in describing babble and it is often best to get them to copy the child's vocalisations and also to note differences compared with their other children. It may also be helpful to determine when the sounds 'baba', 'dada', 'gaga' first appeared (normally at about 6 months); when 'mammam', 'nannan' were used, when speech cadences were evident (both normally at about 8-9 months); and when sentence-like patterns of sounds with complex inflections apparently indicating questions, expostulations, or affection were evident (normally at about 10-11 months). Does he babble in a way that sounds like real conversation even though it does not make sense? Does his babble mostly consist of repetitions of just a few sounds or is the babble varied in character going from one sound to another (about 7-8 months)? Does he 'talk' to himself when playing or when put to bed or is he usually silent? Does he make sounds only to himself or does he seem to vocalise *to* people as if trying to tell them something? Does he try to copy what is said to him (about 9-10 months)?

Although quite a lot is known about the development of vocalisation and babble in normal children (Lewis 1951, Murphy 1964, Rebelsky *et al.* 1967; see also chapter 1), much less is known on the importance of babble in language development. Furthermore, there has been remarkably little study of the development of vocalisation and babble in hearing children with retarded language.

Even so, what little is known suggests that careful attention to the amount and quality of babble may be of some diagnostic importance: clearly it *is* with respect to the profoundly deaf. The vocalisations of the deaf child are normal up to about 6 months (Lenneberg 1964*a* and *b*, Murphy 1964). Between 6 and 9 months there may be subtle changes in the amount of babble and in the range of sounds produced at any one time. By 9 months there will be a loss of vocal quality, the consonants begin to disappear, the vowels become diphthongs and eventually only gutturals and primitive noises remain. This deterioration of vocalisation is a most useful guide to diagnosis.

With other disorders there is less certainty on the significance of babble. Clinical experience of young children and retrospective reports in studies of older children suggest that babble in autism and in developmental receptive language disorders is often either reduced in amount or deviant in quality (Myklebust 1957, Murphy 1964, Rutter *et. al.* 1971). However, apart from an investigation by Ricks (1972) still in progress, there has been no systematic investigation of the matter. The babble of children with a severe developmental disorder affecting word-sound production or with dysarthria may also be abnormal (Lenneberg 1962, 1964a and b) in that there is sometimes a paucity of consonants and an abnormality in vowel sounds.

It should also be said that the type of vocalisation and babble used by the child provides an indication of the level of speech development reached. When a child not yet talking is producing 'sentence' like patterns of sounds with complex inflections, speech cadences and imitative responses, the likelihood (but *not* certainty) is that words will follow soon after, provided language comprehension is also normal. If, however, the vocalisations are non-imitative, are limited in range and contain few consonants, the development of words is not likely to occur for some time.

In short, attention to the quantity and quality of babble provides valuable clues to speech and language development. If a child is slow to talk and shows deficient or deviant vocalisations this is an indication for further investigation and a definite bar to reassuring the parents that if they wait all will be well.

Language Production

In the child who does not talk, it is still necessary to consider whether there is language production using some other medium (Abercrombie 1964). The deaf child and the child with an executive developmental language disorder is usually eager to communicate even when he cannot speak. Accordingly some form of gesture or mime will usually be used. In sharp contrast, the autistic child and the elective mute very rarely use gesture. The mentally retarded child may use a little gesture but it is usually limited in amount and complexity. The child with a receptive developmental language disorder is often socially withdrawn when young but, even so, generally (but not always) uses some gesture.

When language of any sort is being produced, the next question is the *level* of language development. This applies to language in any medium but very little is known about how to measure the complexity of gestural language. The difficulties are quite enough with respect to spoken language so attention will be confined to this.

Complexity of language needs to be considered under at least two separate headings—syntax and semantics. The study of syntactical development has received a tremendous fillip in recent years through the emergence of the discipline of psycho-linguistics. This has caused people to look afresh at the rules of grammar and at the process by which the child learns these rules (Huxley 1969). More than anyone else, Chomsky (1957; 1965) has forced a re-thinking on the syntax of language. His trans-formational approach has led to the development of new methods of measuring language competence (Berko 1958, Fraser *et al.* 1963, Menyuk 1964a). Whereas these provide promise for the future, the initial *clinical* assessment still largely relies on the time-honoured measures of sentence length, use of subordinate clauses, use of qualifying terms such as adverbs, and the extent to which sentences are complete, *i.e.* contain all the appropriate descriptive and connecting words like prepositions, conjunctions, definite and indefinite articles and personal pronouns (McCarthy 1930, 1954, Templin 1957). A consideration of the child's spoken language in these terms can provide no more than a very rough guide to his level of syntactical development, but as an initial guide this is worth having.

In assessing language production, it is again necessary both to obtain an account from the parents and to observe what the child says in the clinic. To get the child to speak it is useful to talk to him about his play with miniature toys and to ask him questions about what he is doing. Another useful technique is to get the child to tell you what is happening in pictures he is shown. Large posters of action scenes are very suitable for this purpose but any interesting pictures may be used. Toddlers are very liable to withdraw in a strange situation and it is important to talk to the parents first to allow the child time to accustom himself to the clinic, then overtures to the child should be friendly but gradual and non-pressuring. It is better to kneel down in order to be on the child's eye-level and often it is preferable to attract the child to approach some interesting toy rather than for the clinician to approach the child. Some children will not talk to a strange person on their first visit to a clinic, in which case it may be useful to allow the mother and child to wait across the room while the examiner does something else. The opportunity may then be taken to listen to what the child says to his mother.

There is considerable variation in the rate at which language is acquired, but the average 18-month-old is likely to be using only one word utterances; in the next few months word combinations will be beginning; at 30 months 2-3 word phrases are typical and by $3\frac{1}{2}$ years the average sentence length should be about 4 words (McCarthy 1954). At first, most sentences are structurally incomplete but by 4 years three-quarters should be complete. Nouns are usually learned first but between 18 and 30 months there is a gradual increase in the proportion of pronouns, adjectives, verbs, prepositions and conjunctions used. Simple sentences predominate throughout the pre-school period but from 3 years onwards there is a very gradual increase in the use of sub-ordinate clauses. The sentences of the average 4-year-old are relatively well-developed as far as grammatical correctness is concerned, but they are nothing like as complex as those of the adult (Rebelsky et al. 1967).

An important question, although not one that can be answered on the basis of clinical observation, is whether language is merely delayed or whether the development of language is also deviant. Curiously, this question has received very little attention up to now. However, a study by Menyuk (1964b) of the grammar of children retarded in speech showed that their grammar was not only delayed in development compared with normal children but it was also different. Obviously, this finding has implications for views on the nature of developmental speech and language disorders.

Semantic complexity, although related to syntactical complexity, needs to be considered separately. Semantics refer to the meaning of words so that development has to be assessed on the child's ability to use words and to express ideas. Some estimate of this may be obtained by getting the child to describe a game, a television programme or an outing, in order to assess the adequacy of his descriptive powers. The child's spontaneous use of words may also be informative. It should be noted whether there is confusion in the use of words with specific and general meanings. For example, does the child use a specific word like 'chimney' to convey a general meaning of anything high up, or conversely, restrict the use of a general term such as 'dog' exclusively to one particular animal? Furthermore, to what extent does the child produce novel utterances and to what extent does he use ready-made phrases he has

41

heard from other people. In autism, to a greater extent than in other language disorders, there is a tendency for semantics to be more severely retarded than other aspects of language. This is frequently concealed by the autistic child's use of echoed or stereotyped phrases which may give a quite misleading picture of his language competence.

A discrepancy between different elements of language competence may also occur with written language. Children with a language delay of whatever kind tend to have mechanical reading skills in advance of their reading comprehension. Occasionally this descrepancy can be extreme as, for example, in a language retarded boy who seemed to have learned to read by virtue of his spending an inordinate amount of time watching television advertisements. He could read fluently at above age level, not only in English but also in French and Latin. However, an analysis of comprehension showed that he understood only a small fraction of what he had read. His comprehension of written language, like his comprehension of spoken language, was severely retarded.

Whether or not language development is delayed is an important point in children who present because their speech is unintelligible. Quite gross disorders of word-sound production may occur in children whose language is perfectly adequate if only one can understand what words the child is trying to pronounce. On the other hand, language delay and word-sound difficulties not infrequently co-exist and, both in planning treatment and giving a prognosis, it is essential to determine the extent to which language is implicated in the disorder.

The child's spoken language should also be examined for abnormal elements such as echolalia or neologisms. Of course, both of these occur as transient phenomena in normal development but their persistence is abnormal. A tendency to echo is most marked in autistic children but it is also fairly common in mentally retarded children and is occasionally present in children with a severe receptive developmental language disorder. Echolalic speech usually indicates a defect in the comprehension of language (Stengel 1964) and reflects the severity of the language disorder (Fay and Butler 1968). A rare condition, described by Beresford (see chapter 13), is characterised by children developing a system of abnormal speech sounds which almost amounts to a deviant language.

A consideration of the social context within which communication occurs is also of diagnostic importance. Deaf children and children with a developmental language

TABLE III

Language production in differential diagnosis

	Use of gesture	Social conversation	Echolalia	Word-sound production
Deafness	+++	++	−	defective
Mental retardation	+	+	++	poor
Autism	−	−	+++	variable
Developmental language disorder	++	++	±	variable/poor
Elective mutism	−	dependent on situation	−	normal

42

disorder usually make full conversational use of whatever language they have. Language may be impaired but communication is not. In contrast, the autistic child, even when he has language, is often handicapped in communication. He is likely to converse by means of limited question and answer. The autistic child tends not to 'chat' and is usually at a loss in a group of people talking together.

Similarly, if the sheer amount of inter-personal communication is considered, the autistic child stands out as one who both speaks little and communicates little. Whereas the mentally retarded child is more likely to make full use of his limited language skills, the autistic child does not do so.

The situation with the elective mute is different again. Characteristically he speaks normally in some situations (usually at home with his family) but rarely or never in others (usually school or anywhere with strangers). The elective mute is not retarded in language. The difficulty is simply in the use of language in certain social situations. Elective mutism should properly be classed with neurotic disorders and is only considered here because of its possible confusion with language retardation proper (see Table III).

Word-Sound Production

Certain aspects of speech have still to be considered. First there is the question of the child's word-sound production—the accuracy with which he is able to articulate words to produce speech sounds (see chapter 2). Careful attention to the quality of the child's speech should enable a differentiation to be made between (a) dysarthria in which either because of a central neurological deficit or because of a local structural defect there is an abnormality in articulation, (b) defective word-sound production secondary to defective sensory in-put, and (c) a *delay* in the normal development of word-sound production. Each of these is associated with a characteristic type of word-sound disorder. For example, children with a high tone hearing loss tend to omit high tone sounds such as 's' and 'th' from their own speech. Disorders of word-sound production have been well described by Ingram (1964, 1969a and b, Ingram and Barn 1961). Their relevance in the present context stems from the clues they may offer to the cause of language delay. In this connection, the characteristic quality of the speech of children with hearing disorders is most important. In addition, the occurrence of dysarthria may alert the clinician to the presence of a neurological disorder underlying the language retardation. Immaturities of speech in the form of consonant omissions and substitutions are common in children with a developmental language disorder and also occur in some autistic children. As part of the assessment of word-sound production, the degree of impairment should be quantified. This is best done by the use of special tests such as those devised by Renfrew (1971) and by Anthony *et al.* (1971). It is necessary to establish the degree of impairment because, of course, certain immaturities of speech are very common in young normal children and are a perfectly acceptable part of normal development.

The child's ability to produce normal speech is dependant in part on his being able to co-ordinate tongue and lip movements accurately and these should always be carefully assessed. As a screening test the child should be asked to move his tongue quickly from side to side and to lick his top lip (Rutter *et al.* 1970). If the speed, smoothness

43

and accuracy of the movements suggest a defect in tongue co-ordination, a fuller examination ought to be carried out. Most attention should be paid to the quality of the movements, as some children with fully normal speech are unable to lick their top lip.

Co-ordination problems in tongue movements may occur in isolation or as part of a general defect in motor co-ordination. One study (Dickson 1962) found that articulation errors were more persistent when they were associated with general clumsiness.

Phonation

Phonation concerns the quality of voicing. There are various local causes of dysphonia, the commonest being chronic laryngitis, but papillomata are also important (see chapter 2). With respect to language disorders, whispering is a common accompaniment to elective mutism and various oddities of voice production are occasionally found in autistic children. However, phonation offers but few clues to the nature of a language disorder.

Rhythm of Speech

Lastly, the rhythm of speech needs to be considered (see chapter 2). The most frequent disorder of rhythm is stammering which is commoner in children who have been delayed in language development and which, like other developmental disorders, is considerably commoner in males (Andrews and Harris 1964). The co-ordination of speaking and breathing may sometimes be impaired in children with autism or with a developmental language disorder, thus giving rise to an abnormality of rhythm.

Other Aspects of Development

The initial clinical assessment of a child referred because he is not yet talking will necessarily involve many functions other than speech and language. However, two—'cognition' and 'socialisation'—require special mention because of their close association with language (Lewis 1963, 1968) and because of their importance in differential diagnosis.

The measurement of cognitive performance is described more fully in chapter 10, so that here only brief mention need be made of the *clinical* assessment of 'cognition'. Obviously, in a child who is not yet talking, it would be absurd to use verbal items to measure intelligence. Motor milestones, too, are of little value in this connection. Nevertheless, much may be learned from questioning the parents closely on the child's use of toys, his patterns of play, his approach to new objects, and the extent to which he can look after himself and help about the home. In observing the child himself, particular attention should be paid to the way he approaches a new situation; to the extent to which he is curious and interested in objects; to his skill in understanding how things work; to his constructional abilities and most of all to the degree of system and logic he uses in finding out how to use or manipulate objects, toys or implements. By these means, a useful rough indication may be obtained of whether or not the child is intellectually retarded as well as slow to speak.

Some evaluation of social and emotional development should also be made in the initial clinical assessment. Social anxiety and shyness is common in children who have a language delay regardless of its cause but there are special features associated with autism and with elective mutism. The mentally subnormal child will be socially and emotionally *immature* but probably not otherwise abnormal in this area of functioning.

Parents should be questioned on the degree to which the child shows his feelings in his facial expression; whether he 'cuddles' and comes for comfort when upset, hurt or tired; whether he responds differently to his parents than he does to other people; whether he is attached to his parents; whether he appears upset when they leave him; whether he runs up to them when they come back; whether he will join in play with other children and whether he has made any 'friends' (*i.e.* individuals of whom he is particularly fond). The first interview with the child provides a good opportunity for observing his relationship with his parents, the way he separates from them and his reaction to meeting strange adults. The young autistic child usually shows a general impairment of emotional responsiveness, a lack of separation-anxiety, a failure to cuddle or come for comfort and a failure to develop enduring personal relationships. It should be added that although this is characteristic of the autistic child of 3 or 4 years, the clinical features change considerably as he grows older. The elective mute is usually normally responsive at home and, indeed, may be over-attached to his parents and unduly dependent on them. Outside home he is generally either inert and unresponsive or he is anxious and very fearful.

Finally, there must be some assessment of the home situation and of parent-child interaction. Is the child left with baby-sitters at all during the day? What are the circumstances (*e.g.* with one familiar adult or with a group of 20 other children under the care of one baby-minder), frequency and duration? When and how much do the parents play or talk with the child? What sort of toys does he have? Does he meet other adults at all (grandparents, friends of the family)? The clinician should also note how the parents deal with the child in the clinic and how they talk to him. Do they show interest in the child and his activities? How do they respond to the child's approaches or vocalisations? What do they do if the child becomes upset? Do they talk to him? Do they cuddle him?

Conclusion

In outlining a skeletal scheme upon which a minimal initial clinical assessment of speech and language might be based, there has been a danger of over-simplification— of making difficult problems of differential diagnosis appear easier than in fact they are, merely by focussing on differences rather than similarities and by de-emphasising ambiguities and overlap. Some of the statements on phenomena have had to be based on clinical descriptions rather than the results of controlled comparative studies and it will have been only too evident that many aspects of language remain relatively uncharted. However, it should also have been made clear that the little we do know, if systematically applied, can carry us well into the process of differential diagnosis before the results of specialised tests are available.

REFERENCES

Abercrombie, D. (1964) 'Language and medium.' *in* Renfrew, C., Murphy, K. (Eds.) *The Child who does not Talk.* Clinics in Developmental Medicine, No. 13. London: S.I.M.P. with Heinemann, p. 22.
Andrews, G., Harris, H. (1964) *The Syndrome of Stuttering.* Clinics in Developmental Medicine, No. 17. London: S.I.M.P. with Heinemann.
Anthony, A., Bogle, D., Ingram, T. T. S., McIsaac, M. W. (1971) *The Edinburgh Articulation Test.* Edinburgh: Churchill Livingstone.

Berko, J. (1958) 'The child's learning of English morphology.' *Word*, **14**, 150.
Carroll, J. B. (1964) *Language and Thought.* Englewood Cliffs, N.J.: Prentice-Hall.
Chomsky, N. (1957) *Syntactic Structures.* The Hague: Mouton.
—— (1965) *Aspects of the Theory of Syntax.* Cambridge, Mass.: M.I.T. Press.
Dickson, S. (1962) 'Differences between children who spontaneously outgrow and children who retain functional articulation errors.' *J. speech Res.*, **5**, 623.
Ekman, P., Friesen, W. V. (1969) 'The repertoire of non-verbal behaviour categories, origins, usage and coding.' *Semiotica*, **1**, 49.
Fay, W. H., Butler, B. U. (1968) 'Echolalia, IQ, and the dichotomy of speech and language systems.' *J. speech Res.*, **11**, 365.
Fraser, C., Bellugi, U., Brown, R. W. (1963) 'Control of grammar in imitation, comprehension and production.' *J. verb. Learning verb. Behav.*, **2**, 121.
Friedlander, B. Z. (1970) 'Receptive language development in infancy: issues and problems.' *Merrill-Palmer Quart.*, **16**, 7.
Furth, H. G. (1966) *Thinking without Language.* New York: The Free Press.
Griffiths, C. P. S. (1969) 'A follow-up study of children with disorders of speech.' *Brit. J. Dis. Commun.*, **4**, 46.
Hammond, J. (1970) 'Hearing and response in the newborn.' *Develop. Med. Child. Neurol.*, **12**, 3.
Herriot, P. (1970) *An Introduction to the Psychology of Language.* London: Methuen.
Huxley, R. (1969) 'Research in language development.' *in* Wolff, P., Mac Keith, R. (Eds.) *Planning for Better Learning.* Clinics in Developmental Medicine, No. 33. London: S.I.M.P. with Heinemann. p. 77.
Ingram, T. T. S. (1964) 'The complex speech disorders of cerebral palsied children'. in Renfrew, C., Murphy, K. (Eds.) *The Child who does not Talk.* Clinics in Developmental Medicine, No. 13. London: S.I.M.P. with Heinemann. p. 163.
Ingram, T. T. S. (1969a) 'Disorders of speech in childhood.' *Brit. J. hosp. Med.*, **2**, 1608.
—— (1969b) 'Developmental disorders of speech.' *in* Vinken, P. J., Bruin, G. W. (Eds.) *Handbook of Clinical Neurology*, Vol. 4. Amsterdam: North Holland. p. 407.
—— Barn, J. (1961) 'A description and classification of common speech disorders associated with cerebral palsy. *Cerebr. Palsy Bull.*, **3**, 57.
Latif, I. (1934) 'The psychological basis of linguistic development and the ontogeny of meaning.' *Psychol. Rev.*, **41**, 55, 153.
Lenneberg, E. H. (1962) 'Understanding language without ability to speak: a case report.' *J. abnorm. soc. Psychol.*, **65**, 419.
—— (1964a) 'Language disorders in childhood.' *Harvard educ. Rev.*, **34**, 152.
—— (1964b) 'Speech as a motor skill with special reference to nonaphasic disorders.' *Monogr. Soc. Res. Child Develop.*, **29**, 115.
—— (1967) *Biological Foundations of Language.* New York: John Wiley.
Lewis, M. M. (1951) *Infant Speech.* London: Harrap.
—— (1963) *Language, Thought and Personality in Infancy and Childhood.* London: Harrap.
—— (1968) 'Language and mental development.' *in* Lunzer, E. A., Morris, J. F. (Eds.) *Development in Human Learning, II.* London: Staples Press. p. 68.
McCarthy, D. A. (1930) *The Language Development of the Pre-School Child.* University of Minnesota Child Welfare Monograph, No. 4. Minneapolis: University of Minnesota.
—— (1954) 'Language development in children.' *in* Carmichael, L. (Ed.) *Manual of Child Psychology*, 2nd edn. New York: John Wiley. p. 492.
Menyuk, P. (1964a) 'Syntactic rules used by children from pre-school through first grade.' *Child Develop.*, **35**, 533.
—— (1964b) 'Comparison of grammar of children with functionally deviant and normal speech.' *J. speech Res.*, 7, 109.
Morley, M. (1964) 'Prognosis in relation to developmental disorders of speech in children.' *in* Renfrew, C., Murphy, K. (Eds.) *The Child who does not Talk.* Clinics in Developmental Medicine, No. 13. London: S.I.M.P. with Heinemann. p. 121.
—— (1965) *The Development and Disorders of Speech in Childhood.* Edinburgh: E. & S. Livingstone.
Murphy, K. (1964) 'Development of normal vocalisation and speech.' *in* Renfrew, C., Murphy, K. (Eds.) *The Child who does not Talk.* Clinics in Developmental Medicine, No. 13. London: S.I.M.P. with Heinemann. p. 11.
Mykelbust, H. R. (1957) 'Babbling and echolalia in language therapy.' *J. speech Dis.*, **22**, 356.
Rebelsky, F. G., Starr, R. H., Luria, Z. (1967) 'Language development: the first four years.' *in* Brackbill, Y. (Ed.) *Infancy and Early Childhood.* New York: The Free Press. p. 289.
Renfrew, C. E. (1971) *Renfrew Language Attainment Scales.* Churchill Hospital, Oxford.
Reynell, J. (1969a) 'A developmental approach to language disorders.' *Brit. J. Disord. Commun.*, **4**, 33.
—— (1969b) *Developmental Language Scales.* Slough, Bucks: N.F.E.R.
Ricks, D. (1972) The Beginnings of Vocal Communication in Infants and Autistic Children. M.D. Thesis, University of London.
Rutter, M., Greenfield, D., Lockyer, L. (1967) 'A five to fifteen year follow-up study of infantile psychosis.' *Brit. J. Psychiat.* **113**, 1183.

—— Graham, P., Yule, W. (1970) '*A Neuropsychiatric Study in Childhood.* Clinics in Developmental Medicine, Nos. 35/36. London: S.I.M.P. with Heinemann.

—— Bartak, L., Newman, S. (1971) 'Autism—a central disorder of cognition and language.' *in* Rutter, M. (Ed.) *Infantile Autism—Concepts, Characteristics and Treatment.* London: Churchill Livingstone. p. 148.

Sheridan, M. (1964) 'Development of auditory attention and the use of language symbols.' *in* Renfrew, C., Murphy, K. (Eds.) *The Child who does not Talk.* Clinics in Developmental Medicine, No. 13. London: S.I.M.P. with Heinemann. p. 1.

—— (1969) 'Playthings in the development of language.' *Hlth. Trends,* **1,** 7.

Stengel, E. (1964) 'Speech disorders and mental disorders.' *in* de Reuck, A. V. S., O'Connor, M. (Eds.) Disorders of Language, Ciba Foundation Symposium. London: Churchill. p. 285.

Templin, M. C. (1957) *Certain Language Skills in Children: their Development and Inter-Relationship.* University of Minnesota Institute of Child Welfare, Monograph No. 26. Minneapolis: University of Minnesota Press.

Worster-Drought, C. (1968) 'Speech disorders in children.' *Develop. Med. Child Neurol.,* **10,** 427.

CHAPTER 4

A Note on the Prevalence of Language Disorders in Young Children

R. C. MAC KEITH and MICHAEL RUTTER

Normal Development

Two-thirds of children say their first single words between 9 and 12 months, the same proportion begin to use phrases between 17 and 24 months and by 2 years of age two-thirds are intelligible to strangers (Morley 1965).

However, there is a wide range of normal, and children who do not reach these milestones at the stated times may still show an essentially normal development. It is a difficult matter to say when a child is so slow to speak that the delay must be regarded as 'abnormal'. It is particularly difficult because many children with speech delay have no recognisable 'disease' and do ultimately speak normally. Yet the eventual acquisition of speech is no guarantee of normality, in that many of the children slow to speak have later educational difficulties (see chapter 15).

In this chapter, an account is given of the prevalence of language delay sufficiently marked to handicap the child. The figures given are conservative and it is probable that a larger number of children have difficulties which, though milder, are still great enough to hinder the child at least temporarily.

Language and Speech Delay

Although there are several studies of children's articulation defects, there are very few epidemiological studies of language delay. The most reliable figures are available from the Newcastle longitudinal study (Spence *et al.* 1954, Morley 1965). In a representative sample of 114 children studied intensively, 6 per cent had a definite retardation of language development at 3 years 9 months, in that they were still using incomplete sentences. At the same age, 11 per cent had speech that was unintelligible. A year later, just prior to starting school, only one child was still using incomplete sentences but 4 per cent remained unintelligible. In a much larger representative group of 944 children studied by health visitors, 10 per cent were unintelligible at 3 years 9 months, 5 per cent at 4 years 9 months and 0.7 per cent at $6\frac{1}{2}$ years. They found a considerable overlap between articulation defects and language delay. The number of school-age children with poor articulation greatly exceeded the number with poor language skills but many of those with defective articulation were slow to speak when younger (Morley 1965).

In short, when children first start at school, some 5 per cent speak so poorly that they are unable to make themselves understood by strangers and 1 per cent (overlapping with the 5 per cent) are seriously retarded in their production of spoken language. These figures are in general agreement with those of the Bristol survey (Herbert and Wedell 1970) which found 1 per cent of children with a handicapping language delay. Boys outnumber girls by 2 to 1 in both the speech disordered and language disordered children.

Specific Developmental Language Disorder

Among the children with *mild* language delays the majority have a specific developmental disorder, but in the group with serious and persisting language problems the proportion is much lower. The best estimate of prevalence is provided by Ingram's surveys in Edinburgh and Aberdeen (Ingram 1963). Speech therapists, educational psychologists, child psychiatrists and audiologists were asked to report children thought to be of average intelligence who had only a few single words at the age of 3 years and only very limited connected speech by the age of 5 years. The estimated prevalence of severe language retardation was 0.71 per 1,000 for Edinburgh and 0.75 per 1,000 for Aberdeen. The Isle of Wight (Rutter *et al.* 1970*a*) figure for developmental language disorders in school age children was closely similar (0.8 per 1,000) so that it may be concluded that the rate is probably slightly less than 1 per 1,000 among school-age children.

Developmental disorders involving a defect in language comprehension ('developmental receptive aphasia') are even rarer still. *Transient* comprehension problems are present in perhaps a quarter to a sixth of children with developmental language disorders (Ingram 1959) but comprehension improves much more rapidly than any other aspect of speech or language. There is no reliable figure for the rate of persistent receptive difficulties but some estimate may be obtained from the fact that in the Newcastle series of 74 children with a developmental language disorder only 2 had marked receptive difficulties (Morley 1965). Clinic studies show that it is, for example, considerably less common than infantile autism (Rutter *et al.* 1971) so that the rate is likely to be less than, and probably much less than, 1 per 10,000.

Intellectual Handicap

At least two and a half per cent of children have intellectual handicap (IQ less than 70) and over half of these show a severe language deficiency or an articulation defect or both—a rate 10 times that in the general population (Rutter *et al.* 1970*b*). Thus, there are some 1½ per cent of children who have intellectual retardation associated with a marked language delay. The most gross language defects are to be found in children with severe intellectual handicap (IQ less than 50) but its prevalence (3.7 per 1,000—Tizard 1966, Kushlik 1968) is far less than that of mild intellectual handicap which, in absolute terms, gives rise to more cases of *moderate* language delay. This is by far the commonest cause of children never learning to talk.

Deafness

Mild hearing loss is a relatively common condition. Thus, Anderson (1967) in an audiometric study of twenty-five thousand children found that nearly 4 per cent had a 20 decibel loss of hearing for two or more frequencies between 250 c.p.s. and 6,000 c.p.s. The number requiring hearing aids is perhaps a twentieth of that—about 2 per 1,000 (Rutter *et al.* 1970*b*), and the number with severe hearing loss even less. Barton *et al.* (1962) found that 0.7 per 1,000 children attended schools for the deaf. Nearly all of these have a serious language deficiency and the rate of marked language retardation due to deafness is probably not more than 1 per 1,000—about the same as for severe developmental language disorders.

Infantile Autism

Infantile autism occurs in some 2 to 4 children per 10,000 (Lotter 1966). In three quarters of cases there is associated intellectual retardation, making the rate of autism in children of normal intelligence about 1 per 10,000. All of these children show language retardation.

Cerebral Palsy

Cerebral palsy occurs in 2 to 3 children per 1,000 (Ingram 1955, Henderson 1961, Rutter *et al*. 1970*a*), of whom a third have an IQ below 50 and about half an IQ below 70. Of the cerebral palsied children with an IQ above 50, about 2 in 5 show language retardation of some degree. Thus, excluding cases with severe intellectual handicap, there are just less than 1 per 1,000 children with cerebral palsy and language retardation, but in most of these the language handicap is mild or moderate rather than severe.

Socio-cultural Language Retardation

There are no reliable figures on the prevalence of socio-cultural language retardation.

Conclusions

The best available estimates suggest that 1 per cent of children come to school with a marked language handicap and a further 4 to 5 per cent may show the sequelae of earlier language difficulties. The commonest condition associated with language delay is intellectual retardation, but deafness, cerebral palsy and developmental disorders are also common, the last two particularly as a cause of mild to moderate language delay. Infantile autism is a less common cause of mild to moderate language retardation but is more important as a cause of severe and persistent language retardation.

REFERENCES

Anderson, U. M. (1967) 'The incidence and significance of high-frequency deafness in children.' *Amer. J. Dis. Child.*, **113**, 560.
Barton, M. D., Court, S. D., Walker, W. (1962) 'Causes of severe deafness in school-children in Northumberland and Durham.' *Brit. med. J.*, **i**, 351.
Henderson, J. L. (Ed.) (1961) *Cerebral Palsy in Childhood and Adolescence: A Medical, Psychological and Social Study*. Edinburgh: E. & S. Livingstone.
Herbert, G. W., Wedell, K. (1970) 'Communication handicaps of children with specific language deficiency.' Paper read at the Annual Conference of the British Psychological Society, Southampton, April, 1970.
Ingram, T. T. S. (1955) 'A study of cerebral palsy in the childhood population of Edinburgh.' *Arch. Dis. Childh.*, **30**, 85.
—— (1959) 'Specific developmental disorders of speech in childhood.' *Brain*, **82**, 450.
—— (1963) *Report of the Dysphasia Subcommittee of the Scottish Paediatric Society*. (Mimeographed report.)
Kushlik, A. (1968) 'Social problems and mental subnormality.' *in* Miller, E. (Ed.) *Foundations of Child Psychiatry*. London: Pergamon. p. 369.

Lotter, V. (1966) 'Epidemiology of autistic conditions in young children. I. Prevalence.' *Soc. Psychiat.*, **1**, 124.

Morley, M. E. (1965) *The Development and Disorders of Speech in Childhood*. Edinburgh: E. & S. Livingstone.

Rutter, M., Graham, P., Yule, W. (1970*a*) *A Neuropsychiatric Study in Childhood*. Clinics in Developmental Medicine, No. 35/36. London: S.I.M.P. with Heinemann.

—— Tizard, J., Whitmore, K. (Eds.) (1970*b*) *Education, Health and Behaviour*. London: Longmans, Green.

—— Bartak, L., Newman, S. (1971) 'Autism—a central disorder of cognition and language?' *in* Rutter, M. (Ed.) *Infantile Autism, Concepts, Characteristics and Treatment*. London: Churchill Livingstone.

Spence, J. C., Walton, W. S., Miller, F. J. W., Court, S. D. M. (1954) *A Thousand Families in Newcastle-upon-Tyne*. London: O.U.P.

Tizard, J. (1966) 'Epidemiology of mental retardation: a discussion of a paper by E. M. Gruenberg.' *Int. J. Psychiat.*, **2**, 131.

CHAPTER 5

Environmental Influences on Language Development

MICHAEL RUTTER and PETER MITTLER

Although we remain largely ignorant concerning the *processes* of language development (see chapter 1), we do know something of the environmental factors which affect the growth of language. These factors may well prove important when language fails to develop and they also have implications for treatment. The treatment of a child who does not talk, or who talks poorly, inevitably involves manipulation of the environment, if only in the therapy sessions. For these reasons, a knowledge of what influences the emergence of spoken language in the normal child is important to those who deal with children retarded in language.

The Meaning of Environment

Environments are usually thought of in broad terms such as institution or home, middle-class or working class, large family or small family. The associations between such variables and language development are discussed later in this chapter, but first it is necessary to consider the effects of more 'fine-grain' variables. Only in this way can we obtain any understanding of *why* children in institutions (for example) are often delayed in language compared with children reared in their own homes. It is not simply the fact of being separated from parents that matters, as it is only in *some* institutions that children are retarded in language. What does make the difference? Is it the lack of face-to-face talk, the high level of meaningless background noise, the lack of play opportunities, the number of caretakers looking after the child, or the size of the family group?

Just as speech and language have to be considered according to their individual components if the nature of speech delay is to be understood (see chapter 3), so environment must be analysed to differentiate the specific features which impinge on the child in a variety of ways. Clinicians frequently talk of the child from a 'deprived' home, but in itself this means little. Is the home deprived in terms of furnishings and decorations, or nutrition, or play opportunities, or conversation or encouragement for the child, or affection or amount of parent-child interaction? The effects of each of these is likely to be rather different.

Specific Influences

Effects on Early Vocalisation

Several studies have shown that both verbal enrichment and social reinforcement can substantially increase the amount of an infant's vocalisation and babble. For example, it has been found that babies vocalise more if they are spoken to only whenever they vocalise. This effect can still be obtained if the speaking is produced on tape without a person present, but the reinforcement is somewhat more effective if there is both a voice and person (Todd and Palmer 1968). Interestingly, vocalisations are apparently not increased by a person's presence alone if he does not speak to the child (Weisberg 1963).

The effects of verbal enrichment were studied by Irwin (1960) in an experiment with 13-to 30-month-old infants. The group was divided into two parts, an experimental group whose mothers read to them for fifteen to twenty minutes per day, and a control group. From 18 months onwards, the experimental group were found to produce more spontaneous babble. It is also possible to influence the type of babble. Routh (1969) showed that contingent reinforcement of vocalisations of two-to seven-month-old infants not only increased sound production but could differentially increase the particular types of vocalisations, namely vowel or consonant sounds.

It appears that mothers talk more to their baby girls than to their baby boys (Moss 1967, Halverson and Waldrop 1970). Whether this has anything to do with the tendency for girls to be somewhat ahead of boys in their later language development (see chapter 1) remains a matter for speculation.

For verbal enrichment to have any value it must have meaning and/or reinforcing properties. Mere increase in vocal noise is not enough. Thus, in a study of institutional babies, Casler (1965) found that the impersonal repetition of a string of numbers had no effect on the babies' developmental progress. He did not examine effects on the rate of vocalisation, but it is likely that similarly negative results would have been found if he had.

These are interesting findings, but it remains to be shown what importance (if any) these gains in babble have for *language* development. The development of babble ordinarily follows a regular and systematic progression (Lewis 1951, McCarthy 1954, Murphy 1964) and babble is often deviant or deficient in children with very severe language impairment (see chapter 3). These findings suggest a possible connection between babble and language. However, in some circumstances language comprehension can develop in the adsence of babble (Lenneberg 1962) and a variety of studies suggest important discontinuities bewteen babbling and language production (Ervin-Tripp 1966, Rebelsky *et al.* 1967). At present, it can only be said that while babble often serves as a useful indicator of language development there is no *necessary* connection between the two. The link between babble and language is complex and requires further study (DeHirsch 1970).

Imitation

Children undoubtedly frequently imitate what is said to them and this constitutes an important phase in their development (Lewis 1951). At first, immediate spontaneous imitations involve little or no comprehension—they merely reflect what is included in a brief memory span. At a later stage, imitation is no longer mechanical, but involves some kind of restructuring or reordering of the material into the framework of the child's level of grammatical skill (Ervin-Tripp 1966). Imitations of this sort provide a reasonable measure of a child's grammatical knowledge.

However, the extent to which young children directly *learn* by imitation is uncertain. They cannot easily be induced to expand the length of their utterances beyond a critical number of words or morphemes. Repeated attempts to induce direct imitation of adult utterances only result in the child repeating his own character-istically truncated version. Imitations (see Brown 1965) usually preserve the word order of the model sentence, but do not increase in proportion to the length of the model. The young child's grammar is relatively resistant to adult models even under constant instruction. Ervin (1964) reported one unsuccessful attempt to replace a child's 'Nobody don't like me' to 'Nobody likes me'. The adult repeated the correct form eight times without success, but at the ninth attempt the child said, 'Oh, I see. 'Nobody don't likes me'. Moreover, imitations only include those elements of adult grammar that are already in the child's repertoire. If the child is not using the '-ing' form it will not usually be possible to elicit it. Thus, the child is likely to say 'Adam fast' in response to 'Adam is running fast'. Imitation is affected by short-term memory, comprehension, 'processing' of the utterance and, in a general sense, by the level both of language and of intellectual development.

Children can sometimes be induced to imitate sentences utilising a somewhat more complex grammar than their original spontaneous productions (Ervin 1964, Miller and Ervin 1964), but the available evidence suggests that, probably, imitation provides only a minor *direct* influence on syntactical development. However, it may well be more important in the learning of vocabulary or in articulation, but this remains to be studied.

Effects on Language Development

For any training to be effective, the child must have reached the stage of biological maturation when language development is possible (Strayer 1930), but given that, in certain circumstances training may well accelerate language development (Luria and Yudovitch 1959, Mueller and Smith 1964). *Which* aspects of training are important in the normal development of language has only been systematically investigated very recently.

Behaviourists have sometimes viewed language as merely another piece of behaviour which develops simply through the process of reward and punishment (Skinner 1953, 1957). Of course, language is behaviour and, like any other behaviour is subject to modification by means of differential reinforcement and other influences on learning (Salzinger *et al.* 1962, Bandura and Harris 1966). But the acquisition of language involves, amongst other things, the learning of various rules of grammar (see chapter 3) and it is by no means self-evident that these are learned by means of reward and punishment. Indeed—at least with normal children—it seems likely that they are not learned in this way.

Brown and Hanlon (1970) studied parental approval and disapproval in relation to children's utterances. They found that reinforcements were not primarily linked with the grammatical form of the utterance: rather, they were linked to the truth value of the child's statement, or sometimes to the correctness of the word-sound production. For example, the sentence 'Mama isn't a boy, he is a girl' was followed by the mother saying 'That's right' in approval of the child's concept of mother as female in spite of syntactic errors in the statement. Contrariwise, the child's assertion that 'There's the animal farmhouse' was followed by the mother's 'No, that's a lighthouse' —responding to the content of the statement, not to its syntactic correctness. Only three families were studied so that generalisations are not yet warranted, but it seems that reinforcement may be important with respect to phonetic and semantic development but not to syntactic development.

The importance in language training of the way in which adults talk to children has been studied experimentally (Cazden 1966, Brown *et al.* 1969). In Cazden's study, negro children aged 28-38 months attending a day centre were divided into three groups. In the first experimental group, the children received forty minutes per day of intensive and deliberate expansions of their statements for a period of three months. The adult echoed what the child said but filled in the missing functions to make a complete sentence: if the child said 'Dog bark', the adult would reply, 'Yes, the dog is barking', the rationale being that the child would learn the correct grammar for what he had said. In the second experimental group, the adult produced an equal number of well formed sentences, but avoided using expansions: in reply to the child's 'Dog bark' he might say 'Yes, he's mad at the kitty'. The third group (which served as a control) had an equal time in the experimental play room, but no verbal stimulation.

Contrary to the author's predictions, the children in the second group made most progress in language. The expansion group also made more progress than the control children, but not as much as the modelling group. At first sight this seems paradoxical, in that both the expansion and modelling group received the same amount of language stimulation, the difference being that the expansions were more explicitly linked to the grammar of the child's own utterances. Among the possible explanations are (1) the lack of novelty in expansions may depress the child's interest in what the adult says, (2) the expansions may misinterpret the child's intended meaning, so misleading the child in a way which interferes with his learning, and (3) the modelling provides more semantic information for the same syntactic experience.

Whatever the correct reason, these preliminary findings suggest that in normal children with a normal language competence, a rich, varied and informative verbal interchange without direct modification of the child's own utterance provides the best stimulus for syntactical development. Unfortunately, very little is known about the best stimulus for semantic and phonetic development (which may be different from what is required for the growth of grammar) and next to nothing is known about what is needed when there is defective language competence, or deviant (as distinct from delayed) language development. What very limited evidence there is suggests that in cases of deviant development more direct techniques of speech training may have a place in treatment (see chapter 17). The advantages of specific phonetic training remain to be established (Wilson 1966).

Wider Environmental Influences

The discussion so far has been concerned with the effects of specific types of environmental intervention. Greater knowledge about these effects should aid our understanding of the mechanisms involved in environmental influences on language development, but at present we have made little progress in that direction. We should now consider the consequences for the child who is reared in different types of environment.

Institutional Care

Many studies have shown that prolonged institutional care frequently has a profoundly depressing effect on language development (Haywood 1967, Tizard 1969). The effects are demonstrable even in infancy (Brodbeck and Irwin 1946, Provence and Lipton 1962) and persist throughout childhood accompanied by a similar depression of verbal intelligence. Similar results are seen with children reared at home in circumstances where there is a gross lack of verbal stimulation (Gordon 1924, Asher 1935, Wheeler 1942, Jones 1954). To a considerable extent, the retardation is reversible by improving the quality of institutional care with particular attention to adult-child interaction (Tizard 1964, Yarrow 1964). However, temporary and partial remediation of deprivation (either in the institution or at home) is of very limited benefit (Skeels *et al.* 1938, Eisenberg 1967). Children removed from poor institutions and adopted in very early childhood have a good prognosis for language as well as for other aspects of development (Haywood 1967). Furthermore, in institutions where adequate stimulation is provided, the children are not retarded (Yarrow 1964, Tizard 1971). This is an important finding as it demonstrates that it is the nature of care which is important for language development and *not* whether the child remains at home with his parents.

It is not known how early remedial measures need to be provided in order to be effective. Obviously, the longer the depriving circumstances have lasted the more difficult it will be to reverse the language retardation. Nevertheless, it would be quite wrong to assume that if language has not developed by 5 years of age (or at any other age) it is too late to provide treatment. There is one famous case of a 6-year-old girl, mute and performing at a severely retarded level on IQ tests when discovered, having lived in isolation up to that time in a dark attic with a mute mother. She was given intensive language training (as well as medical treatment for rickets and other therapies) on a residential basis and made a remarkable recovery. At follow-up she was apparently linguistically, emotionally, and intellectually normal, although somewhat behind in her schoolwork (Mason 1942, Davis 1947). Obviously, it would be foolhardy in the extreme to suppose that such a good outcome would be the usual result, but the point is that recovery is sometimes possible even after such prolonged and severe deprivation, provided that there is total removal of the depriving circumstances.

The relationship between the quality of institutional care and the presence of language retardation emphasises that it is the nature of the child's environment (rather than separation from parents as such) which is important. This is also indicated by the generally good development of kibbutzim children (Kohen-Raz 1968). Institutions differ from ordinary homes in many respects (Tizard 1969) and which features are important for language development are not known with any certainty. However, one of the most striking deficiencies of most institutions is the paucity of adult-child interaction of any kind (Rheingold 1960, 1961) and doubtless this is one important factor.

Institutional rearing as such is not sufficient to explain language retardation and a much more detailed analysis is required to identify and isolate the 'fine-grain' environmental variables involved. Institutional environments often involve a constant background of people and of noise from television and radio. This in turn brings

56

about a difficulty for the child in distinguishing relevant foreground from irrelevant background. It is only rarely that he is talked to at close quarters, and there is usually all too little opportunity for close conversational interchange in which the child can use the reaction of the adult speaker as feedback to help him regulate his behaviour. Moreover, as Spradlin (1968) points out, it tends to be non-verbal rather than verbal behaviour which is reinforced by patterns of institutional living (King *et al.* 1971). Which of these various influences associated with an institutional upbringing is most important for language development has still to be established.

Family Structure

Although there are few consistent associations between family size and early speech development (Rebelsky *et al.* 1967), there are strong associations with verbal intelligence. Several large scale studies have shown that children in large families have lower scores on tests of vocabulary and verbal IQ than do children with only one or two brothers or sisters (Nisbet 1953, Douglas 1964, Douglas *et al.* 1968). The same association applies to reading ability which requires skills in written language (Rutter *et al.* 1970), but not to non-verbal intelligence or mathematics which do not include language skills. Thus, the association applies specifically to abilities associated with competence in higher language functions. The association with family size is not explicable in terms of social class differences and can be found even in professional families, although the association is not as marked as in the working class population.

Furthermore, the association between large family size and verbal skills is not accountable in terms of genetic influences; though genetic factors are certainly important in the development of language functions (Mittler 1969) they cannot account for the association with family size. As family size is associated with verbal skills, but not with non-verbal skills, this could reflect a hereditary mechanism only if either (a) verbal skills have a high genetic component whereas non-verbal skills do not, or (b) if highly verbal parents restrict the size of their families whereas parents of high non-verbal skills do not. The first possibility can be ruled out by the evidence that perceptual and spatial abilities have at least as strong a genetic loading as verbal abilities (Meades and Parkes 1966, Vandenberg 1968, Mittler 1971). There is no direct evidence on the second possibility, but it seems inherently unlikely.

Rather, it seems more probable that the association between family size and language skills is a function of family conditions in early childhood—the verbal difference between children in small and in large families is maximal by eight years of age. It has been suggested that a child's growth of vocabulary is affected by the extent to which, when learning to talk, he comes into contact with other pre-school children whose small vocabularies and elementary grammar offer little verbal stimulation, rather than with adults whose language is richer and more varied (Nisbet 1953, Douglas *et al.* 1968). In keeping with this view is the finding that children's vocabulary scores fall as the number of pre-school children in the family increases (Douglas *et al.* 1968). In large families there is probably less intensive interaction and less communication between parents and children. On the other hand, it may be the *clarity* of the language environment, rather than its complexity, which is the key variable. In a study of tape recordings of family conversation in the home, Friedlander (1971) found that the presence of sibs tended to lead to a tumultous clamour in which several people spoke at once at different levels. Perhaps this kind of linguistic chaos makes language acquisitions more difficult in large families. However, this supposition is based on very little evidence, and there is need for further study of differences in family interaction according to family size, as well as studies relating such differences to language development.

Children of Multiple Births

A special instance of unusual family structure occurs in twins and other multiple births. Twins and triplets start speaking several months later than singletons (Day 1932, Howard 1964) and the Dionne quintuplets (Blatz *et al.* 1937) were not using words until 22 months of age. Characteristically, children of multiple births make more use of gesture and mime to communicate than other children and quite often they have a jargon which is intelligible only to their co-twins. The retardation in spoken language persists throughout the pre-school years as shown by an overall poverty of vocabulary, immature grammar and primitive sentence constructions, shorter utterances, and a more limited use of spoken language for abstraction and conceptualisation. In the school years, the language deficit is evident in the verbal intelligence scores which are lower than those for singletons. The non-verbal intelligence of twins may be slightly below average, but the difference is small and appreciably less than that for verbal skills.

Using the Illinois Test of Psycholinguistic Abilities, Mittler (1970) compared 200 four-year-old twins with 100 singleton controls of the same age and social background. At the age of 48 months, twins showed an average retardation of 6 months of language development. Analysis of the ITPA profiles did not indicate any characteristic pattern of linguistic disability; the results could be explained most parsimoniously in terms of an overall immaturity of language development. There were no differences between identical and fraternal twins. As in Day's (1932) study, an attempt was made to control for non-verbal intelligence. The twins showed average, or above average scores on non-verbal tests; and were only marginally inferior to the singleton controls. The language retardation could not therefore be explained in terms of an overall intellectual deficit, however slight.

When the results were examined in the light of social class differences, it was clear that language retardation in relation to controls was far greater in middle class than in working class twins. Twins from social classes I and II differed from comparable singleton controls by 9 months of language age; the gap was reduced to 4 months for social class III, and reached insignificant proportions (2 months) for social classes IV and V. These findings suggest that middle class twins are more vulnerable in terms of language development than working class twins. Reasons for this are far from clear, but it is possible that middle class twins, by virtue of the 'closed communication system' of the twin situation (Zazzo 1960), are somehow less able to take advantage of the facilitating language environment conventionally associated with the middle class home.

The delay in onset of speech in twins is not usually great enough for the children to be referred for failure to speak. Although during the pre-school period they lag well behind in language development, most twins start speaking by 18 months of age. Day (1932) found that the average vocabulary for twins at 24 months of age was 55 words. Nevertheless, some language impairment is often evident and this requires explanation.

Twins and triplets are frequently of low birth weight and short gestation, and are subject to a greater than usual risk of perinatal damage. This may be a minor factor in the really small babies, as there is a slight (but significant) tendency for the lighter twin to have a somewhat lower verbal reasoning score than his heavier partner (McKeown 1970). However, even when there is a weight difference of at least 0.9 kg, the verbal IQ difference is only some three points, so that this is unlikely to be more than a minor contributory factor.

As in any other child, genetic factors play an important part in the determination of language development in twins. But, genetic factors probably play no part in the impaired language of twins compared with singletons, and overall, non-genetic factors are probably more important in language development than in the development of general intelligence (Mittler 1969). The importance of post-natal influences is most strongly shown by the finding that the verbal intelligence of twins whose co-twin was still-born, or who had died in early infancy, is only half a point below that of singletons (Record *et al.* 1970). In contrast, when both twins survived their score was 4.5 points below other children.

It is not known with certainty quite what these postnatal influences are. Probably one important factor is the one already discussed with respect to family size—*i.e.* there is less parent-child interaction and communication than in single births. Twins and triplets receive a higher proportion of verbal interchange from those of their own age than singletons. This tendency is much increased by the tendency for twins and triplets to have a jargon or 'secret language' which is only understood by their co-twin (Zazzo 1960). It seems that the language of other pre-school children provides a less satisfactory stimulus than that of adults.

'Deaf Environment'

It might be thought that the lack of spoken language in the environment of a hearing child brought up by deaf parents is likely to have a profoundly depressing influence on linguistic development, but Critchley (1967) has shown that this is not necessarily so. Of 4 children in this situation studied, one showed some language impairment and a second showed an articulation pattern similar to that seen in deaf children. The other two children appeared normal. Apparently, the parental use of gesture and sign provides an important stimulus to communication, and oral stimuli may be provided by others. The hearing child of deaf parents may, in fact, have more linguistic experience than other children through his having to act as interpreter for the family and make contact for them.

Bilingualism

The effects on language development of learning two languages, appear to differ according to whether the children are true bilinguals learning both languages from the outset, or whether they are basically monolinguals who have to learn a second language because their first language is not the accepted tongue for the region in which they live. Most studies have been of the latter type (Darcy 1953, Soffietti 1955), and these show that the children who have to learn a second language tend to have a smaller vocabulary and perform somewhat less well on tests of verbal intelligence than monolinguals. However, in these cases there are many factors other than bilingualism which are operative. The second language may be learned in pidgin form, there may be social barriers and prejudice involved in the differences between the two language cultures, and subcultures which have to learn a second language may be socially deprived. On the other hand, when children are truly bilingual there may even be linguistic and cognitive advantages associated with the learning of two languages—possibly associated with greater conceptual flexibility (Peal and Lambert 1962).

From the comprehensive studies of Smith (1935a and b, 1949, 1957), it appears that bilingualism does *not* delay the early development of speech, that it is better if children learn each language from a different source, and that the later linguistic handicaps are most evident in the intellectually dull child. Bilingualism is not a cause of failure to develop speech, and whether the possession of two languages rather than one constitutes an advantage, or disadvantage, depends on the social context, on the abilities of the child, on the extent to which he is truly bilingual and on whether he is taught mainly in his preferred language.

Social Class

Numerous studies have shown that working class school-age children show an inferior language performance to middle class children (McCarthy 1954, Templin 1957, Lawton 1968); this difference also applies to tests of vocabulary knowledge and verbal intelligence (Douglas *et al*. 1968). The social class differences with respect to the age of starting to speak, and to the speed of development of syntactic and semantic competence in language, are quite small. Indeed, in many respects, even slum children are not significantly retarded in *early* language development. Accordingly, social class influences are only of minor importance with regard to the main topic of this book—children referred because they are retarded in speech development. But the differences are of major importance with regard to the wider topic of language skills, especially in relation to educational performance where the working class child is particularly at a disadvantage.

To some extent, these findings are probably due to differences in general intelligence (which is substantially under the influence of genetic factors). Only a few studies have attempted to partial out or control for IQ when investigating social class differences in language functioning. Nevertheless, it seems that there are important social differences in language usage even after IQ has been taken into account.

These differences in usage are most marked with respect to abstract functions and to the *way* in which language is used, rather than to language competence as such. For example, working class children describing a picture make more use of 'exophoric' pronouns to refer to something not actually mentioned by name, whereas middle class children use more nouns. Thus, a middle class child might say 'three boys are playing football and one boy kicks the ball and it goes through the window ....', whereas a working class child might say 'they're playing football and he kicks it and it goes there ....' (Hawkins 1969). The middle class children are thereby more specific and more elaborate in a way which is intelligible without the immediate context. In contrast, what the working class child says is less explicit, makes more assumptions, and is only fully understandable in context.

In the same way, middle class mothers have been found to be more explicit and informative than working class mothers when teaching their child and when answering their questions. Middle class families more often use language to express ideas and concepts and they tend to do so in a way which is precise and takes less for granted (Hess and Shipman 1965, Robinson and Rackstraw 1967, Brandis and Henderson 1970). It is clear, then, that there are links between the ways in which parents talk to their children and their children's skills and style in language usage. So far it has not been shown that this is a causal relationship, but, at least in part, it probably is.

Bernstein (1965), whose work has been most influential in this area, has described the differences in terms of what he calls an 'elaborated' and a 'restricted' code or style of speaking. An elaborated code is one where the speaker selects from a relatively extensive range of syntactic alternatives to express ideas or concepts in such a fashion that the message could be understood in its own right without knowledge of the speaker or the social context. In contrast, a restricted code is one where the range of syntactic alternatives is severely limited and where the understanding of the message is largely dependant on a knowledge of the speaker, the circumstances in which he spoke, and the social setting of the conversation.

It should be noted that each code is preferable to the other for some purposes. For example, in a group which share certain values and experiences, phrases which have an implicit meaning to those in the know (a restricted code) may aid a sense of solidarity and may also be a more economical use of words. In-jokes and shared references in a family or a group of friends may serve this purpose. On the other hand, a restricted code is not suitable for exploring logic, conveying fine discriminations in ideas, or teaching new concepts. For this reason, an elaborated code is much more effective for educational purposes. The distinction between the codes is not an absolute one, but Bernstein's thesis is that in certain social groups (such as in many working class settings) there is such a preponderance of restricted code usage that language involving an elaborated code fails to develop adequately.

Of course, the fact that some working class individuals make little use of an elaborated code does not necessarily mean that they do not have one available. Indeed, Robinson (1965), in an ingenious series of experiments, has convincingly shown that working class children who were normally restricted code users could be induced to use *some* features of the elaborated code by giving them a formal task in which the elaborated code was more appropriate (writing a letter to someone in authority).

Nevertheless, what is still not at all clear is the extent to which the social class differences refer to language *competence*, rather than to the ways in which language is used to communicate. Bernstein (Gahagan and Gahagan 1970) has been quite explicit that he has been concerned only with usage and not with availability, but his theories have often been misleadingly extended from linguistic codes to linguistic abilities. Social class differences are only really striking with respect to vocabulary, higher order language functions concerning abstraction and conceptualisation, and the use of language as a medium for the accurate transmission of precise information. In terms of the relevance of language for cognitive development, these abilities are, of course, crucial, but it is important not to confuse these semantic and cognitive skills with syntactic performance and even less with syntactic capacity.

Nevertheless, language is essentially a social skill and it seems highly likely that the style of communication which Bernstein calls an 'elaborated code' follows a developmental course. Glucksberg and Krauss (1967) have described an experiment in which two children were seated on either side of an opaque screen. Each child had in front of him a series of unusual designs. One child then had to describe the design he had picked up in such a way that his companion could recognise it from an identical display. Children under the age of 6 years were hopeless at this task; they used phrases such as 'It goes like this' (which was, of course, meaningless to the other child who could not see what the first child was doing). Older children were more likely to give informative descriptions such as 'It's like a boat' or 'It's like a hat'. This development in the skills of referential communication has some surface similarity to the development of an elaborated code.

Bernstein's attempts to work out a detailed model of the ways in which social organisation and social relationships might affect the development and use of language, have opened up important new avenues of thought concerning environmental influences on language development. Much has still to be learned about this topic, especially with regard to developmental issues. For example, to what extent does someone who fails to *use* an elaborated code also have difficulty in *understanding* an elaborated code?—the important distinction between language comprehension and production emphasised throughout this book. How far does the usage of particular linguistic codes reflect their availability and the individual's linguistic competence in different codes? To what extent does failure to use an elaborated code impair its development? At what age does code usage tend to become established and how far can this be altered later?

Implications for Therapy

In discussing environmental influences on language development, we have been restricted to areas where systematic studies have been conducted, and it is important to note some of the influences we have not considered which may also be important. For example, it is likely that the amount of interest parents show in what their children say, the degree to which they encourage him to express his ideas and join in conversation, and the extent to which they convey to him the importance of his verbal contribution, are equally influential. But these factors have not been systematically evaluated. Understanding, confidence, and social participation are all important elements in the growth of language. Other chapters (see chapter 1 and 3) have emphasised the way in which comprehension of language usually precedes language production and the important link between make-believe play and language. Although not proven, it would seem to follow that when pretend play and understanding of speech are impaired, attempts should be made to aid their development as a crucial part of speech therapy. Studies of deaf children suggest that aiding communication in any medium whether it be speech, mime or gesture, is likely to promote language, and it need not be thought that if gesture is helped speech will suffer: the converse is more likely to be true.

It is not easy to apply the findings on environmental influences to speech therapy, as much will depend on the nature of the child's handicap. What is quite clear, however, is that language training has much to offer even before words are present (Greene 1967). In deciding which therapeutic approach to follow, perhaps the most crucial distinction to make is between the 'objective' and 'effective' environment (Rutter and Sussenwein 1971). If parents keep talking to a child in complex and interesting sentences, 'objectively' there is a rich and varied language environment. If, however, the child is deaf, to all intents and purposes the 'effective' environment is barren and unstimulating. Similarly, if the child has a defect of language comprehension, long complex sentences merely create confusion and the child may just 'shut off'. Yet again, if the child is autistic or withdrawn, social and language opportunities will not impinge on him unless deliberate efforts are made to intrude, to ensure he pays attention and to make the stimuli interesting. In short, what matters is that the environment be meaningful and available to the child, taking into consideration his particular handicaps. Therapy needs to determine both what environmental influences he needs *and* how to make these available to him. Children with disorders of perception, or of language comprehension, are unlikely to respond to the environment in the same way as normal children, and any therapeutic programme should take this into account.

The therapist also needs to know the extent to which language is *deviant* as well as delayed (Menyuk 1964, 1969, Morehead and Ingram 1970). Although little studied to date, it seems that some children who are slow to speak differ in the *way* that speech develops as well as in its timing. Furthermore, although in the normal child syntactical skills (or competence in grammar) tend to develop in close conjunction with semantic skills (or competence in the meaning of words; *see* Herriott 1968, 1970), these two aspects of language are distinct (Suci 1969) and, particularly in cases of abnormal development, they may be affected differentially. The implications of these findings for treatment remain uncertain, but for the present if should not be assumed that what helps development in the normal child is necessarily needed by the child with a language defect or disorder. Treatment programmes may have to be oriented specifically to one type of handicap (*e.g.* Conn 1971).

This is relevant to a consideration of the value of pre-school programmes for the child who is slow to speak, or whose linguistic usage is poor with respect to educational needs (Pines 1968, Starr 1971). Is a more structured environment, or more specific language teaching, necessary to encourage the development of speech and language in children with language delay? Some suggest that a good nursery school for normal children provides the best environment, but others argue that children from a very deprived background, with a defect in language comprehension, deviant language development, or possibly just a severe language delay, are unable to profit from an environment which provides only general verbal 'stimulation'. Because of their handicaps, they neither perceive environmental stimuli normally nor do they take up the opportunities for interaction. Perhaps the most extreme protagonists of this view are Bereiter and Engelman (1966) who advocate highly formal teaching methods designed to provide instruction in a graded programme of language acquisition. Most workers have advocated less rigidly formal methods than these, but there is some evidence that programmes need to be directly focussed on the children's specific defects (Haywood 1967, Weikart 1967).

Much further research is needed into the types of pre-school provision which are most effective for children with linguistic handicaps. Certainly, merely providing 'more of the usual' stimulation is not likely to be adequate, and advising the parents to 'keep talking to him' is of little benefit. Similarly, interaction with other children is of limited value in itself. Adults seem to play a more important rôle in furthering language development than do other children, and it follows from this that sending speechless children to nursery schools in the hope that they will 'learn from the others', may be more an act of faith than judgement unless specific efforts are directed to obtaining the desired verbal interaction. Free play and opportunity to experiment are valuable, but on their own they are of little use to children handicapped in language comprehension or linguistic usage who have not yet learned to profit from such opportunities.

Conclusions

While there is ample evidence that a child's language development is influenced and modified by environmental circumstances, we are only just beginning to find out which circumstances have which effects by means of which mechanism. Until these mechanisms are understood, we should be cautious in loosely ascribing 'language difficulties' to 'social deprivation' or to any other broad and global entity. It should also be recognised that children with biological handicaps tend to be more susceptible than normal children to adverse environmental influences. Many language disorders have more than one main determinant. When we have learned more about these complex interactions, and about which specific features of the environment influence which particular aspects of language development and in what way, we shall be in a stronger position to plan a rational and sound programme of treatment.

REFERENCES

Asher, E. J. (1935) 'The inadequacy of current intelligence tests for testing Kentucky mountain children.' *J. genet. Psychol.*, **46,** 480.
Bandura, A., Harris, M. B. (1966) 'Modification of syntactic style.' *J. exp. Child Psychol.*, **4,** 341.
Bereiter, C., Engleman, S. (1966) *Teaching Disadvantaged Children in the Pre-School.* Englewood Cliffs, N.J.: Prentice Hall.
Bernstein, B. (1965) 'A socio-linguistic approach to learning.' *in* Gould, J. (Ed.) *Penguin Survey of the Social Sciences.* Harmondsworth: Penguin Books. p. 144.
Blatz, W. E., Fletcher, M. I., Mason, M. (1937) 'Early development in spoken language of the Dione quintuplets.' *in* Blatz, W. E., Chant, N., Charles, M. W., Fletcher, M., Ford, N. H. C., Harris, A. L., McArthur, F., Mason, M., Millichamp, D. A. *Collected Studies on the Dionne Quintuplets.* Toronto: University of Toronto Press.
Brandis, B., Henderson, D. (1970) *Social Class, Language and Communication.* London: Routledge and Kegan Paul.
Brodbeck, A. J., Irwin, O. C. (1946) 'The speech behavior of infants without families.' *Child Develop.*, **17,** 145.
Brown, R. (1965) *Social Psychology.* New York: The Free Press.
—— Cazden, C., Bellugi-Klima, U. (1969) 'The child's grammar from I to III.' *in* Hill, J. P. (Ed.) *Minnesota Symposia on Child Psychology*, Vol. 3. Minneapolis: University of Minnesota Press. p. 25.

—— Hanlon, C. (1970) 'Derivational complexity and order of acquisition in child speech.' *in* Hayes, J. R. (Ed.) *Cognition and the Development of Language*. New York: John Wiley. p. 11.

Casler, L. (1965) 'The effects of supplementary verbal stimulation on a group of institutionalised infants.' *J. Child Psychol. Psychiat.*, **6**, 19.

Cazden, C. (1966) 'Subcultural differences in child language.' *Merrill-Palmer Quart.*, **12**, 185.

Conn, P. (1971) *Remedial Syntax*. I.C.A.A. Occasional Papers, No. 1. London: Invalid Children's Aid Association.

Critchley, E. (1967) 'Language development of hearing children in a deaf environment.' *Develop. Med. Child Neurol.*, **9**, 274.

Darcy, N. T. (1953) 'A review of the literature on the effects of bilingualism upon the measurement of intelligence.' *J. genet. Psychol.*, **82**, 21.

Davis, K. (1947) 'Final note on a case of extreme isolation.' *Amer. J. Sociol.*, **52**, 432.

Day, E. J. (1932) 'The development of language in twins. II' *Child Develop.*, **3**, 179, 298.

DeHirsch, K. (1970) 'A review of early language development.' *Develop. Med. Child Neurol.*, **12**, 87.

Douglas, J. W. B. (1964) *The Home and the School*. London: Macgibbon & Kee.

—— Ross, J. M., Simpson, H. R. (1968) *All our Future*. London: Peter Davies.

Eisenberg, L. (1967) 'Clinical considerations in the psychiatric evaluation of intelligence.' *in* Zubin, J., Gervis, G. A. (Eds.) *Psychopathology of Mental Development*. New York: Grune & Stratton. p. 502.

Ervin, S. M. (1964) 'Imitation and structural change in children's language.' *in* Lenneberg, E. H. (Ed.) *New Directions in the Study of Language*. Cambridge, Mass.: M.I.T. Press. p. 163.

Ervin-Tripp, S. (1966) 'Language development.' *in* Hoffman, L. W., Hoffman, M. L. (Eds.) *Review of Child Development Research, Vol.* 2. New York: Russell Sage Foundation. p. 55.

Friedlander, B. Z. (1970) 'Receptive language development in infancy: issues and problems.' *Merrill-Palmer Quart.*, **16**, 7.

Gahagan, D. M., Gahagan, G. A. (1970) *Talk Reform: Explorations in Language for Infant School Children*. London: Routledge & Kegan Paul.

Glucksberg, S., Krauss, R. M., (1967) 'What do people say after they have learned to talk? Studies of the development of referential communications' *Merrill-Palmer Quart.*, **13**, 309.

Gordon, H. (1924) Mental and Scholastic Tests among Retarded Children. London: Board of Education Pamphlet, No. 44.

Greene, M. (1967) 'Speechless and backward at three.' *Brit. J. Disord. Commun.*, **2**, 139.

Halverson, C. F., Waldrop, M. F. (1970) 'Maternal behavior towards own and other preschool children: the problem of "ownness".' *Child Develop.*, **41**, 839.

Hawkins, P. R. (1969) 'Social class, the nominal group and reference.' *Lang. Speech*, **12**, 125.

Haywood, C. (1967) 'Experimental factors in intellectual development: 'the concept of dynamic intelligence.' *in* Zubin, J., Jervis, G. A. (Eds.) *The Psychopathology of Mental Development*. New York: Grune & Stratton. p. 69.

Herriot, P. (1968) 'The comprehension of syntax.' *Child Develop.*, **39**, 273.

—— (1970) *An Introduction to the Psychology of Language*. London: Methuen.

Hess, R. D., Shipman, V. C. (1965) 'Early experience and the socialization of cognitive modes in children.' *Child Develop.*, **36**, 869.

Howard, R. W., (1964) 'The language development of a group of triplets.' *J. genet. Psychol.*, **69**, 181.

Irwin, D. C. (1960) 'Infant speech: effect of systematic reading of stories.' *J. speech Res.*, **3**. 187.

Jones, H. E. (1954) 'The environment and mental development.' *in* Carmichael, L. (Ed.) *Manual of Child Psychology*. 2nd edn. New York: John Wiley. p. 631.

King, R. D., Raynes, N. W., Tizard, J. (1971) *Residential Care of Children: Sociological Studies in Institutions for the Handicapped*. London: Routledge & Kegan Paul.

Kohen-Raz, R. (1968) 'Mental and motor development of Kibbutz, institutionalized and home-reared infants in Israel.' *Child Develop.*, **39**, 490.

Lawton, D. (1968) *Social Class, Language and Education*. London: Routledge & Kegan Paul.

Lenneberg, E. H. (1962) 'Understanding language without ability to speak: 'a case report.' *J. abnorm. soc. Psychol.*, **65**, 419.

Lewis, M. M. (1951) *Infant Speech*, 2nd edn. New York: Humanities Press.

Luria, A. R., Yudovitch, F. (1959) *Speech and the Development of Mental Processes in the Child*. London: Staples Press.

McCarthy, D. A. (1954) 'Language development in children.' *in* Carmichael, L. (Ed.) *Manual of Child Psychology*, 2nd edn. New York: John Wiley, p. 492.

McKeown, T. (1970) 'Prenatal and early postnatal influences on measured intelligence.' *Brit. med. J.*, **3**, 63.

Mason, M. K. (1942) 'Learning to speak after years of silence.' *J. speech Res.*, **7**, 295.

Meades, J. S., Parkes, A. S. (Eds.) (1966) *Genetic and Environmental Factors in Human Ability*. Edinburgh: Oliver & Boyd.

Menyuk, P. (1964) 'Comparison of grammar of children with functionally deviant and normal speech.' *J. speech Res.*, **7**, 109.

—— (1969) *Sentences Children Use*. Cambridge, Mass.: M.I.T. Press.

65

Miller, W., Ervin, S. (1964) 'The development of grammar in child language.' *Monogr. Soc. Res. Child Develop.*, **29**, 9.

Mittler, P. (1969) 'Genetic aspects of psycholinguistic abilities.' *J. Child. Psychol. Psychiat.*, **10**, 165.

—— (1970) 'Biological and social aspects of language development in twins.' *Develop. Med. Child Neurol.*, **12**, 741.

—— (1971) *The Study of Twins*. London: Penguin Books.

Morehead, D. M., Ingram, D. (1970) 'The development of base syntax in normal and linguistically deviant children.' *Papers and Reports on Child Language Development*, No. 2. California: Stanford University Press.

Moss, H. A. (1967) 'Sex, age and state as determinants of mother-infant interaction.' *Merrill-Palmer Quart.*, **13**, 19.

Mueller, M., Smith, J. O. (1964) 'The stability of language age modifications over time.' *Amer. J. ment. Defic.*, **68**, 537.

Murphy, K. (1964) 'Development of normal vocalisation and speech.' *in* Renfrew, C., Murphy, K. (Eds.) *The Child who does not Talk*. Clinics in Developmental Medicine, No. 13. London: S.I.M.P. with Heinemann. p. 11.

Nisbet, J. (1953) 'Family environment and intelligence.' *Eugen. Rev.*, **45**, 31.

Peal, E., Lambert, W. E. (1962) 'The relationship of bilingualism to intelligence.' *Psychol. Monogr.*, **76**, (27).

Pines, M. (1968) *Revolution in Learning*. London: Allen Lane.

Provence, S., Lipton, R. C. (1962) *Infants in Institutions*. New York: International Universities Press.

Rebelsky, F., Starr, R. H., Luria, Z. (1967) 'Language development: the first four years.' *in* Brackbill, Y. (Ed.) *Infancy and Early Childhood*. London: Collier-Macmillan. p. 289.

Record, R., McKeown, T., Edwards, J. H. (1970) 'An investigation of the difference in measured intelligence between twins and singletons.' *Ann. hum. Genet.*, **34**, 11.

Rheingold, H. L. (1960) 'The measurement of maternal care.' *Child Develop.*, **31**, 565.

—— (1961) 'The effect of environmental stimulation upon social and exploratory behaviour in the human infant.' *in* Foss, B. M. (Ed.) *Determinants of Infant Behaviour, Vol.* 1. London: Methuen. p. 143.

Robinson, W. P. (1965) 'The elaborated code in working class language.' *Lang. Speech*, **8**, 243.

—— Rackstraw, S. J. (1967) 'Variations in mothers' answers to children's questions as function of social class, verbal intelligence test scores and sex.' *Sociology*, **1**, 259.

Routh, D. K. (1969) 'Conditioning of social response differentiation in infants.' *Develop. Psychol.*, **1**, 219.

Rutter, M., Tizard, J., Whitmore, K. (1970) *Education, Health and Behaviour*. London: Longmans.

—— Sussenwein, F. (1971) 'A developmental and behavioural approach to the treatment of preschool autistic children.' *J. Autism Childhd Schiz.*, **1.** 376.

Salzinger, S., Salzinger, K., Portnoy, S., Ekman, J., Bacon, P., Deutsch, M., Zubin, J. (1962) 'Operant conditioning of continuous speech in young children.' *Child Develop.*, **33**, 683.

Skeels, H. M., Updegraff, R., Wellman, E. L., Williams, H. M. (1938) A Study of Environmental Stimulation: an Orphanage Preschool Project. University of Iowa Studies in Child Welfare, **15**, no. 4.

Skinner, B. F. (1953) *Science and Human Behaviour*. New York: Macmillan.

—— (1957) *Verbal Behaviour*. London: Methuen.

Smith, M. E. (1935a) 'A study of some factors influencing the development of the sentence in preschool children.' *J. genet. Psychol.*, **46**, 182.

—— (1935b) 'A study of the speech of eight bilingual children of the same family.' *Child Develop.*, **6**, 19.

—— (1939) 'Some light on the problem of bilingualism as found from a study of the progress in mastery of English among preschool children of non-American ancestry in Hawaii.' *Genet, Psychol. Monogr.*, **21**, 119.

—— (1949) 'Measurement of vocabularies of young bilingual children in both of the languages used.' *J. genet. Psychol.*, **74**, 305.

—— (1957) 'Word variety as a measure of bilingualism in preschool children.' *J. genet. Psychol.*, **90** 143.

Soffietti, J. P. (1955) 'Bilingualism and biculturalism.' *J. educ. Psychol.*, **46**, 222.

Spradlin, J. E. (1968) 'Environmental factors and the language development of retarded children.' *in* Rosenberg, S., Koplin, V. H. (Eds.) *Development in Applied Psycholinguistic Research*. Riverside N. J.: Macmillan. p. 612.

Starr, R. H. (1971) 'Cognitive development in infancy and assessment, acceleration and actualization.' *Merrill-Palmer Quart.*, **17**, 153.

Strayer, L. C. (1930) 'Language and growth: the relative efficacy of early and deferred vocabulary training, studies by the method of co-twin control.' *Genet. Psychol. Monogr.*, **8**, 209.

Suci, G. T. (1969) 'Relations between semantic and syntactic factors in the structuring of language.' *Lang. Speech*, **12**, 69.

Templin, M. C. (1957) *Certain Language Skills in Children*. Minneapolis: University of Minnesota Press.

Tizard, B. (1971) 'Environmental effects on language development: a study of residential nurseries.' Paper read at The British Psychological Association Annual Conference, Exeter, April, 1971.

Tizard, J. (1964) *Community Services for the Mentally Handicapped.* London: O.U.P.

—— (1970) 'The role of social institutions in the causation, prevention and alleviation of mental retardation.' *in* Haywood, H. C. (Ed.) *Socio-Cultural Aspects of Mental Retardation.* New York: Appleton-Century-Crofts. p. 282.

Todd, G. A., Palmer, B. (1968) 'Social reinforcement of infant babbling.' *Child Develop.*, **39**, 591.

Vandenberg, S. G. (1968) 'The nature and nurture of intelligence.' *in* Glass, D. C. (Ed.) *Genetics.* New York: Rockefeller Press and Russell Sage Foundation. p. 3.

Weikart, D. P. (1967) *Preschool Intervention.* Ann Arbor, Mich.: Campus Publications.

Weisberg, P. (1963) 'Social and non-social conditioning of infant vocalization.' *Child Develop.*, **34**, 377.

Wheeler, L. R. (1942) 'A comparative study of the intelligence of East Tennessee mountain children.' *J. educ. Psychol.*, **33**, 321.

Wilson, F. B. (1966) 'Efficacy of speech therapy with educable mentally retarded children.' *J. speech, Res.*, **9**. 423.

Yarrow, L. J. (1964) 'Separation from parents during early childhood.' *in* Hoffman, M. L., Hoffman, L. W. (Eds.) *Review of Child Development Research, Vol.* 1. New York: Russell Sage Foundation. p. 89.

Zazzo R. (1960) *Les Jumeaux: le Couple et la Personne.* Paris: P.U.F.

CHAPTER 6

The Assessment of a Child in a Speech Clinic

T. T. S. INGRAM and ANN HENDERSON

In the past, speech therapists have been expected to undertake the diagnosis as well as the management of children who suffer from speech disorders. Yet a high proportion of children referred to speech therapists suffer from diseases which directly affect the structure or the function of lips, tongue and palate, or they suffer from conditions which are the primary causes of their speech difficulties, *e.g.* mental defect or hearing loss. Many show psychiatric abnormalities which may be primary or secondary to their speech defects (McGrady 1968).

Children referred to any hospital speech clinic are found to suffer from a wide variety of diseases. Some of these are relatively common, *e.g.* Down's syndrome and cerebral palsy; others are much rarer, *e.g.* myasthenia gravis, congenital dystrophia myotonica, congenital nuclear agenesis. In addition, many children with predominantly psychiatric or social problems are referred to the speech clinic because their parents are reluctant to seek help on other than strictly medical grounds, and their family doctors are well aware of this.

In these circumstances, it is unrealistic to expect a speech therapist to diagnose children as well as to treat them. The speech therapist is entitled to expect that children referred to her have been fully assessed from the medical standpoint. The doctor who assesses the child should have some knowledge of speech defects. Unfortunately, very few medical schools educate their undergraduates about speech disorders and it is difficult even for medical officers of health and school medical officers to obtain postgraduate education in this field, though an increasing number of courses are being made available.

In many cases, the detailed assessment of a clinical or educational psychologist can be invaluable to the speech therapist in indicating the intelligence quotients (IQs) of the child and, more importantly, the particular disabilities from which he suffers. The psychologist has an increasing number of comprehension, cognitive development and performance tests, the results of which are of great value to the speech therapist working with a child with the aim of improving his speech.

It is important that the assessment of a child with a speech disorder should be regarded as one that merits a team approach—though the team may differ in content according to the nature of the child's speech disability—with the paediatrician as the constant member of the team, and here we wish to consider his rôle in more detail.

The Medical Assessment

Whenever possible, the speech therapist should see the child before the doctor. This serves as an occasion for the speech therapist to meet the child and to put the parents and child at ease before the medical examination. It also allows the speech therapist to make observations about the child's behaviour, language and articulation, which are of great help to the doctor when he comes to the stage of interviewing the parents and examining the child more formally. The doctor (not white-coated) elicits the formal history, examines the child, and then discusses the case with the speech therapist and decides with her on what further investigations are required and on the subsequent management.

The order in which the history is taken varies from paediatrician to paediatrician. This paediatrician likes to begin with the family history and ask about neurological disease, congenital deformities, any history of mental defect, speech disorders, left handedness, ambidexterity or hearing defect in all known relatives. The family history is deliberately introduced early so that parents may have a chance of thinking about it subconsciously or consciously during the rest of the interview—experience has shown that they often remember important details before leaving the clinic.

A rather informal social history is obtained. Questions are asked about the father's employment and his relationship with the child, and it is very often at this point that the real nature of the problem underlying the child's referral to the clinic comes to light, though it is then quietly ignored so that it can be discussed in more detail once the child's own case history has been considered.

The mother is asked about her reproductive history, the number of her conceptions, the number of abortions, the number of still births, neonatal deaths and infant deaths, and the health of her other children. A history of her pregnancy, labour and delivery is obtained, particular attention being paid to any history suggestive of rubella infection in pregnancy, pre-eclampsia, antepartum haemorrhage or hydramnios. A history of the labour is obtained (though not relied on) and the mother is asked to give an account of the delivery and the child's neonatal state. Since in Scotland a high proportion of mothers are delivered in hospital, these details are usually supplemented by notes obtained from the relevant maternity hospital.

The mother is asked about the state of the child when she took him home, about his sleep, feeding, the presence or absence of fits, his alertness, and her feelings about him.

Developmental Diagnosis

A developmental history is obtained. In spite of the fact that it has been shown that mothers' memories become less accurate as they and their children grow older, it is remarkable to find how much detail an intelligent mother can remember about her child's development. Occasionally she will come carrying a 'baby book' which is still more helpful. The paediatrician asks her questions according to the Gesell schedules of motor, linguistic, adaptive and social development.

Motor development comes first. The mother is asked about postural control: when did the child first hold up his head; sit with support and without support; crawl (either on his hands or knees or shuffling along on his bottom); walk holding with a hand and without support; when did he first walk upstairs, when downstairs.

Manipulation is another aspect of motor behaviour. The mother is asked when did the child first reach for objects; when did he first drop objects (a milestone most mothers remember quite accurately); and when did he first pick up things using a thumb and forefinger.

She is asked about the development of his adaptive behaviour: when was the child toilet trained by day, when by night; when could he undress himself except for small buttons and when could he undress himself completely; when could he dress himself and when could he manage his top button, tie and laces.

The child's feeding history is elicited: when could he first take a biscuit to his mouth by hand; when could he first use a spoon and when a fork. Usually, mothers remember when their child was first able to use a knife and fork. Often they can remember when he was able to manage a tricycle and a bicycle. Questions are asked about play, such as what does the girl do with her dolls, what does the boy do with plastic soldiers, or what do they do with 'Lego'.

We are not in favour of proformata. In fact it is possible to take the developmental history using symbols (see Fig. 1). The advantage of this system over proformata is that when particular points of importance arise (*e.g.* school difficulties) they can be discussed expansively at the time of history-taking and not left until later. Developmental history-taking must be systematic—but the use of proformata leads to rigidity in history-taking (and in the doctor's thinking). This system allows history-taking which is both systematic and flexible.

It is more difficult to obtain milestones of social development, but many mothers do remember when their child first looked at them and smiled (usually during feeding) and can recall when he began to recognise other members of the family, and also when he began to co-operate in play with other children. If the child is of school-age, the relationships between him and his teacher and his class-mates are obviously of interest and should be asked about. Often during this type of history-taking, a fairly accurate idea of the child's intelligence can be obtained.

Following the history of motor, adaptive and social behaviour, a history of the child's health is usually obtained. Particular emphasis is put on the occurrence of upper respiratory tract infections in infancy and early childhood, especially if these are associated with otitis media. Direct questions are asked about the child's hearing and vision and whether convulsions have occurred or not. A note is made of immunisations against vaccinia, diphtheria, tetanus, whooping cough and poliomyelitis.

It is not uncommon to find that mothers who have previously regarded upper respiratory tract infections with middle ear disease as 'minor complications of teething' suddenly realise that the child may have been hard of hearing for years—and all too often he has.

After the details of the child's medical history have been elicited, a detailed history of his speech development is taken. Useful information on the child's first vocalisations is rarely given, but most parents know when the child really began to babble ('ma', 'da') in sequence and can tell you when he said his first 'proper words'. They can very often make a guess at the time when the child first joined words together and when he said his first 'proper sentences'. It is useful to ask about the intelligibility of speech because parents are quite good at remembering when the child was first intelligible to his mother, his brothers and sisters, his father, neighbours, and to strangers.

Parents can often give quite a good account of the nature of the child's difficulties.

	age 4/52	age 5/12	age 7/12	age 9/12	age 10/12
Motor (posture)	holds up head	sits with support	sits without support	crawls	bottom crawls
	stands holding on	stands un-supported	walks with support	walks without support	does not walk unsupported
	cannot sit with support		18/12 ... 24/12 stairs walked		

Manipulation	reaches for objects with right hand, not with left		voluntarily drops objects	pincer grasp

Speech	4-5/12 babble Ma/Da	13/12 sp. proper words	18/12 phr. phrases	24/12 sen. sentences
Intelligibility	13/12 sib.	18/12 M. mother	30/12 F. father	32/12 neighbour
Adaptive Feed	12/12 hand	15/12 spoon	20/12 fork	20/12 knife and fork

Undress	4 (small buttons - 5)
Dress	5 (small buttons - 6) laces - 7
Toilet	(2-ish) (4-ish) D. day N. night
Tricycle	2, pedal same - 2½ - 3

School Progress	yes = ✓ no = (✓)	jig-saws	Lego	meccano	play

Social				
	looked and recognised mother	S = smiled at mother and anyone	SM = smiled at mother discriminately	
	Fam = recognised other members of family			
	Recognises : neighbouring children sibs	neighbouring adults aunt/uncle	strangers	
	Nursery: friends - yes = ✓ trouble with other children = (✓)			
	School: friends - yes = ✓ difficulties = (✓)			
	Teacher: - OK = ✓ trouble = (✓)			

Fig. 1. These symbols, many devised by the late Professor Charles McNeil but never published, are some of those in use in the speech clinic of the Royal Hospital for Sick Children, Edinburgh. Ages are very approximate.

They recognise stammer, hesitation and blocking quite readily. They can usually give a list of sounds which are omitted or substituted in the Developmental Speech Disorders syndrome They can usually tell the examiner whether the speech defects are consistent or inconsistent (in general, speech therapists use this term to denote the child who may use a sound in a certain position correctly one day and not the next—rather than the child who consistently omits the sound in a medial or final position); and, for example, they may note that an 'l' sound is 'all right in the middle of a word but he can't say it at the beginning of a word'. It is usually possible by history-taking to ascertain if there are difficulties in language as well as in articulation. Parents will tell the examiner that 'He has words but cannot say them' or 'He just has not got the words to say what he means', and they are particularly good at noting a child's inability to recall specific names, as is found in nominal dysphasia.

Questions should always be asked about the child's comprehension of spoken language, the ages at which he was first able to obey simple commands, more complicated commands, and the age at which it was possible to hold prolonged conversations with him. It is often useful at this point to ask for information about the ability of older children to understand what they read and to obtain details of educational progress.

Information obtained from parents varies in its reliability. Some mothers can give a very detailed account of the child's motor, linguistic, adaptive and social development in infancy and in early childhood. Others, especially those with large families, are vague. As noted by Neligan and Prudham (1969a and b), the older the child (and the longer after the events she is asked to recall) the less accurate the mother's dates for milestones tend to become. Nevertheless, great stress is laid on history-taking in our speech clinic in Edinburgh and sometimes the parents' account is almost diagnostic, as in the cases of typical infantile autism, elective mutism, mental retardation, ataxic or dyskinetic cerebral palsy and acquired dysphasic disorders.

The history obtained from the parents should always be supplemented by accounts from other sources. Women who have been delivered under anaesthesia, for example, are very often quite unaware of the fact that their child suffered a period of apnoea immediately after birth. Visiting is often restricted in fever hospitals and it is always worthwhile asking for notes of illness which required admission to hospital. (For example, one child with obvious language difficulty suffered from a transient, mild right hemiparesis following a convulsion which complicated measles at the age of eighteen months. This was unknown to his parents.)

Reports from nursery supervisors are particularly valuable in giving an indication of how the child responds to other children in a situation outside the home. The reports of teachers of children of school-age are particularly valuable in indicating the extent to which speech is a social and educational handicap and also in indicating specific difficulties encountered in the learning situation. A high proportion of school-age children referred to the speech clinic have had psychological testing carried out by local authority educational psychologists and their reports are always sought, as are those of any speech therapists who have treated the child in the past.

The Physical Examination

The physical examination of patients referred to a speech clinic must be carried out with the same care as patients referred to the general neurological clinic. As indicated above, a huge variety of different disorders may be encountered and it must always be remembered that the parents' complaint of the child having a speech defect may be a cover for concern about other aspects of his physical or behavioural development.

As far as general behaviour is concerned, a great deal will have been learnt about the child if he has been in the same room during history-taking and playing actively with a nurse or speech therapist. The level of his activity, what toys he chooses and what he does with them, the degree of his independence and the amount of his vocalisation will all have been observed. Very often, by the time the history is taken and the child has been observed, a provisional diagnosis has been made. For example, dysphonia, speech dysrhythmia, and retarded speech development (whatever its cause) are relatively easily identified if the child vocalises freely. Characteristic patterns, such as those found in high-tone hearing loss or in velar incompetence or inadequacy of the nasal airway are also easily recognised. The suspicion that the child may be deaf is often aroused during this period of history-taking and inspection of the child, for he may fail to respond to environmental noises which attract the attention of other people in the room. The child's hand preference during play will have been observed. Unfortunately, a high proportion of children referred to the speech clinic, particularly those with retarded speech development, are immature in other aspects of behaviour and tend to cling to their mothers or sit on their mothers' knees and may fail to vocalise at all during history-taking and examination. Even in these circumstances, however, one has learnt something about the child's ability to relate to people other than his mother.

A general physical inspection is carried out with the particular aim of recognising stigmata characteristic of the various known clinical syndromes associated with mental defect, *e.g.* Down's syndrome, Hurler's syndrome, De Lange's syndrome and the presence of complete transverse palmar creases, abnormalities of the external ears, the mouth, tongue or palate. The head size is routinely measured, though children are not routinely undressed before they come into the examination room.

The first part of the examination is devoted to confirming the developmental status of the child as described by the parents during history-taking. Motor milestones elicited by examination may be divided into two types. Firstly there are positive motor milestones. These consist of the child's voluntary control of posture and of manipulation. At 7 or 8 months he should be sitting without support. At 13 to 18 months he should have learnt to walk without support. Shortly afterwards he should be able to climb stairs on his feet, and he should be able to descend stairs before the age of 2. By 3 he should be running without flexing his shoulders. At 5 he should be able to stand on one leg for ten seconds with his eyes open, and by 7 he should be able to stand on one leg with his eyes shut for ten seconds. At 10 he should be able to stand on one leg with the contralateral heel placed on the standing knee with his eyes shut.

At 7 or 8 months the child should be able to release the grasp and drop things instead of having to throw them out of his grasp if he wants to be rid of them. At the age of about a year he has accurate pincer movements which allow pellets to be picked up between the thumb and forefinger. By the age of 3 he should be able to put his hand repeatedly one on top of the other with considerable rapidity, and by the age of 4 he should be able to make rapidly alternating movements of pronation and supination of the forearms and 'piano playing' movements of the fingers on request. From this age onwards, manipulation is tested more by observations carried out in the course of studies of adaptive behaviour, *e.g.* when he uses a spoon for feeding or a pencil for drawing.

By negative milestones of motor development we understand those manifestations of immature motor behaviour which disappear as the child grows older. For the most part, these consist of reflexes characteristic of infancy which disappear as the higher nervous centres in the hemispheres develop. The classical example of a reflex of this type is the Moro reflex, in which a sudden movement of the newborn child results in a brisk extension of all four limbs and then a slower return to the semiflexed posture characteristic of the newborn. This reflex gradually becomes less brisk in the normal child from the age of about 3 months and it is very unusual to find it in a healthy baby after the age of 5 months. Another, similar reflex is the stepping reflex; tilting the newborn baby to and fro in the erect position results in reflex reciprocal stepping movements of the lower limbs so that the child appears to 'walk' either on a flat or vertical surface. This reflex becomes progressively more difficult to elicit after the age of 6 or 8 weeks and is normally absent by the age of 12 weeks. In children whose higher nervous centres fail to develop, these reflexes persist because they are not inhibited as they should be. Thus it is not too uncommon to find stepping reflexes in children who suffer from cerebral diplegia at 18 months or 2 years, and in children with dyskinetic cerebral palsy this reflex is found at even later ages. Of particular importance in the speech clinic are the feeding reflexes. The rooting reflex, in which the head turns towards a stroking stimulus on the cheek directed towards the mouth, normally becomes inhibited in the second half of the first year.

In the newborn, the lip reflex (which consists of mouth opening and tongue protrusion in response to a stroking stimulus on the lip) changes usually between the ages of 6 and 12 weeks, so that the mouth continues to open but the tongue is no longer protruded. In a proportion of patients, however, especially those with a personal and family history of tongue thrusting, this facet of the reflex may be elicited even at the age of 3 or 4 years. Tongue thrust associated with mouth opening usually disappears towards the end of the first year of life in normal children, but it may persist in children who suffer from cerebral palsy and in a few children with immature patterns of feeding and speech sound production.

In the young child, involuntary associated movements during voluntary activity tend to be very marked. Thus, if a child of 6 months grasps an object firmly in one hand, flexion movements of the digits and thumb will be observed in the contralateral hand. This tendency to involuntary associated movements tends to diminish as children grow older and as the higher nervous centres exert their inhibitory influence to a progressive degree. This is the basis of the tests of reflex activity described by Fog and Fog (1963). They describe two tests. In the first a child is asked to exert enough pressure to open bulldog clips of various resistances and the behaviour of the contralateral hand is observed. (By the age of 10, involuntary contralateral associated movements of the hand are very slight, if present at all.) In the second test, the 'Foot-hand Test', the child is asked to walk with his feet inverted, *i.e.* on the outside edges of his shoes. Children under the age of 5 show marked supination of the forearms often accompanied by extension at the wrist, extension of the digits, and extension at the elbows. From the age of 5 onwards there is a rapidly decreasing tendency to extension at the elbows, though pronation of the forearms diminishes less rapidly and disappears completely only by the age of 10 years, or later in healthy children.

Other, less well standardised tests can be employed to elicit associated involuntary movements. A particularly potent test is one where the child is asked to make a fist with one hand and then extend his flexed digits against resistance. Up to the age of 7, very little resistance to voluntary extension produces involuntary extension of the contralateral digits, and even up to the age of 14, powerful resistence to extension of the digits and the hand being tested results in some extension of the contralateral digits. Another test, which might be described as the 'inverted Fog test', is to ask the child to walk on the inner borders of his feet, in which case there is a marked tendency to pronation of the forearms and flexion of the wrists and semiflexion of the fingers which disappears rather later than the supination observed when children are asked to walk on the outside edges of their shoes. Tests of neurological maturation are followed by tests of laterality. Eyedness is tested by asking the child to look through a telescope or kaleidoscope, the instrument being placed in first the right hand and then the left hand. Handedness is tested by asking the child to throw a ball, to catch a ball, and to break a spatula or small wooden stick using two hands with the forearms pronated (the operative hand is almost invariably the dominant one on other tests and the degree to which the contralateral hand is used gives some indication of the extent of lateralisation). Footedness is tested by asking the child to kick a ball placed centrally between the two feet and to step onto a chair or step, the leading foot being regarded as the dominant one.

There follows a formal neurological examination during which an informal assessment of intellectual functions and speech is made. The child is asked about his orientation in time, space and person. He may be asked to give a brief account of his trip from home to the hospital and this gives an opportunity for assessing, to some extent, his ability to express himself using spontaneous spoken language and the degree to which he comprehends what he is being asked to do. Commonly, merely listening to the speech gives the diagnosis. The presence of 'cleft palate speech', which may be due to cleft palate, submucous cleft palate or the palatal disproportion syndrome, is easily identified. Hyporhinophonia, most often attributable to enlarged adenoids, is equally easy to identify, especially—as so often happens—if it is accompanied by profuse nasal discharge and mouth breathing.

The fundi should always be examined because the retinal pigmentation that occurs with rubella retinopathy is typical and very frequently associated with hearing impairment and encephalopathy. Moreover, occasionally one can identify the early signs of the cerebromacular degeneration described by Speilmeyer and by Batten (1914) before dementia occurs (Foster and Ingram 1962). Visual acuity should always be tested. A great many children with speech difficulties are referred by teachers who attribute the childrens educational problems to their speech difficulties when in fact it is their vision which is defective. Strabismus may remain unrecognised for a long time unless it is looked for carefully, and it is necessary to study eye movements in all patients.

Eye movements and movements of the face are likely to be defective in the Moebius' syndrome (nuclear agenesis) and in some types of cerebral palsy. The movements of the face should be studied when the child smiles, whistles, or blows his cheeks out to command, and during spontaneous emotional expression, for if the hemispheres are involved it may only be in these latter functions that obvious asymmetries are observed.

In our clinic, the doctor routinely tests hearing in a rough-and-ready way by asking the child to repeat numbers spoken behind him in a whisper. The ear drums are inspected routinely. Formal audiometry should be carried out sooner or later whether or not there is doubt about the child's hearing, but rough-and-ready tests of the type described do indicate the patients in whom hearing testing seems to be relatively urgent.

Great attention is paid to the structure and function of the lips, tongue and palate and to the organs closely related to them, such as the teeth, the pharynx and the adenoids. During routine examination of the throat, it is usually possible to assess the degree of voluntary and involuntary palatal movement. The range and co-ordination of voluntary tongue movements can be tested fairly readily in older children by asking the child to put his tongue out to the maximum extent, withdraw it to the maximum extent, and put it into either cheek, and then to ask him to alternately protrude and intrude it as rapidly as possible. Sensation of the tongue and palate to touch is readily tested by touching these structures with a blunt probe and observing the reaction.

Further examination consists of assessing the degree of voluntary movement of the limbs, the co-ordination of these movements and the ability to carry them out rapidly. Further, one examines the tendency to involuntary movements, as described above, using the Fog and similar tests. It is also often very valuable merely to ask the child to run rapidly up and down a corridor, watching his associated movements and listening to his footsteps. If there is assymmetry of movement or excessive involuntary movement this is almost always manifest in a difference in the sound of his footsteps and the amount of the associated involuntary movements in his upper limbs. Muscle tone is examined by 'flapping' the limbs and assessing the degree of the stretch reflex. The biceps, triceps, knee and ankle jerks are tested, and the plantar responses examined; sensation is examined, though not usually in great detail.

A detailed examination of the upper respiratory tract is made so that the size of the tonsils and any enlargement of the related cervical glands are noted. It is not generally realised, but it is often possible to pulpate the adenoids of patients by pushing one's fingers rapidly behind the soft palate. This has to be done quickly in order to avoid distress, but the results of this examination are rewarding.

Ancillary investigations which may be ordered by the paediatrician are numerous. They include x-ray palatography, in which soft tissue radiographs are obtained of the child when his palate is at rest, when he says 'n', and when he says 'e' or 'i' (when the palate should be closing off the nasopharyngeal orifice). Not only do these x-ray pictures demonstrate the range of palatal movement, but they also give a clear indication of the size of the adenoids and whether these should be removed. Pure tone audiometry is almost routine in the clinic, and a high proportion of patients are referred to psychologists for intelligence testing or to psychiatrists for a full assessment of the degree to which they are emotionally disturbed. Others are sent to the ear, nose and throat department for fuller assessment of the significance of abnormalities found on otoscopy or examination of the pharynx. Yet others are referred directly to plastic surgeons if there is obvious evidence of gross palatal disproportion which might be corrected by plastic surgery. Young, very immature children are often referred to the speech therapist and occupational therapist in the hospital who run a pre-nursery group for children with immature behavioural patterns. Frequently, the doctor writes to the Medical Officer of Health asking if some priority could be given for nursery placement in local nurseries which are designed to cater for normal children.

In many children with mild retardation of articulatory development unassociated with language disorder, a period of further observation may be required without further investigations being undertaken. In more complex or severely affected patients, the speech therapist makes much more detailed studies of the child's speech abnormalities so that an accurate diagnosis may be achieved. In such complex cases, it is only after the speech therapist has completed her studies of the child's language and articulatory development that a definitive plan of management is made.

The Rôle of the Speech Therapist in the Speech Clinic

The speech therapist assesses speech and language processes. This evaluation is achieved by using special tests and assessment scales and observing the speech used by the child in play and in communication with adults. Additional information may be supplied by parents and teachers, and others who know the child. Only those tests and procedures which are important in the assessment of speech and language development are included in this chapter.

Ideally, the assessment starts as the child and parents enter the waiting room. Samples of speech and language may often be obtained in these circumstances more easily than in the more formal clinical situation. The behaviour of the child can be observed unnoticed and the parent-child relationship can be studied in the relatively informal situation outside the clinic.

The child can often be seen in the relative privacy of the speech therapy room before the doctor's history-taking and examination. Sometimes he will come into the room alone and a brief assessment may be carried out with the minimum of distraction. If he is not ready to do this, parents and siblings are invited to join him.

During the initial assessment, a formal situation is strictly avoided, and the therapist may come down to the child's level, physically as well as metaphorically: a small child may not be able to see an adult's face when the adult is standing. Toys and books may be casually introduced, with the speech therapist sitting beside the child so that words can be addressed directly to him or whispered in his ear.

An appraisal of auditory abilities is followed by simple instructions designed to test comprehension. During conversation a brief assessment of articulation is made. Expressive language is assessed for information and grammatical content. Play and general behaviour is observed carefully, but the therapist does not write much down at this stage as it tends to formalise the situation.

A skilled listener easily recognises specific abnormal patterns of speech. Hyporhinophonia, hyperrhinophonia, or rhinolalia mixta indicate defective palatal function. Omissions, distortions or substitutions of specific groups of sounds may be caused by dysarthria or anatomical irregularities. All bilabials or all alveolar sounds may be affected, indicating problems of lip movement or tongue tip articulation respectively. Abnormal voice production may be due to laryngeal problems or hearing loss. Confusion of consonants which are acoustically similar, or distortion of vowels which have high frequency components, suggest auditory problems. The 'open-syllable' may be used, with no word endings. All speech sounds may be produced further forward in the mouth than is normal with anterior articulation. The Edinburgh Articulation Test (Anthony et al. 1971) is useful when distinguishing deviant patterns of articulation from articulation immaturity.

An interview of 15 to 20 minutes may be necessary to assess the nature and extent of the speech problems presented by the child. It is seldom that it provides sufficient information for the accurate diagnosis of the speech disorder. However, in this preliminary interview, additional information may be obtained. The response to auditory stimuli in the form of voice and complex tones is assessed, and auditory discrimination is tested using 'A Picture Screening Test of Hearing' (Reed 1960). Articulation is assessed using the Edinburgh Articulation Test. From the results obtained, an 'articulation age' can be quickly calculated, and by referring to the Qualitative Assessment Sheet, the nature of the articulatory errors can be ascertained. Ability to imitate movements of the tongue and lips is examined, as is the ability to repeat sounds in isolation or in series. Comprehension is studied by noting the response given to commands of increasing length and complexity. A brief test of expressive language skills is then given using the Action Picture Test (Renfrew 1970). The results of the assessment are evaluated and reported to the doctor, together with other relevant information gleaned from parents or general observation.

In a proportion of patients, for example those suffering from the Specific Developmental Speech Disorder syndrome which affects articulation without any obvious impairment of language functions, further investigations may not be felt to be indicated though periodic observation is usually required. In other cases, a much more detailed assessment of the child's articulation and speech functions is needed. The speech therapist's investigations may be supplemented immediately. Studies of the home and school background are made by a medical social worker, the assessment of intelligence by an educational psychologist or clinical psychologist. Radiological examination—for example, palatography—supplements the information gained about palatal movement from clinical examination and from listening to the child's speech.

The full assessment by the speech therapist usually takes place on a different day, in view of the amount of time required, and the fatigue which many children show by the time they have been subjected to a medical examination and associated studies.

Diagnosis of the Nature of the Speech Abnormality

Speech and language problems may have more than one cause. Further specialised investigations are often necessary. The observations of all the people involved in the initial assessment of the child are taken into consideration before further detailed studies are recommended.

Auditory functions may require further examination. Routine audiometry may be done using earphones or the free-field method. Electroencephalographic audiometry, impedence audiometry, tests of auditory fatigue and response to filtered speech may be required.

Auditory attention may be defective. In this case, consistency of response to auditory stimuli is studied. Responses to verbal and non-verbal auditory stimuli may be observed, and systematically analysed.

A study of responses to amplification may be made. This may improve awareness of sound, assist comprehension, aid learning of speech, or do none of these things. 'Conditioning' procedures may be possible using touch, vision or hearing, with varying reliability, and require careful evaluation.

Comprehension may need further investigation and the specific tests used for this purpose are described in Appendix I (see also chapter 9). The child may recognise familiar noises, voices, speech sounds, words or phrases. He may be primarily visually orientated and show ability to lip-read, he may respond to gesture and learn from visual presentation. On the other hand, it may be necessary for him to handle toys, letter shapes and touch the speaker's face before he can learn to understand speech. The way in which he learns requires careful study.

Verbal and non-verbal language may be assessed and observed from different points of view. Inner language may be demonstrated non-verbally through the use of gestures and in various forms of play showing use of specific concepts, ideas and categorisation abilities. Non-verbal expressive capacities can be judged from the way in which he uses his voice, jargon, shouting and screaming, and the way he manipulates others to express his wants.

Other specific linguistic skills may be assessed, appertaining to reading, writing spelling and calculation. The formal language tests used routinely by the speech therapist are indicated in Appendix I.

When evaluating the results of these investigations, it may be necessary to take into account the quality of behaviour shown and, in particular, motor activity and personal control. Exploratory activity may be normal or the child may not move at all unless directed. The quantity of random purposeless movements, degree of perseverance, distractibility, and quality of social perception may be relevant.

When studying speech, anatomical and functional abilities are of prime importance. Voice quality and the ability to sustain laryngeal tone may affect the results. Articulation may vary in spontaneous conversation, repetition, reading and reciting from memory, and with general fluency. It is important to take a comprehensive view of the problems.

A brief elaboration of some features of the differential diagnosis of speech disorders follows.

Where a problem of reception of acoustic information is severe, it is important to ensure that no aspect of the input remains uninvestigated. Hearing loss may render the child deaf so that he cannot distinguish the spoken word: 'On the other hand, the peripheral hearing mechanism can be anatomically intact but the brain function may be abnormal central to the cochlear nuclei. There are a variety of clinical variations of response to sounds in affected children. Basically two types are recognised depending on the consistency or inconsistency of response to sounds' (Taylor 1966). It is also important to recognise the child with some peripheral impairment and associated central disorder, in view of the different management problems involved.

The child with a disability in achieving complex muscle co-ordinations may have a reduced phonemic vocabulary. He may omit those distinctive features which are for him most difficult and substitute those which he can produce most easily. In sequential production of phonemes adjacent features influence each other and articulation will tend to show erratic use of phonetic sounds as they occur in varying phonetic sequences.

Another condition which may give rise to phonetic variation of a different type is a fluctuating deafness. Where this is found to occur, it is important to check the hearing at regular intervals and to keep a record of the serial audiograms, as this condition may be alleviated by appropriate medical or surgical treatment.

These are just a few of the problems which may emerge. There are many others; for example, the stammerer with a language disorder, the child with a cleft palate and hearing loss, the dyspraxic child with some intellectual impairment, and the child with language impairment associated with autistic features.

Wherever a therapeutic programme is necessary, it is essential to have the most thorough assessment possible in order to ensure that the programme is based on firm ground, or much time will be wasted and the therapy may even be valueless.

Tests of Learning, Comprehension, Language and Articulation

Assessment procedures described in Appendix I were selected on the basis of their general use with speech defective children who come to the Speech Clinic of the Royal Hospital for Sick Children, Edinburgh.

Vocabulary tests and reading tests, used with older children, have not been included, nor have tests which shed light on the pre-linguistic and conceptual skills of the younger child, such as those of Piaget. Procedures for assessing palato-pharyngeal competence, fluency and diadokinetic skills have not been discussed, in view of their specific application. Comprehension tests devised with hearing impaired children in mind are likewise omitted. Methods of linguistic analysis of speech are discussed in chapters (3 and 9).

The Communication Evaluation Chart is mentioned here as it covers many aspects of development which a speech therapist would wish to assess. It is based on the development patterns of children from infancy to five years of age and was designed, using sources from Gesell, Binet and Cattell, to give a rough determination of language and performance levels.

The language development section lists the normal child's capacity to use 'language' at three monthly intervals up to 36 months and at 4 and 5 years. The items include co-ordination of speech musculature, hearing acuity, auditory perception, acquisition of vowels and consonants and the growth of receptive and perceptive language. The parallel scale indicates normal development of the average child's motor co-ordination, visual acuity, figure-ground discrimination, spatial relationships, visual and motor perceptual skills. The use of this scale enables the therapist to evaluate results and designate where a child is functioning in comparison with the normal on both verbal and non-verbal activities, and is a useful screening tool in selecting whether a child requires speech therapy, more detailed assessment of his verbal skills, or full investigation by the assessment team.

The Vineland Social Maturity Scale is another valuable assessment tool, for the social maturity of the child is an important facet of his development and may affect his speech acquisition.

All tests should be considered in their rôles of valuable tools for diagnosis and assessment. It is the aim of the therapist to amass as much information as possible which may be directly relevant to the child's presenting speech problems and future management. It is not enough to know that a certain type of disorder is present. It is even more important to know how a child is learning and as a result what type of treatment will benefit him most—auditory training, lip-reading, group or individual work, articulation therapy or language therapy, remedial help at school, or a combination of these. It is necessary therefore to conduct diagnostic trials of therapeutic procedures and evaluate the child's response to specific therapeutic methods in many cases.

Throughout the course of the speech disorder the help of the doctor is invaluable, as is the information from all other members of the assessment team. A speech disorder is not a static condition. It may improve or alter in its presenting characteristics. It may even deteriorate. Prompt investigation from the medical team is important in all such cases. The speech therapist and the doctor can work together to help parents, teachers, and others involved in the management of the child. This is the ideal state of affairs and thoroughly to be recommended. (For illustrative case histories see Appendix II).

REFERENCES

Andrews, G., Harris, M. (1964) *The Syndrome of Stuttering.* Clinics in Developmental Medicine, No. 17. London: Spastics Society with Heinemann.

Anthony, A., Bogle, D., Ingram, T. T. S., McIsaac, M. W. (1971) *The Edinburgh Articulation Test.* Edinburgh: Churchill Livingstone.

Batten, F. E. (1914) 'Familial cerebral degeneration with macular change (so-called juvenile form of family amaurotic idiocy).' *Quart. J. Med.,* 7, 444.

Brimer, M. A., Dunn, L. M. (1963) *Manual for the English Picture Vocabulary Test.* Slough, Bucks.: N.F.E.R.

Fog, E., Fog, M. (1963) 'Cerebral inhibition examined by associated movements.' *in* Bax, M., Mac Keith, R. (Eds.) *Minimal Cerebral Dysfunction.* Clinics in Developmental Medicine, No. 10. London: Spastics Society with Heinemann, p. 52.

Foster, J. B., Ingram, T. T. S. (1962) 'Familial cerebro-macular degeneration and ataxia.' *J. Neurol. Neurosurg. Psychiat.,* 25, 63.

McGrady, H. J. (1968) 'Language pathology and learning disabilities.' *in* Myklebust, H. R. (Ed.) *Progress in Learning Disabilities,* Vol. 1. New York: Grune & Stratton.

Neligan, G., Prudham, D. (1969a) 'Norms for four standard developmental milestones by sex, social class and place in family.' *Develop. Med. Child Neurol.*, **11,** 413.
—— —— (1969b) 'Potential value of four early developmental milestones in screening children for increased risk of later retardation.' *Develop. Med. Child Neurol.*, **11,** 423.
Reed, M. (1960) *Reed Test of Auditory Discrimination.* London: Royal National Institute for the Deaf.
Renfew, C. (1964) *Word Finding Vocabulary Scale.* Abingdon, Berks.: Abbey Press.
Reynell, J. (1969) *Reynell Developmental Language Scales.* Slough,Bucks.: N.F.E.R.
Richards, C. M. (1967) 'A test of understanding the spoken word.' *Brit. J. Disord. Commun.*, **2,** 124.
Taylor, I. G. (1966) 'Hearing in relation to language disorders in children'. *Brit. J. Disord. Commun.*, 1 1.
Watts, A. F. (1964) *The Language and Mental Development of Children.* London: Harrap.

CHAPTER 7

Hearing Loss and Hearing Behaviour

J. A. M. MARTIN

Out of the wide variety of conditions which may contribute to absent or delayed spoken language, deafness is probably the most important and best recognised single factor. Many children have been diagnosed as mentally retarded, aphasic, emotionally disturbed or plain naughty when more careful investigation would have demonstrated hearing loss.

History

The detailed opinion of the parents should be sought. They have countless opportunities to reach intuitive decisions about their child's hearing ability and, though sometimes unable to rationalise their opinion, their views must command respect. The infant may continue to sleep undisturbed by the noise around him, children playing, dogs barking. He may not startle when heavy objects are accidentally dropped or doors banged. Later he may fail to recognise meaningful noises made near him. Mother getting the meal ready or preparing the bath may not precipitate a joyful excited reaction from her child if he cannot see what she is doing. The child may show surprise or even fright when he suddenly sees someone standing near his cot or pram, not having heard the advance warning of approaching footsteps, and a comforting voice in the dark carries no solace. When comprehension of spoken language begins to be shown by the child's ability to look around on request for a person or pet, to fetch a toy or carry out other simple errands, the parents will remark upon the deaf child's failure to show such behaviour. Children with certain rare forms of disorder of language acquisition in which hearing loss is not a significant feature may behave in the same way to spoken requests.

Detection of Hearing Loss

The earliest possible diagnosis can be achieved by the parents, but it is surprising how long a severe hearing loss can escape detection. Screening tests were therefore introduced by a number of local Health Authorities in an effort to ensure that the deaf child was discovered early. Authorities vary in their approach, some endeavouring within the limits of their facilities to screen every child, some restricting their attention to the children who can be demonstrated as being 'at risk'. This concept was developed by Sheridan (1962) who, being well aware of the lack of personnel and the wide range of potential handicap, considered that it was more effective to concentrate on children who were particularly prone to some handicapping condition. The most significant aetiological factors for hearing loss might be summarised as a family history of deafness, maternal rubella, anoxia or jaundice occurring during birth and the neonatal period, and subsequently meningitis. Other factors would include the giving of ototoxic drugs to the mother during pregnancy or to the young child.

A child who is late in learning to talk or who shows defects of spoken language outside normal developmental limits will also be 'at risk' of having a hearing loss.

The Screening Test

The optimum age for screening hearing is a month or so either side of 9 months. At this age the infant can be expected to hold his head up and to sit unsupported with good control of movements of the head and neck.

A typical screening test consists of administering a variety of 'meaningful' sounds in a quiet, not unduly reverberant room. The child sits comfortably on his mother's lap and an assistant sits facing the child to attract his attention from wandering around the room and to assess response. Slight alterations of behaviour, changes of facial expression and movements of the eyes and eyelids may all be evidence of hearing response, but it may require a highly skilled observer to evaluate these in the presence of random behaviour. There is much to be said for the less experienced relying on a clear localisation response alone, which can be detected from behind by the tester.

The sounds usually employed are the quietest rustling of cellophane paper, the gentle stroking of the rim of a china cup with a metal teaspoon, the slightest agitation of a rattle made of brittle plastic containing two or three small glass beads, and voice sounds. These latter include the gentle whispering of the child's name, quiet vocalisation of one or two vowel sounds such as 'ooo—ooo' and of consonant sounds such as 'sss' or 'ts-ts-ts'. This repertoire of sounds is made about 5ft. away from the child at an angle of 45° behind and level with his ear, so that whilst he cannot possibly see, it is easy for him to localise the source. The sounds are not always presented for the first time to the same ear, but both the side and the rate of presentation are varied so that there is no fixed pattern of testing.

In a screening test of this nature the result is recorded simply as pass or fail, and there is no attempt at assessment of degree of hearing loss if this is thought to be present. The child who fails more than one or two individual tests must be referred for more detailed examination. Younger children can be tested so long as due allowance is made for their inability to control head movement in the erect posture, for their more limited localisation abilities and for their reduced auditory spatial world.

Screening tests are subsequently carried out by many Health Authorities during the first year of school entry when the child may be 5 or 6 years old. The technique involves the use of a pure tone audiometer and measurement of the child's threshold of hearing.

Assessment of Hearing Loss

Diagnostic techniques for measuring the degree of hearing loss will vary with the age of the child. There is no hard and fast limit here and one, not infrequently, is obliged to fall back on techniques used for a child some months or years younger. This may be particularly appropriate in the mentally retarded child.

Under 1 Year

The technique is essentially as described under screening tests. The child who does not respond to screening levels needs the sounds to be made progressively louder.

This is best done first by bringing the sound source nearer the ear and, in the continuing absence of response, by increasing the intensity of the noise. It is always necessary to avoid letting the child see one's hand or the sound-making apparatus, or touching or stimulating the child through any sensation other than hearing. Squeakers, rattles and bells, the loudly spoken voice, xylophone, drum and the pure tone free field audiometer are all used. The tester must always have in mind the overall loudness level of the different stimuli (a portable sound level meter is invaluable), and the need to evaluate the child's hearing for low and high pitched sounds.

Over 3½ Years

A considerable number of children can be conditioned at this age to join in some simple game such as the 'Go' game of the Manchester school (Ewing and Ewing 1944). The child transfers a brick from a box or knocks down a skittle when he hears the tester call out behind him. The result can be more precise in terms of frequency and intensity if a free field audiometer is used, particularly if it becomes part of the play situation. It may be necessary first to condition the child visually as well as by ear if there is a severe degree of loss and this is done by letting the child see the xylophone or the drum being struck. Sounds can then be made progressively quieter behind the child, or the free field audiometer used. Children who have just reached their second birthday may respond to this form of testing whilst five-year-olds may stubbornly refuse. A child who has given satisfactory responses in free field can usually be tested in the more formal pure tone techniques using earphones and bone conductors, but many are apprehensive and one may have to wait some months before they will accept them.

Speech. Every child who shows some understanding of the spoken word should in addition have his hearing tested by speech. The simplest method is by asking the child to point to a named picture or object placed in front of him. Picture cards remain a useful method for children who are reluctant to use their own voices in the presence of strangers, and the Reed series of single syllable words in which either the vowels or consonants may be confused with the names of other pictured objects is particularly valuable. There are a wide variety of word lists available in addition to the Reed series mentioned; the Kendall Toy Test, the Manchester Junior word list, the Fry list and so on (Dale 1962, Watson 1967). It is essential in all tests of this nature to discover if the child knows the words being used and the value of picture cards is that he can identify them before the test begins.

1 Year—3½ Years

This is the difficult age, when children are no longer reacting in the simple manner of the 8 month infant, nor yet able to co-operate with the requirements of a conditioning technique.

Reliance is placed on distraction, much as for the infant. He sits on his mother's lap or by her side, and his attention gently held by some activity of the assistant which must be neither too absorbing, nor of a nature which precludes the examiner from deciding whether the child is moving his head to watch what is going on in front of him, or is half-turning to the sound stimuli. Normally hearing children can be particularly difficult. After they have turned once or twice they may lose all interest in the noises and concentrate only on what is before them: some partially hearing children will behave the same way. The severely deaf child however is so unused to hearing sounds that he takes much longer to inhibit his responses and a reasonably accurate threshold can be determined.

Clinical Examination. Once hearing tests have been completed and the opportunity taken to observe the child's general behaviour, his attention and alertness, and the quality of motor activity; the ears, nose and throat should be examined. This is the appropriate time to look for tell-tale stigmata of genetic syndromes such as broadening of the root of the nose, heterochromia of the iris, poorly formed cheek bones or mandible and so on. The external ears and meati are examined for abnormalities of shape and size, and to exclude wax and foreign bodies as a possible cause of hearing impairment. Detailed examination of the tympanic membrane may reveal the presence of middle ear abnormality by changes in colour of the drumhead, evidence of fluid, retraction, scarring or perforation. Such examination should never be omitted (though it not infrequently is), and abnormalities referred for otological opinion.

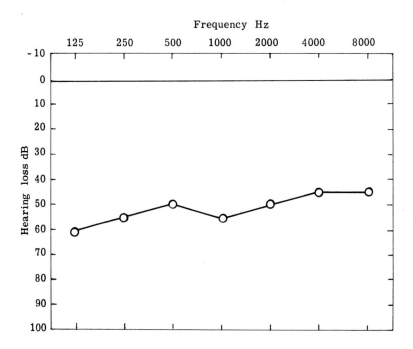

Fig. 1. Audiogram showing flat loss of the order of 50 dB. This child was in an E.S.N. school; her hearing was thought to be normal until she was seen at age 15 years.

Partial and Intermittent Hearing Loss

Many children are diagnosed incorrectly as having normal hearing when there is a degree of hearing loss sufficient to impair language development or to cause defective speech. The errors occur in three main ways and may not be discovered until long after the child has reached school age.

Intensity

In Fig. 1 there is a loss of hearing so that the threshold lies at the 50dB level. A child with a loss of this magnitude is easily classed as having no significant loss because the tester is unaware of the loudness levels of the sounds which he is using as test stimuli. It is not generally realised that the rustling of cellophane paper may reach over 60dB at 3ft. from the ear, or the quiet clinking of a small bell may peak at 70dB. A portable sound level meter is an indispensable tool in every clinic where free field measurements of hearing are made. In screening tests, the conditions laid down for the examination must be rigorously adhered to, such as the manner of eliciting the sounds, the test sounds used, and the distance they are made from the child.

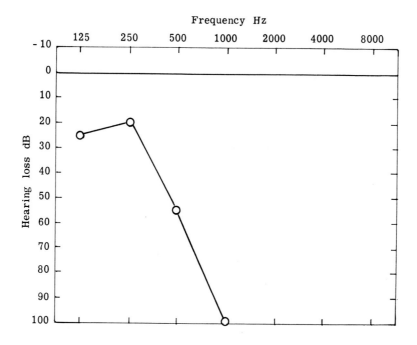

Fig. 2. Audiogram showing profound hearing loss in the frequencies from 1kHz upwards with virtually normal hearing at 125Hz and 250Hz. This child was considered to have normal hearing until the age of 6 years.

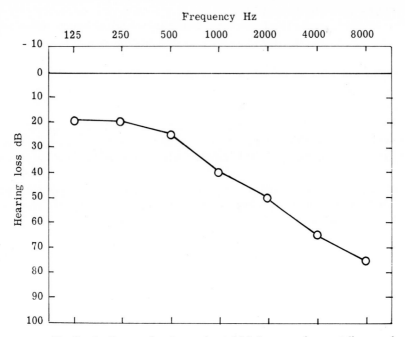

Fig. 3. Audiogram showing moderate high frequency loss; not discovered until the age of 11 years, when the child's education was suffering severely.

Frequency

Fig. 2 shows a severe high tone loss. It is not unlike that of some children who have suffered a severe asphyxiating episode at the time of birth. A more frequently encountered and less extreme degree of loss could be indicated by Fig. 3 and the problem is essentially the same. The energy distribution of most test sounds is concentrated in the lower frequencies. In high tone loss some of the test articles could be as little as 10dB above normal threshold and a hearing response gained. The 'high frequency' rattle, made of brittle plastic and containing three or four tiny glass beads, and high pitched speech sounds of the 's' and 'ts' variety should be used. One cannot remain content that significant impairment has been excluded until there is a response to the 4000Hz frequency of the free field audiometer at 40dB. If there is any doubt of the child's hearing ability he should be re-examined until this is obtained.

Variation

In middle ear involvement, characterised by secretory otitis media, there are episodes of hearing impairment with intervening periods of normal hearing. Hearing tests carried out at these times will fail to reveal any significant loss. It may be that one of these tests is the school audiometric examination, and the class teacher is understandably reluctant to argue against such evidence of normal hearing unless he is aware that hearing loss can be intermittent, variable and a common occurrence in the primary school years. Careful examination of the tympanic membranes will lead one to suspect this very common condition, estimated by Watson (1969) at an incidence of 3-4 per cent in 5-year-old children. Tuning fork tests or comparison of air conduction threshold audiograms with those for bone conduction should reveal a considerable gap between the two, there being no loss for bone conduction. The acoustic impedance meter, an investigation now being more generally used, measures the increased stiffness (or resistance to deformation under pressure) of the drumhead, and the degree of negative pressure in the middle ear space.

Psychogenic deafness occurs in children and its more extreme manifestations are readily suspected. When it is moderate in degree it may not be possible to identify the real nature of the condition until two or three visits have shown inconsistent results. It is usually a reaction to stress which may arise at school or within the family, and may be seen in pre-school age children. In all forms of psychogenic hearing loss, it is wise to assume the presence of an underlying organic loss until this can be disproved.

Problems in the Hearing Test

In the young child, the necessity for free field techniques introduces acoustic, developmental and psychological problems which render the investigation of hearing a very much more sophisticated procedure than is generally recognised (Martin 1971). It is beyond the scope of this chapter to enter into the nature of these problems, and discussion will be confined to consideration of the way in which diagnostic errors arise in the clinical assessment of the child's hearing.

In the majority of children it is usually not difficult to answer the question 'Is there a hearing loss?' with some degree of certainty, and to estimate the threshold for sounds of different frequency. As with any other sense modality, the testing of hearing is dependent on the response of the subject and cannot be divorced from it. It is possible to construct from the factors *Hearing* and *Response*, which may be present or absent, a Table of four combinations, two of which will give an accurate indication of hearing ability, whilst the other two will be false (Table 1). 'Hearing Absent' is not synonymous with total deafness, but indicates that the intensity of the sound stimulus is below the individuals threshold.

The ideal of all test procedures is to elicit a response from a sound stimulus if hearing is present, and to have no response if the subject does not hear the sound. If a sound is made correctly, in the right conditions, and the child does not respond, the only interpretation allowable is that he has not heard it. Most of us, if sufficiently introspective, would admit to a curious tendency to explain away certain responses, or their absence, but preconception or bias must be held in check. The more sophisticated tester, well aware of exceptions to the rule just stated, needs to be particularly wary of this tendency, and to be ready at any time to change his opinion if subsequent results are inconsistent. The consequences for the child are too severe to behave otherwise.

TABLE I

Accuracy of diagnosis of hearing loss

HEARING	RESPONSE	
	Present	Absent
Present	true	false
Absent	false	true

The combinations of hearing and response shown in Table 1, which give a true indication of the presence or absence of hearing, need no discussion. Mistakes are made however, and clinically children are thought to have good hearing when they have not, or to be deaf when their hearing is within normal limits.

Hearing Absent

The deaf child who has apparently responded to the hearing test gives a false diagnosis, and the response must result from factors other than the sound stimulus. The most common is vision and the child may respond because the tester has allowed himself or the test article to be seen. Even when the tester remains well behind the child's field of vision, visual clues creep in. The observer glances momentarily at the person making the sound; the child sees this and turns to the appropriate side to find out what is going on, and a response is scored. The tester's presence may be revealed by reflections of light dancing around the room from the sun shining off the rattle, or his shadow attracts attention as he moves about behind the child. The child may respond for yet other reasons. The tester may inadvertently touch the child's clothing or a strand of hair. The child may feel his breath or a tiny puff of air from the squeaker pointed the wrong way, or detect the whereabouts of the tester by the perfume of the hair dressing or other cosmetic.

Hearing Present

The possibilities of error which arise in this group suggest that our concept of the hearing process is inadequate. Clinical understanding of hearing and its disorders does not extend beyond the cochlear nuclei, but analysis must clearly extend beyond consideration of peripheral hearing and elicitation of response if there is to be understanding, however approximate, of normal hearing behaviour and its disorders.

Identification. Hearing, if it is to be of any value to us, means more than the detection of sounds at threshold. There is the process of discrimination, comparing sounds with those that have been heard before, and the isolation and recognition of sound patterns as being meaningful, called 'comprehension hearing' by Whetnall and Fry (1964). These processes will be referred to as *identification*.

Decision. One of the major difficulties in testing children arises from their ability to withold any overt response. It is for this reason that it is very much easier to assess hearing in the eight month infant than in a two-year-old, and this difficulty continues until complete co-operation is forthcoming. The decision to respond or to inhibit a response may vary throughout the test procedure and is a difficult factor to control, some children being able to reduce the examiner to complete impotence by their lack of co-operation.

Profiles of Hearing Behaviour

The four factors—Hearing, Identification, Decision and Response—may either be present or absent. The total number of combinations is sixteen, only eight of which have meaning in the biological, rather than the logical sense. There is a large potential for observer error to be borne in mind; the response may be minimal or transient or unrepeatable. The child may be hungry, sleepy, angry or uncomfortable. The mean level of noise in the test room may be high, and peaks of noise may occur as outside activity filters through. Until the test situation is approached with the knowledge, precision and skill, and the unhurrying attention to detail which characterise the experienced surgeon in the operating theatre, mistakes will continue to be made, and unfortunately even then.

In the remainder of the discussion on hearing behaviour the following symbols will be used:

H the activity and response of the peripheral sense organ—middle ear, cochlea and auditory nerve—to a sound above its threshold of stimulation: **h** indicates the absence of hearing where the threshold, be it normal or pathologically raised as in various forms of deafness, has not been reached for that particular sound.

I the ability to identify and to recognise the nature and quality of a sound, to locate its sound source, to attach meaning to the sound. It is a shorthand symbol covering a wide variety of physiological and psychological functions, many of which are not understood. Its absence is indicated by **i**.

D there needs to be initiation of motor activity to produce a visible response. After a certain age this will be entirely under voluntary control so that there is the decision to respond. Its absence, **d**, is the failure to reach a decision to respond.

R the observable response typically seen in the child turning his head to locate the source of sound. The absence of response is indicated by **r**.

(The various profiles of hearing behaviour indicated by combinations of **H, I, D, R**, and their absence is summarised in Table II, and may be encountered in the normally hearing subject and in certain pathological states.)

The Normal Child

In the neonate and during the first few weeks of life the state of hearing is shown in profile (5), **H i d R**, a purely reflex 'startle' response. Inhibition is a normal, sophisticated response, seen in profile (3), **H I d r**. Once the sound has been identified there is no intention of responding again, behaviour typical of the alert intelligent child which can be demonstrated under 12 months old. The child who has been overtested comes into this category, his response pattern possibly going through the stages Profile (P)4 → P1 → P3. It sometimes happens that older children, up to the age of five or six years, are persistently unco-operative, shown also by profile (3), **H I d r**. These children are excessively shy, cling to their mothers, do not utter a word in the clinic, and are

91

TABLE II
Profiles of hearing behaviour

Profile no.	Hearing	Identification	Decision	Response	Diagnosis	Observer error
1	+	+	+	+	true	
2	+	+	+	—	false	usual
3	+	+	—	—	false	may be
4	+	—	+	+	true	
5	+	—	—	+	true	
6	+	—	—	—	false	may be
7	—	—	—	+	false	yes
8	—	—	—	—	true	

unresponsive to all hearing tests. It may be virtually impossible to exclude a partial hearing loss and the clinician must be wary of his exasperation faced by such intractable behaviour.

EEG audiometry of the evoked response type has an invaluable part to play in the investigation of such children. This is a technique of pure tone threshold audiometry which gives a high level of correlation with the standard audiometric procedures in adults and school-age children. It can also be used in younger children, some degree of sedation often proving necessary. The details which follow are derived from the work of Beagley and Knight (1967) and Beagley and Kellogg (1969). The EEG trace is obtained from electrodes fixed to the vertex and to some convenient reference point such as the ear lobe. Tone pulses of fixed intensity and frequency are administered. A computer, under precise time control, sweeps for one second and summates the EEG voltages at 1024 points during this period. Three hundred milliseconds after the onset of the sweep the tone pulse is released, and the resulting evoked potential is also measured and summated by the computer. This process is repeated every 1.25 secs. until a sufficient number of stimuli, perhaps 60, have been presented and the resulting evoked response wave form recorded. The evoked cortical response before summation is so small that it is almost impossible to detect in the general wave form. As progressively more pulses arrive, the computer adds successive responses until the characteristic wave form becomes clearly visible. The background cortical activity is more random, and the negative and positive wave forms tend to cancel out, or to summate more slowly than the evoked response.

Patients in whom one cannot rely upon accurate responses, including the non-organic type of hearing loss and in simulated deafness or malingering, children who cannot readily be assessed by existing methods, especially where there is marked non-co-operation, and children with other handicaps such as visual defect or mental retardation are the most suitable for this technique.

The infant reared in an institution may be typified by profile (6), **H i d r**. Sounds have never been directed to him personally in sufficient quantity and have failed to acquire meaning, so that identification cannot take place. The infant up for adoption may be peculiarly difficult to evaluate, and a normal home—the very condition which is essential to the development of his hearing capabilities—may be denied him because he is suspected of being deaf. Severe mental retardation may produce the same effect in the older child.

Children with handicaps other than deafness may be physically incapable of making a response, as in profile (2), **H I D r**. A child with a severe form of cerebral palsy may be suspected of deafness because he has not started to talk and yet the sensory side may be intact. If he is unable to hold his head up in the sitting position, he cannot be expected to turn his head from side to side to locate the source of sound. Far from being deaf, he may have excellent discrimination for a wide vocabulary of words, detected in the older child by noticing that his eyes point to the object named out of a small selection placed on the table in front of him.

Disorder of Hearing Behaviour

The most difficult problems in diagnosis arise in the group of children aged two years and over in which hearing is present but who have not started to talk. Identification of sound may be normal as shown in profile (3), **H I d r**, or absent as in profile (6), **H i d r**. These profiles may serve to indicate the combination of factors which differentiate between expressive and receptive aphasia respectively for those who use this terminology. Autistic children may be included under profile (3), in which identification of sound occurs but the decision is made not to respond. Their hearing behaviour can present a complex pattern of unresponsiveness and apparent deafness (Rutter *et al.* 1967). In some a sensory, disorder is suspected in which there is failure of identification and recognition shown by profile (6), **H i d r**. Before non-responsive children of whatever type can confidently be considered to have a hearing loss, it is necessary to examine their reactions to sensory stimuli for other modalities. This may be done by blowing gently on the child's cheek or touching his hair, or by deliberately allowing the sound producing material or some other visually more stimulating object to come into the field of vision. Absence of response impairs the reliability of the hearing assessment.

In children who have reached the level of co-operation required, and in adults, pure tone audiometry indicates the presence of hearing loss and measures the alteration from normal threshold. The usual technique is to give a test tone well above threshold intensity, and to reduce it progressively until no response is obtained. An intermediate stage can be clearly observed in three-year-olds who are able to take part in the conditioning type of audiometry. When the tone is reduced below a certain level, the conditioned response is not made, although the child has given evidence of having heard the sound in other ways. The sound has become so attenuated that it is not sufficient to trigger a newly learned response and the state of indecision can be seen. The procedure can be indicated schematically: $P1 \rightarrow P3 \rightarrow P8$.

In screening tests of hearing, and in all children being tested whose co-operation cannot be relied upon, it is essential to reverse this procedure, starting with very quiet sounds, and increasing the loudness level until a response is obtained. This is the only way to overcome the factor of inhibition, and to obtain a quantitative measure of hearing loss if present. Prolonged testing, from a pedantic desire to determine the threshold within the nearest 5dB, may have the same effect. Consistency and reliability rather than precise determination are the more important criteria.

93

REFERENCES

Beagley, H. A., Kellog, S. E. (1969) 'A comparison of evoked response and subjective auditory thresholds.' *Int. Audiol.*, **8**, 345.

—— Knight, J. J. (1967) 'Changes in evoked auditory response with intensity.' *J. Laryng. Otol.*, **81**, 861.

Dale, D. M. C. (1962) *Applied Audiology for Children*. Springfield, Ill.: C. C. Thomas.

Ewing, I. R., Ewing, A. W. G. (1944) 'The ascertainment of deafness in infancy and early childhood.' *J. Laryng. Otol.*, **59**, 309.

Martin, J. A. M. (1971) 'Problems of diagnosis of hearing loss in the young child.' *Proc. roy. Soc. Med.*, **64**, 571.

Rutter, M., Greenfield, D., Lockyer, L. (1967) 'A five to fifteen year follow-up study of infantile psychosis. II. Social and behavioural outcome.' *Brit. J. Psychiat.*, **113**, 1183.

Sheridan, M. D. (1962) 'Infants at risk of handicapping conditions.' *Mth. Bull. Hlth. Lab. Serv.*, **21**, 238.

Watson, T. J. (1967) *The Education of Hearing-handicapped Children*, London: University of London Press.

—— (1969) 'Indentification and follow-up of children with exudative otitis media.' *Proc. roy. Soc. Med.*, **62**, 455.

Whetnall, E., Fry, D. B. (1964) *The Deaf Child*. London: Heinemann.

CHAPTER 8

Attention and Feedback

KEVIN MURPHY

Introduction

Under normal circumstances, language development in children begins from and through speech. Spoken-language usually demands that the user will have adequate hearing, the bases of developing discrimination and comprehension, together with the ability to focus these three elements upon sounds which could provide linguistic cues. Focussing hearing is commonly described as listening. There are numerous definitions of listening but, in the main, they agree on three fundamental criteria. These are that the attention must be focussed on auditory stimuli and that the attentive focus will lead to perceptual and cognitive function. In other words, we have (a) auditory acuity; (b) auditory attention; and (c) auditory concepts. These three aspects of auditory behaviour cannot lead to language learning in the absence of a fourth and separate element, namely (d) language processes. This is the ability to submit auditory concepts to the brain's language centres in order to develop language discrimination, comprehension and usage.

Even today, there are still people who are amazed to discover the existence of failure to comprehend or develop language in the presence of an otherwise normal ability to develop non-linguistic auditory concepts. We still find children with language failures wrongly labelled 'deaf', 'mentally subnormal' or 'psychotic', as though these three areas of disability can be the only relevant causes of language disorder. However, the first point this chapter will emphasize is the fact that without auditory attention there can be no prospect of *any* auditory learning, much less of language learning except as an artificially acquired skill.

Auditory Attention

In the presence of normal hearing, auditory attention is needed for the following:

(1) for auditory response;

(2) for auditory discrimination (which describes the use the individual makes of his auditory acuity);

(3) for the encouragement of continued vocalisation;

(4) for auditory decoding and encoding;

(5) for consequent vocabulary acquisition;

(6) for cognitive processes associated with the 'language acquisition process': (4, 5 and 6, together with auditory recall, form the basis of the individual's development of auditory concept);

(7) for social readiness;

(8) for continued social contact, basic to language usage and hence to growth;

(9) for the process of self-monitoring, which is basic to accurate expression of needs, emotions, or cognitive processes.

With these factors in mind, we can see that minor degrees of auditory dysfunction, relatively minor degrees of hyperkinesis or hyper-distractability, immaturity leading to the domination of auditory state by visual function, psychological, neurological or metabolic disorders leading to modification of external or internal attention, can all modify the climate for normal language development. As Meyerson (1956) says: 'Human beings spend more time in listening than in any other activity and yet we do not know how an individual learns to listen or how this function develops.' While this may have been an adequate description of the state of knowledge up to 10 to 15 years ago, much more is now known about auditory attention and certain aspects of its development, though it is still true to say that we know far more about factors which prevent or modify such development than those which assist or encourage it.

The individual who has worked with children affected by language disorders knows that they often have severe problems in the focussing of attention and also that they tend to find certain patterns of language discrimination, decoding, encoding and recall to be particularly difficult. To some extent, this set of problems may be more easily understood if we recognise what is involved in listening. The speech of others will only develop meaning for the child who listens to it if he hears it often enough for decoding to occur. The child will not be able to speak (as distinct from vocalise) until encoding develops. The processes of decoding and encoding cannot occur unless the child is capable of a kind of split-level attention, both aspects of which must focus simultaneously on external stimuli and on previously acquired codes. Recall in such circumstances demands a rapid and accurate deployment of short-term memory, and cannot occur unless the association between current events and previous experience can be made. In other words, when we attempt to focus a child's attention on sound, the amount of actual attention required is at least twice as great as would be required for simple decoding if we intend the child to use this decoding for purposes of expression. For example, many speech therapists find that the cerebral palsied child has considerable problems of auditory attention if he knows that he is immediately expected to respond to auditory stimuli by speaking. It appears that in such cases the focussing of attention on expression has acted as a barrier to a similar focus of attention on reception. In one's own experience it is only too apparent that any distraction of attention can modify the ability to concentrate on what one is saying. Listening to oneself is essential for accurate speech and is based on auditory feedback.

What Occurs in the Child's Auditory Feed-back System?

By auditory feedback I mean not just the simple monitoring of sounds but the whole process which eventually allows the child to produce accurate comprehensible and meaningful speech. It involves many processes which I shall now outline.

(1) Incoming sound is received auditorily and transmitted to the primary auditory area of the cortex.

(2) Such transmissions are stored.

(3) Repeated sounds are decoded in relation to prior experience of sound.

(4) Vocalisation occurs as a biological phenomenon.

(5) Stimulation or need provokes continued vocalisation.

(6) As the anatomical structures develop, the infant is able to produce an increasing

range of vocalisations and, as a result, is compelled to select from this repertoire. By the age of eight or nine months, we see the infant beginning to group his utterances into patterns of 'sentence-like chunks' (Weir 1962) with characteristic melody and phonetic structures. Sounds which have occurred randomly in earlier infancy are now grouped into patterns which approximate more closely to those of the adult. We assume, therefore, that encoding occurs. Following encoding, the infant scans the store, selects from it, probably rehearses it or organises it for accuracy and brevity, and then produces it.

(7) He listens to himself to ensure that what he says is what he intended to say, *i.e.* resembles his decoded material and, as an accurate representation of his encoding selection, conveys as clearly as possible what he wants to say.

When the child is talking to adults (as distinct from children), one can observe the throes of composition. He half begins a sentence, halts, begins again, gives it partial expression, sprinkles it liberally with verbal condiments, an assortment of 'ums', 'ahs', and 'ers' and a profusion of gestures before satisfying himself that he has developed an approximation to the kind of pattern used by the adult. Watching children talking together in circumstances where the presence of the adult does not intrude, the pattern of speech tends to greater spontaneity and there is less evident searching for structures. If, for instance, the incidence of such pause markers as 'um', 'ah' and so on is counted, child conversation with peers (in the three to seven year range) will be seen to contain less than half the amount used in conversation with adults. Whether or not this phenomenon relates to rôle play on the part of the child, it is clearly an index of the extent to which auditory feedback is an integral part of conversation.

The maturation of serial store and sequential decoding is a prerequisite for the development of linguistic skills. Against such stored codes incoming auditory cues are evaluated, leading to further decoding or a new serial store. From this store, encoded material is selected for vocal expression. Problems of discrimination, recognition, code analysis and linguistic organisation prior to vocalisation may result in the modification of skill in language usage. We now know that problems of discrimination produce severe difficulties in attention and also in the stimulation and monitoring of utterance. In the case of children with psychological problems which affect the ability to identify between self and not-self, one wonders how they can ever be sure whether events are real or imaginary. When, in such cases, is an event not an hallucination? In such circumstances, decoding and encoding would seem to be quite impossible, and this phenomenon might well provide a partial explanation for the presence of echolalia in such children. Such a hypothesis would appear even more plausible in those cases where echolalia is accompanied by inability to formulate speech spontaneously.

Attention and Language Learning

There are other features of attention which are essential to language development apart from the process of auditory feedback which has just been discussed. Some outline of the underlying processes of language development is required in order to illustrate the significance of features of attention. Because these processes are described in several other chapters (see especially 5 and 15), the present summary is deliberately selective and abbreviated.

(1) The infant's attention must focus on sounds which are heard clearly, consistently, and with a certain degree of continuity.

(2) Auditory stimuli must be related to an awareness of all other relevant events as a basis for concept formation. Such concept formation requires more than intelligence; unless the child can focus his attention simultaneously on the relevant sensory stimuli such associations will be impossible. For instance, if the hierarchy of sensory dominance is insufficiently developed, auditory attention may well be blocked or distracted by visual or kinaesthetic stimuli. It follows, therefore, that during the period of maturation in which auditory inputs are dominated by the other senses, the growth of auditory associations will be slow. However, from about the age of six months, the blending of sensory inputs should facilitate a more rapid growth of integration of auditory cues and hence of audio-visual or audio-kinaesthetic learning. From this age onwards, we may expect to see a more rapid maturation of auditory awareness and hence of auditory concepts.

(3) In the early stages of concept formation, events develop significance partly by repetition and partly by the extent they relate to, or satisfy, needs and wants.

(4) During the early period of concept formation the infant makes sounds and hears the sounds he produces. If he cannot hear them there is grave danger that without artificial aids he will cease to use his voice. He learns that the sounds he makes are signals which seem to affect his environment and also to satisfy his needs and wants.

(5) Satisfaction of needs and wants is generalised from the events which produce the satisfaction to the sounds associated with these events. The infant quickly learns to associate his sounds and those of others with such satisfaction. Social learning occurs when he discovers a relationship between the fact that he produces sounds and that others respond, or perhaps more significantly, that the sounds made by others encourage him also to make sounds.

(6) Such learning leads to the recognition that sounds are another medium by which information can be exchanged. Learning of speech and language demands, therefore, a social situation in which needs and wants are satisfied. The rate of learning will depend to some degree on the extent to which such events are affected by vocalisation.

(7) In addition to the social factors outlined above, these social relationships must have a certain emotional character before the child will want to understand spoken language and to talk.

(8) Given the right socio-emotional climate, the development of perceptual and cognitive functions and of language are inextricably inter-related. Growth in cognition assists language development. Language development and usage assists cognitive function. The continued exercise of cognitive skill leads to its further improvement.

(9) As has already been stated, the feedback systems facilitate a process of matching our own vocalisations against those of others. Although the quality and quantity of vocal models presented to the infant are crucial to development, without an adequate feedback system the matching process will be severely or totally handicapped.

Attitude and Attention

The clinician who is in daily contact with disturbed children will probably consider discussion of attitudes to be almost a work of supererogation. And yet the focus of attention can be seen to be vulnerable to modification of attitudes to oneself and the community. Attitude to others demands, and to a considerable extent is derived from, attitude to oneself. In this sense, spoken language is inextricably involved in the growth of self-awareness. As Lewis (1968) has pointed out: 'The child's acts and the expression of his emotions evoke verbal approval or disapproval from others. As a result he becomes more clearly aware of his behaviour and attitudes as set beside those of other people. He realises that he can provoke co-operation, resistance or approval and begins to appreciate that he is as much the object of the behaviour of others as they are of his. In the end he comes to recognise that he also is the object of his own behaviour. If we combine with this the quality of the child's social relationships and his development of some ethical criteria we have reached an organisation of personality factors which are intrinsic to adult living and learning.'

Not only is language usage vulnerable to social stress, but as we have already seen, in its turn it is potential source of stress, particularly in the presence of modification of its normal function. Without language, the freedom to accept and learn from environmental opportunities is seriously threatened. Without language, the absorption or dissemination of information not only modifies the rôle of the child but undermines the social structure in which he develops. Without spoken language the child is prevented from developing and displaying the attitudes described above.

Selective Processes and Attention

The organisation of attention is a selective process. Early selective processes are dependent on the anatomical structures which are relatively constant. This constancy does not compel us all to use our brains in the same way. The selection from presented auditory or visual stimuli, its organisation and direction, differs for every individual and, in that associations are based on prior personal experience, there are obvious differences in the selection of emotional and cognitive associations stimulated by the sensory inputs. There are at least two selective mechanisms involved, one at the level of selective awareness and the other at the level of selective association. These two selections are then passed through a third process which selects the response pattern. Such response patterns may begin as inhibition or minimal response and range in their extent from gross startle, or other loco-motor activity, to the relative sophistication of vocal function. These responses used in early childhood tend to self-reinforcement and so to persist into adulthood. For this reason, the early selective processes, upon which the maturing brain mechanisms are based, are crucial to both the type and extent of such mechanisms or structures.

The notion of attention has now become an acceptable area of research and its bibliography is extensive. We have briefly studied problems of selectivity in the infant. Our project investigated the effect of reverberatory conditions on infant listening and we gained the impression that infants' auditory selective processes are affected by reverberation. Infants' ability to listen appeared impaired when the extraction of meaningful noise from meaningless background noise was rendered too difficult.

99

One form of selective difficulty appeared when the signal presented was too close to background noise in intensity, frequency and time. Such a situation commonly arises when the signal is masked by the presence of its own echo.

The relevance of the selective process as one aspect of attention becomes more apparent if we look at four primary levels involved in decoding and encoding all speech sounds.

Acoustic Selection

By eliminating extraneous or irrelevant sounds the auditory inputs are simplified in terms of quantity but amplified in terms of significance. Information reduction, the control of redundancy, leads to increased information.

Phonetic Selection

This is a process of feature abstraction by means of which the recognition and analysis of loudness, pitch and temporal sequence is facilitated.

Grammar and Syntax

The infant's own coding processes are related to the overheard speech of others. Such relation depends on the developing skill of language analysis and the generation of rules of syntax which eventually become the basis for adult pattern. Such processes of analysis clearly have a selective basis.

Semantics

The significance of the spoken signal requires comprehension as well as analysis of its structure. Certain elements in the signal have to be correctly selected for such comprehension to occur.

Whether the brain is involved in refinement, feature abstraction, the generation of linguistic hypotheses or the organisation of conceptual processes, the attention must be focussed. When the development of language demands the simultaneous organisation of all these features it becomes even clearer that the structuring and use of attention requires a considerable degree of skill.

Feedback and Emotional Development

Earlier in the chapter, the discussion of feedback processes was predominantly concerned with self-monitoring—listening to one's own utterances, observing their social significance and building coding skills. Because feedback is one method of attending to all the consequences of communication, there is a danger that emotional aspects will be ignored in favour of those elements already described. As we have already stated, the inter-relationship between the individual and the environment is the classic route to intellectual growth. If, within the term 'environment', we include social contacts, then it becomes more apparent that emotional growth is to be expected also and that, in fact, we would find it impossible to separate either intellectual or emotional components from the development of personality structures. If we accept that language is a link between the individual and the environment which encourages or assists the growth of personality, we may regard it as a kind of social nourishment. Just as, in the past, nourishment and socio-economic conditions have been related, we now see researchers seeking to relate language quality and socio-economic features. We recognise that mal-nourishment may create conditions in which the ability to absorb nourishment will be impaired.

The infant is not passive. His social rôle produces certain necessary satisfactions in the family. In fact, the whole family (and particularly the mother) have certain needs which the infant normally satisfies. When such satisfactions do not occur, the family is effectively deprived, the social environment is contaminated, the seeds of stress are sown and hence the prognosis for language is increasingly impaired. In particular there is danger, as Lillywhite and Bradley (1969) pointed out, that communication failure may well result in the withdrawal of 'verbal stimulation and affection and perhaps bring about the substitution of anxiety, over-solicitousness, over-protection, harshnsse or rejection'. If the child's attitude to life is to be kept in a healthy balance between introversion and extraversion, it is clear that the psychological climate of the home is of considerable significance. It is clear also that the development of social skills, of which language is only one, demands a social climate in which learning of such skills is encouraged and assisted. In turn, such learning demands a pattern of attentive behaviour, the experimentation with social-emotional rôles and attitudes, their evaluation in the light of social reaction, and their adoption or rejection as the bases of developing behaviour patterns and personality structures.

Lewis (1968) emphasises another consideration when he deals with orectic development. He rightly emphasises that the emotional aspects of life are also a function of learning and maturation. The progressive organisation of the emotions, personality structures, social, aesthetic and ethical criteria are said to be aspects of orectic development. Russian research has claimed that the development of language facilitates emotional development (Luria 1961). Even the naming of emotions seems to encourage discrimination of them, and such discrimination will ideally lead to their direction and control. As Lewis says: 'Language development may well play an important part in stimulating and maintaining the motivation to undertake and persist in particular patterns of behaviour.' To paraphrase Lewis, we differentiate between pleasure *in* usage and pleasure *from* usage. Pleasure in usage seems to be akin to preening, or 'Look at me, see how clever I am'. Pleasure from usage would relate to the development of insight, of conceptual growth, of the maturation of intellectual processes. In other words, we differentiate between 'learning how' and 'learning that'. Both of these elements of pleasure are important to the notion of feedback.

It becomes increasingly apparent, therefore, that therapy with children suffering from language disorders must be directed almost as much to the home as to the child. In fact, in many cases, therapy may well begin through and from the home and particularly through the mother. We cannot expect feedback to occur unless the social stimuli emanating from the child provoke responses which he or she can identify. The child who is prevented from communicating adequately not only suffers from frustrations commonly recognised and acknowledged by therapists but is deprived of a basic need, a source of comfort and security and, perhaps most important, a source of self-expression and therefore of the feedback process which underlies the development of self-realisation and self-identification. Without these last two qualities, the mechanism by which a child recognises his own existence and social function may be so severely impaired as to prevent any real social contact or manipulation of the environment.

Feedback from the Environment

We have stated that listening during conversation implies a two-fold direction of attention. The first direction is to the speaker himself and the second is to the person to whom he is speaking. The converse is also true. During the process of self-monitoring, the speaker speaks both to himself and to his listener. The acts of speaking and of listening are dual spans in the bridge of social activity. They are, therefore, vulnerable to those aspects of social structuring which are basic to inter-personal relationships. A recent report by Lloyd and Kay Meadow (1969) illustrates the above point. Conducting a survey of some social aspects of deafness, they asked a deaf couple about the vocal function of one of their children with normal hearing. The mother stated that, by the age of nine months, her infant had ceased to vocalise to attract attention; instead, he waved or banged the side of his cot. In spite of his normal hearing and normal potential for speech, his failure to use his voice in the home was so apparent to the parents, they presumed he had recognised that, being deaf, they could not respond to vocal signals! It would probably be more accurate, however, to relate this situation to modified feedback and consequent lack of vocal reinforcement similar to the cases one meets of parental neglect or institutionalisation.

Maturation and Attention

We tend to relate the rate of progress in audio-vocal function to the general pattern of maturity of the child. In this context, Lenneberg (1967) made an interesting point when he claimed a close relationship between the constancy of development in normal children of a fixed sequence for 'certain important speech milestones'. He sees in this development a 'remarkable synchronisation of speech milestones and motor development milestones'. Though the steps of progress he describes are necessarily superficial within the range which he selects, there appears a stability in the pattern of general maturation. Lenneberg stresses, quite rightly, that these aspects of progress must not be regarded simply as neuro-motor in origin. Even so, the majority of child observers have noted that, although the whole process of maturation has predictable stages, within this pattern the balance between the development of voice and that of other skills varies from time to time. For instance, the focus of attention on learning to walk may lead to diminution in the amount of vocalisation with consequent temporary delay in vocal progress. One sees similar trends in the balance between vocalisation and more general loco-motor activity. Concentration on reaching, climbing, and crawling, especially in the early learning phases, seems temporarily to exclude, or at least diminish, vocal activity.

The report by Moray (1969), in which he summarises research on auditory attention, tends to support the earlier statements of Luria (1961) and Masland (1958) concerning the interdependence of various areas of the brain. This becomes particularly important when they refer to auditory attention alone, especially in their emphasis on the importance of the association fibres of the brain. When Masland was discussing various areas of the brain in which pathology could give rise to language disorders, he made an interesting statement which differentiated between speech development and speech initiation. He said: 'Whereas the areas and structures outlined above are clearly involved in the elaboration of speech, it is by no means established that they are involved in such more abstract activities as attention, consciousness, concept formation, and the initiation of speech.'

Models of Language Development

In creating a structure which illustrates the development of language, we can deliberately simplify. The child begins to learn *from* the environment *that* the voice is a signal, *to* use it as a signal and *how* to use it. Such an analogy may be followed throughout the development of the articulatory, phonological, sequential, syntactical and numerous other features upon which spoken language depends. Because there are so many situations and conditions which can modify the progress and quality of development, there is considerable danger in looking too closely for a set pattern or even for a rate of growth which is common to all children. Hence, identification of features upon which prognostic or diagnostic statements can be based is difficult and still needs extensive research.

Recent reports from psycholinguistic conferences have shown us that irrespective of geographical distribution or of the mother tongues employed, all normal infants seem to have a basic inborn skill in language acquisition described by Chomsky (1961, 1965) as Language Acquisition Device, (LAD), or by Katz (1966) as Language Acquisition System (LAS), or by Slobin (1966) as the Language Acquisition Process (LAP). Interesting and helpful as these papers are, they refer only to language potential and in some ways illustrate the old discussions that used to occur about 'Nature or Nature' as bases of intelligence. In making this comment one is in danger of implying that the writers mentioned above are not concerned with language acquisition from the environment. This, of course, is not the case. All three have written copiously about the growth of language in relation to language environments. In other words, a balance is postulated between the inborn selective and creative process and the sensory information provided by the environment. The information supplied from the environment has its own selective function. The pre-speech vocalisations of infants are said to be vested with meaning by the parents, depending on the language structure within which they occur. From such reinforcements, one may see a natural basis for a vocabulary selection and for the development of strings of single words, by which the language maturation of children was judged at one time.

Recourse to the most elementary textbook on language acquisition, however, will illustrate that research into vocabulary length is, at best, of dubious significance in terms of language structures. Three commonly reported researches into the development of such structures are those of Brown and Frazer (1964), Ervin (1964) and Braine (1963). All three collected records of the speech of two-year-old children and, though their methods were different, their results were remarkably similar. Without going into their systems of classification, we can see two clear conclusions: the *first*, that the utterances had a structure which could be classified in all three cases; the *second*, that these classifications show a language balance present in all children studied which was so different from the adult model that it was statistically impossible for that particular structure to have been imitated from adults. In other words, the structure formulation used by each child, though derived from adult vocabulary, was different from the adult model.

My interest is not so much in the difference between adult and child models as in the similarity from child to child and the fact that even by two years of age there are clear language structures present. Structure recognition or structured formulation occurs in the first two years of life, and by the age of three to three-and-a-half has covered a large proportion of our basic linguistic rules. The amount of information so developed is of such magnitude and complexity that it has been shown to be too much for the infant to derive directly from heard speech. It is for this reason that the linguistic postulates of a Language Acquisition Device, System or Process seem such a valuable hypothesis.

Because the child needs language models and, of course, acquires his vocabulary upon which such models are constructed from heard speech, some reference is necessary to aspects of word recognition. Hirsh (1967) describes the steps required for word recognition as Detection, Discrimination, Recognition or Identification and Comprehension. He says: 'That the sounds of a word must be audible in order that thay may be processed further is too obvious to dwell on, but it is this dimension of audibility that is most affected by various kinds of hearing loss.' It is also true to say that this dimension of audibility is most vulnerable to factors of attention.

The development of a receptive structure upon which a language model can be based demands a certain consistency of receptive function for purposes of discrimination and also for purposes of attention. In this particular regard, the mild fluctuating hearing impairment associated with a conductive hearing disorder may well prove to be an important factor. A fluctuating loss of the conductive type does not only attenuate but also distorts the signal. Both attenuation and distortion vary in severity throughout each attack and also from attack to attack of conductive dysfunction. In a child with immature language structures, such a situation is bad enough, but in a child with a peripheral hearing loss or a language disorder the addition of a conductive overlay may well create insuperable difficulties in auditory detection. Any condition which threatens auditory attention will threaten the growth of a mature language model. Thyroid imbalance, relatively slight modification of protein metabolism, of sugar absorption, of hyperkinesis, have all been inculpated in relation to attention modification and also in relation to language delay. The clinician interested in understanding the problems of his patients with speech and language disorders must examine the processes of feedback and attention.

REFERENCES

Braine, M. D. S. (1963) 'The ontogeny of English phrase structure: the first phrase.' *Language*, **39**, 1.
Brown, R., Fraser, C. (1964) 'The acquisition of syntax.' *Monographs of the Society for Research in Child Development*, **29**, (1), 43.
Chomsky, N. (1961) 'On the notion 'Rule of Grammar'.' *in* Jakobsen, R. (Ed.) *Structure of Language and its Mathematical Aspects. Proceedings of the 12th Symposium in Applied Mathematics*. Providence, R.I.: American Mathematical Society. p. 6.
—— (1965) *Aspects of the Theory of Syntax*. Cambridge, Mass.: M.I.T. Press.
Ervin, S. (1964) 'Imitation and structural changes in children's language.' *in* Lenneberg, E. (Ed.) *New Directions in the Study of Language*. Cambridge, Mass.: M.I.T. Press.
Hirsh, I. J. (1967) 'Perception of Speech.' *in* Graham, A. B. (Ed.) *Sensorineural Hearing Processes and Disorders*. Boston, Mass.: Little, Brown. p. 129.
Katz, J. J. (1966) *The Philosophy of Language*. New York: Harper and Row.
Lenneberg, E. H. (1967) *Biological Foundations of Language*. New York: John Wiley.
Lewis, M. M. (1968) *Language and Personality in Deaf Children*. Slough, Bucks.: N.F.E.R.

Lillywhite, H. S., Bradley, D. P. (1969) *Communication Problems in Mental Retardation*. New York: Harper and Row.

Luria, A. R. (1961) *The Role of Speech in the Regulation of Normal and Abnormal Behaviour*. London: Routledge & Kegan Paul.

Masland, R. L. (1958) 'Higher cerebral functions.' *Ann. Rev. Physiol.*, **20**, 54.

Meadow, L., Meadow, K. P. (1969) 'Dealing with deafness.' *Talk*, No. 52.

Meyerson, L. (1956) 'A psychology of impaired hearing.' *in* Cruickshank, W. M. (Ed.) *Psychology of Exceptional Children*. London: Staples Press.

Moray, N. (1968) *Listening and Attention*. Harmondsworth. Middx.: Penguin Books.

Slobin, D. I. (1966) 'The acquisition of Russian as a native language.' *in* Smith, F., Miller, G. A. (Eds.) *The Genesis of Language*. Cambridge, Mass.: M.I.T. Press.

Weir, R. (1962) *Language in the Crib*. The Hague: Mouton.

CHAPTER 9

Psychological Assessment of Language Abilities

PETER MITTLER

Introduction

The conventional intelligence test was not designed to be diagnostic, though Binet always hoped that it would be: 'After exposing the child's intellectual deficits, let us at once proceed to remedy them', he wrote in 1909. It is a pity that until comparatively recently this advice has been ignored. Intelligence tests were used increasingly as instruments of classification and prediction and came to be used as the basis for administrative decisions about placement and selection. Although they are anything but inefficient for this purpose, they are insensitive to the specific needs of special education. Their continuing use has exposed psychologists to some harsh criticism from teachers in special education—perhaps not without good reason. The psychologist who confines himself to tests such as the Binet or Wechsler scales is usually accused of telling the teacher what he already knows—namely, that the child is or is not suitable for the kind of school or class in which he finds himself. The tests do not provide the kind of detailed diagnostic information which the teacher needs to help him to plan a remedial programme for the child.

These examples from intelligence and intelligence-testing apply with equal force to language, perception, learning and memory. The task facing educational psychology in the coming decade is to devise diagnostic instruments and assessment techniques which will provide a more penetrating analysis of the many skills and abilities which are involved in each of these global terms (Mittler 1970a and b). A modest beginning has already been made. In the field of intelligence, the new British Intelligence Scale (Warburton et al. 1970), which is now under construction at Manchester University, is probably the most ambitious multifactorial test yet devised; it consists of subscales concerned with verbal items (vocabulary, comprehension, information); reasoning (induction, operational thinking, matrices); creativity; memory (auditory, visual); number; and spatial abilities (visual spatial and block designs). The subscales and subtests take account of recent work in developmental psychology, particularly the important contribution of Piaget to our knowledge of cognitive development.

Similarly, the Frostig Developmental Perception Test (Frostig et al. 1964) represents an attempt to identify and isolate specific perceptual skills, such as Eye-Motor Co-ordination, Figure Ground Perception, Form Constancy, Position in Space and Spatial Relations. Although there is some doubt whether these abilities are really distinct, since some 45 per cent of the variance of the test is still accounted for by a general perceptual factor (Ward 1970), the scale does represent a useful model which allows the psychologist to differentiate between different aspects of perception. Moreover, the test is backed up by a parallel remedial programme which contains activities and exercises designed to help the child to overcome specific perceptual disabilities.

It should not be thought that all the complex skills contributing to intelligence, perception or language can be assessed by psychometric methods alone. Although only a few of the relevant abilities can be sampled by means of a test, this should at least provide certain clues about other possible areas of deficit. These can then be investigated by experimental methods of studying the single case, as advocated by Shapiro (1970). Standardised tests can tap only a small sample of the many skills involved; it is important not to assume that a comprehensive assessment has been carried out when all that has been done is to administer 'the' relevant test. Although this may, in many cases, provide useful information, full assessment of language abilities involves the use of a wide range of assessment techniques, including some for which there may not be normative data. Fully comprehensive assessment of speech and language functions is fortunately rarely needed, since this would involve a complete description in terms of phonology, morphology, syntax and semantics. Nevertheless, specialists in these aspects of language should be available for the assessment of at least some language disordered children.

Language as a Group of Skills

Progress in the teaching of language skills depends on the ability to consider language not merely as a single global entity but as composed of a large number of specific skills and abilities. This may be important in relation to patients with a language disorder as some of the processes involved may be less impaired than others. It may be possible to use these as the basis of a programme of language teaching. Very little work has been done along these lines so far, though some promising developments are being reported.

These processes can usefully be considered as similar to those found in dealing with perceptual stimuli as a whole. Stimuli have to be taken in, identified, sorted, and given individual meaning; in other words, we should consider input, integration, output and feedback. Thus, the following conditions have to be present for effective language functioning (Eisenson 1966). The subject has to (a) be able to receive stimuli produced in sequential order; (b) maintain a sequential impression of the message so that its components can be integrated into a pattern; (c) scan the pattern from within in order to categorise the data and compare it with an existing store, and (d) to respond differentially to perceptual impression.

The best known attempt to identify and isolate constituent language abilities can be found in the Illinois Test of Psycholinguistic Abilities. This test (which will be more fully described below) is based on a model first proposed by Osgood (1957), distinguishing between processes, channels and levels, and consists of 10 subtests each concerned with a different aspect of language. But it would be unrealistic to suppose that a psychometric instrument could sample more than a few aspects of language skills.

The Development of Comprehension

Although there is by now a monumental literature on the development and use of language in young children, research has been almost exclusively concerned with what children say rather than with what they understand. This is a curious placing of the developmental cart before the horse, since it is generally agreed that comprehension precedes production of language by quite a considerable period. If we assume that language represents a series of hierarchically organised skills, it seems curious to be as pre-occupied as we have always been with expressive aspects of language, since these depend to a large but unknown extent on the prior development of receptive abilities.

Experience of children with delayed language development forces us to cast around for means of assessing comprehension. The mother of such a child will almost invariably assure you that 'he understands everything you say'; a moment's reflection will indicate that such a statement is unlikely to be true. The processes and mechanisms by which we try to 'follow' what another person is saying involve a guessing strategy in which we combine what cues we can get from the speaker with our pre-existing expectations of what we think he is going to say. Furthermore, we supplement linguistic cues with visual and situational prompts, such as the speaker's facial expression, amount of eye contact, use of gesture and so forth. The halting, ungrammatical and generally chaotic nature of spontaneous spoken language normally puts such obstacles in the way of comprehension that it is surprising that children learn to understand language as well as they do.

A child with a partial hearing loss may be unable to hear consonants but, depending upon his store of language, may get the gist of what is being said by 'filling in' consonants that he cannot hear. Readers of certain Eastern languages have to learn to do without vowels, and are forced to guess which word is intended merely from a knowledge of the consonants, plus what information they can derive from a situational context. The very young child between about 18 and 24 months of age is in a similar position. He knows, from frequent examples, the context within which a large number of single words is normally spoken, but this is not to say that he is equal to the task of decoding a long and syntactically complex sentence, even though he may 'know' and be able to identify each individual word of the sentence. The child who goes to sit at the table in response to the mother saying 'Get ready for your dinner', is not really proving his comprehension of her utterance as a whole; he may have understood no more than the word 'dinner', and might have reacted similarly, though perhaps with some surprise, if she had said 'dinner your for ready get'. If comprehension is to a large extent a matter of guesswork, then it seems reasonable to suggest that the less intelligent child is at a considerable disadvantage in the task of comprehending spoken language. This is because he lacks a sufficiently wide range of experience against which to compare new utterances; similarly, he may be less receptive to the exceedingly subtle and minimal cues which utterances normally contain, and which facilitate the discriminations on which adequate comprehension depends.

Although very little information is available, we can probably assume that the developmental processes underlying comprehension of single words have their origins in the wider communication contexts within which utterances occur. We are told that babies 'understand' the word 'No' as early as 9 months, but it is difficult to be sure whether it is the word that is understood or whether the baby stops whatever he is doing because the adult also looks cross, or raises his hand, or shouts. Eventually, of course, we finish with a conditioning process which has succeeded in linking the word 'no' with a series of possible consequences; once this happens, it might be enough merely to say the word in an unemotional or neutral fashion. However, this does not seem to happen very often.

But are we justified in speaking of comprehension once the child begins to react consistently to specific utterances? Obvious examples are the child who claps his hands in response to the word(s) 'Pat-a-Cake', or who obediently waves his hands following 'say bye bye'. These behaviours presumably develop on the basis of fairly simple conditioning processes, which may be highly specific to certain individuals and only occur in certain situations. It is only later that they come to be generalised, but we are almost entirely ignorant about the way in which these processes develop.

The subnormal child is at a particular disadvantage because he is less skilled than a normal child in indicating that he has failed to understand. Normal people develop a wide repertoire of behaviour to indicate that they are either partly or wholly failing to understand a speaker. They may look puzzled or sceptical, ask the speaker to speak more slowly or distinctly, or ask for clarification of the meaning of a word or sentence. Subnormal children tend to retain an unchanged facial expression if they do not understand, so that the speaker has to make continuous checks to ensure that he is being understood. A teaching programme might begin by providing him with multiple visual and situational cues, but then gradually removes these prompts and leaves him with nothing but the linguistic message to decode. We might also suggest the obvious corollary of teaching him to emit non-verbal, as well as verbal, signals of non-conprehension. He might, for example, be taught to frown or look puzzled or to signal non-comprehension in sign language if necessary. This may be more acceptable than teaching the child to say 'I don't understand'.

Assessment of Comprehension

How then can we assess comprehension? It is not difficult to test for comprehension of single words, and standardised tests are available for this purpose. Perhaps the best known is the Peabody Picture Vocabulary Test (Dunn 1959). This test merely requires the child to point to one of four pictures in response to a stimulus word spoken by the experimenter. The number of words correctly identified can be compared against available norms, and expressed in terms of a vocabulary age, percentile equivalent or IQ. The test begins at a 21 month level, and usually presents few difficulties of administration, since the child merely has to be able to select one of four pictures by pointing. It is a useful test to administer at the beginning of an assessment session, though results must be interpreted with caution. Although the test shows acceptable levels of reliability, it does not always correlate well with other language tests such as the Illinois scales (Carr *et al.* 1967), or with a test of general intelligence such as the Wechsler (Shaw *et al.* 1966). To use it as an intelligence test may therefore be misleading; it is, however, of interest as a simple measure of vocabulary recognition, yielding a vocabulary age. Shortened English versions are also available, though only from a 3 year level upwards (Brimer and Dunn 1962).

One of the difficulties of tests of the Peabody type is finding visual referents which provide an equal amount of information to the child. The very young or the very handicapped child may point to the most interesting picture of the four, or the one that provides the most novelty. It is almost impossible to hold visual variables constant, so that one picture does not prove to be more salient or prominent to the child than any other. If the child is correct, then we can safely assume that he knows the word being tested; if he points to the wrong picture, or appears to be pointing quite randomly, then we do not really know whether this is because he does not know the word, or because he cannot carry out the visual search operations necessary to enable him to look at each picture successively; furthermore, he might be unable to integrate the visual scanning task with the verbal signal from the examiner. (In other words, he might have difficulties in cross-modal coding, or in short term memory.) Most commonly, however, the very young child tends to point to the picture that first captures his attention, and sometimes does so even before the examiner has had a chance to say the stimulus word.

The Peabody test is merely the most obvious instance of our ignorance of the psychological processes underlying what appears at first sight to be a commonplace task. In fact, we have not begun to study all the relevant variables involved in tests of this kind, and there is reason to be dissatisfied with most tests that purport to measure comprehension of language, but which depend heavily on the need to scan visual material and then to make fairly complex discriminations in which the relative prominence of auditory and visual cues is difficult to control.

Similar problems arise when we ask a child to carry out comprehension tasks using small toys and other three dimensional material. Here again, such items as 'put the spoon in the cup' or 'give me the car' are highly predictable, and are just the kind of actions which the child might carry out even if no instructions had been given. (Toys have the additional disadvantage of being too interesting, so that a child might become so absorbed in playing with them that he is not really listening to the examiner asking him to carry out certain actions.) He might therefore be correct because most of the commands might be guessed by chance, or he might be wrong for any of the reasons discussed earlier, but also because the test has become too much of a play situation for him.

These sources of error or bias must not be exaggerated, but it is also important not to assume that a child's failure is due to lack of comprehension when other variables may be involved which have not been adequately controlled in the test, and which generally remain uninvestigated, For this reason, it is necessary to ask the child to carry out fairly unexpected actions with the test material, though this too may have the disadvantage of violating too many pragmatic expectations. If, for example, one is investigating the child's comprehension of prepositions, he may not expect you to say 'Put the spoon *under* the cup', and conclude that you must obviously be asking him to 'Put the spoon *in* the cup'.

It is apparent, therefore, that the listener trying to understand a message is dealing not only with the language used by the speaker but also with a very large number of communication cues. If we want to assess the extent to which a child understands language, we should try as far as possible to exclude as many non-linguistic cues as possible. To some extent, this is bound to be an artificial exercise, since the child normally has so many non-linguistic cues available to help him. But these cues will obviously vary considerably from one situation to another, so that it seems important to try to differentiate between linguistic and non-linguistic information and, in particular, to vary the nature of the linguistic input in a systematic manner.

Work is now in progress in the Hester Adrian Research Centre to develop a sentence comprehension test. This test was originally devised with Angela Hobsbaum at Birkbeck College, London, and has now undergone various modifications. The child is presented with four examples of 15 types of sentence of varying complexity and grammatical structure. His task is to identify which of three or four pictures corresponds to the sentence spoken by the examiner. Each picture illustrates an alternative grammatical interpretation. Thus, in response to the sentence '*The cat is sleeping*', the child is showing pictures of a *dog* sleeping, and also of a cat *playing* with a ball of string, *i.e.* the noun and the verb have been systematically varied. Similarly, in response to the sentence '*the girl is cutting the cake*', the child is shown the following pictures.

> The girl is cutting the cake (stimulus).
> The boy is cutting the cake (subject varied).
> The girl is eating the cake (verb varied).
> The girl is cutting the loaf (object varied).

Other sentence types tested include comparatives and superlatives, past and future tenses, passives, negatives, plurals, prepositions and embedded clauses.

Data are now available on 150 normal nursery school children between 34 and 45 months (Hobsbaum 1970); the test has also been administered to samples of severely subnormal (SSN) children matched for mental age (MA) with the normal controls (mean MA 3-7). Order of difficulty was very similar for normal and subnormal children (rho = 0.78), suggesting that the test is measuring comparable processes in the two groups. It also shows acceptable levels of test reliability (Mittler and Wheldall 1971).

This test is still at the research stage and is mentioned mainly in order to illustrate the difficulty in differentiating between comprehension of language and the child's response to the total communication situation of which language forms only one element. It is important to bear in mind that failure on a test is no proof of inability to perform a cognitive task; it is possible that the child has not adequately understood what is required of him, that he has been distracted by an irrelevant feature of the test situation, or that he is in a general sense inattentive to the task. When dealing with mentally handicapped children, we cannot assume, as we usually do for normal children, that they are attending to or understanding our instruction, or that they are interested in carrying it out. In this sense, we need to pay special attention to the complexity of the language which we use in testing or talking to children with intellectual or linguistic handicaps.

The Revised Illinois Test of Psycholinguistic Abilities

The main diagnostic test available for the assessment of language abilities is the Illinois Test of Psycholinguistic Abilities. An experimental edition of the test was published by McCarthy and Kirk (1961), and has been widely used in research and remediation (see summaries of research by Bateman (1965) and Kirk (1968). A revised edition of the test has now become available in Britain (Kirk *et al.* 1968, Paraskevopolous and Kirk 1969).

111

The test is based on a model of communication processes first proposed by Osgood (1957). Basically, the model distinguishes between (a) channels of communication, (b) levels of organisation and (c) psycholinguistic processes. The model aims to provide a specification for all the processes and all the levels that appear to be involved in both understanding and speaking a language, but the scale includes only 10 subtests (and 2 supplementary tests). Each test can be scored in terms of raw score, language age and standard score; a total language score can also be derived.

(a) Channels of Communication

The term channel refers to various combinations of stimulus input and response output; the two channels incorporated in the test are auditory-vocal and visual-motor. Thus the auditory-vocal channel is characterised by auditory input (from the tester) and vocal output (from the child).

(b) Levels of Organisation

Two levels are postulated: first, the representational level, which requires mediation and interpretation of symbolic aspects of language involved in understanding, speaking or thinking about language; second, the automatic level in which 'the individual's habits of functioning are less voluntary but highly organised and integrated' (Paraskevopoulos and Kirk 1969)—these include visual and auditory sequencing and skills involved in 'closure', such as the use of appropriate morphological inflections.

(c) Psycholinguistic Processes

The main psycholinguistic processes involved in language are receptive,—the ability to understand or recognise what is seen or heard; expressive—skills necessary to express ideas either vocally or by gesture; and association processes, which involve the internal manipulation of percepts, concepts and linguistic symbols.

A psycholinguistic ability is, therefore, defined as 'a given process, at a given level, via a given channel'. The 12 subtests will now be briefly described. More detailed descriptions, together with information about reliability and validity are contained in the test literature.

Tests at the Representative Level

(1) *Auditory Reception*. This involves the ability to understand simple sentences, in the form 'Do (noun) (verb)?', and requiring a 'yes' or 'no' response, or gesture (*e.g.* 'Do dogs eat?' 'Do dials yawn?'.)

(2) *Visual Reception*. The child is shown a stimulus picture followed by four comparison pictures. His task is to select the one that is 'like' the stimulus picture on the previous page. Only a pointing response is required.

(3) *Auditory Association*. A test of the familiar verbal analogies type: 'I cut with a saw, I bang with a ....'; 'Soup is hot, ice cream is ....'.

(4) *Visual Association*. A test requiring the child to relate concepts presented visually. He has to choose an alternative most closely corresponding to a stimulus picture presented on the same page (*e.g.* sock with shoe, hammer with nail).

(5) *Verbal Expression*. The subject is shown a simple object (ball, brick, envelope, button) and asked to say as much as he can about it. Scoring is in terms of the number of discrete, relevant concepts expressed.

(6) *Manual Expression*. The child is shown pictures of common objects and asked to mime the appropriate action (*e.g.* guitar, telephone).

Tests at the Automatic Level

(7) *Grammatic Closure*. This test essentially samples the child's ability to use inflectional and morphological aspects of grammar. It requires the child to complete a visually illustrated statement with an inflected word. Among the inflections sampled are regular and irregular forms of the plural, past tense, comparatives and superlatives.

(8) *Visual Closure*. The child has to identify common objects from an incomplete visual presentation. Objects are partially hidden amongst others.

Tests of Sequential Memory

(9) *Auditory Sequential Memory*. A modified digit repetition test, but presented at two digits per second.

(10) *Visual Sequential Memory*. Sequences of non-meaningful figures have to be reproduced from memory.

Two Supplementary Tests

(11) *Auditory Closure*. A test of organising processes at the automatic level. The child is asked verbally to fill in the missing parts of a truncated word (bo/le, tele/one).

(12) *Sound Blending*. Similar to auditory closure, except that the child has to identify a word when the individual parts are spoken at half second intervals (f-oot, d-i-nn-er).

Normative and reliability data are presented in detail for each subtest and for each of the age levels between 2½ and 10 years of age. Although the test is open to a number of psychometric criticisms (*e.g.* Weener *et al.* 1967), and can also be faulted for failing to take account of advances in developmental psycholinguistics, particularly the work of the generative grammarians (Chomsky 1965, Smith and Miller 1966, Lenneberg 1967, Rosenberg 1970), it does nevertheless provide a useful if not comprehensive model of language behaviour and allows the clinician to study constituent aspects of language behaviour and to draw up a profile of a child's relative assets and deficits so that he can design a corresponding programme of remedial education. In other words, it does not stop at mere assessment.

An extensive literature has been built up around the experimental edition of the test, testifying not only to its psychometric credentials, but also to its possibilities as the basis for a remedial programme (Bateman 1968). A small number of British studies suggest that American norms can probably be used in this country, though a complete restandardisation seems desirable (Phillips 1968, Mittler and Ward 1970). The revised edition of the test has not yet been extensively tried out, and few reports have so far appeared; a study by Marinosson (1970*a* and *b*), (described in greater detail in chapter 11), suggested that matched groups of normal, educationally subnormal (ESN) and SSN children obtained similar ITPA profiles, with the significant exception of the two sequencing tests on which SSN children appeared to show marked and specific deficits. Other studies on the use of the revised ITPA on normal children are now in progress in Manchester and elsewhere (Hatch and French 1971, Smith and Marx 1971).

Other Language Scales

A variety of other language tests have been published in recent years. Some are designed for individual administration, others are essentially developmental scales which a trained observer can use to help him make a rough estimate of the stage which a child has reached in various areas of language functioning.

1. *Individually Administered Normative Tests*

(a) *The Reynell Developmental Language Scales* (Reynell 1969). The Scales have normative data based on children between the ages of six months and six years, but were designed from the outset with the needs of handicapped children in mind. They distinguish between receptive and expressive aspects of language. The Verbal Comprehension Scale (A) requires mainly a simple pointing response or the manipulation of appropriate play materials. The child is required to point to objects or pictures which have to be identified or manipulated according to instructions of gradually increasing complexity. There is an alternative form of the Comprehension Test (B) for use with physically handicapped children who cannot pick up or even point to toys. The expressive tests aim to elicit samples of the child's spoken language in free conversation and in response to standard materials, and to score these in terms of structure, content and vocabulary. The RDLS is of particular value in the assessment of children whose language development is immature or uneven, and for whom more precise information is needed than that provided in general tests of language development. The distinction between receptive and expressive skills is a particularly important contribution towards assessment. It has not been available long enough for validation or subpopulation studies to be carried out on a large scale, but a dissertation by Rogers (1971) suggests that severely subnormal children produce substantially lower receptive than expressive scores.

(b) *The Renfrew Language Attainment Scales* (Renfrew 1971). The Renfrew Scales are primarily designed to help speech therapists and other experienced examiners to assess relevant aspects of language and speech in children between 3 and 7 years. They consist of the following tests.

ARTICULATION ATTAINMENT TEST. This test is designed to 'provide a standardised estimate of the extent to which use is made of all the English consonants.' The test makes use of 38 words containing 100 consonants, and is phonetically balanced in so far as each consonant is represented with the same frequency as in everyday speech. Spontaneous naming of the objects in pictures is required, as well as serial counting and imitation of phrases.

WORD FINDING VOCABULARY. This scale assesses the ability of children to find words, as distinct from recognising them in association with pictures (as in the Peabody tests). The items are modified from those originally used by Watts (1944), and call for the identification of parts of the body, the naming of objects and shapes, the use of common and proper nouns, verbs, prepositions and other parts of speech.

ACTION PICTURES. This test is designed to stimulate the child to give short samples of spoken language for purposes of a simple grammatical analysis. The child is shown 9 pictures illustrating common activities, and asked questions designed to elicit the use of present, past and future tenses in regular and irregular forms, singular and plural nouns, and simple and complex sentence constructions. The test is separately scored in terms of information and grammar.

A TEST OF CONTINUOUS SPEECH. A sample of continuous speech is elicited by first telling the child an interesting story, illustrated by suitable pictures (The Bus Story), and then asking him to tell the story to the examiner. Scoring criteria are in terms of information and sentence length.

Some of the Renfew tests have been under constant development and modification for a period of years, and data are available on a large number of children tested in various parts of Britain. Although problems of scoring and interpretation remain, the tests promise to be a useful addition to the better known and more ambitious scales already described.

(c) *The Michigan Picture Language Inventory* (Lerea 1958, Wolski 1962). The Michigan Inventory represents an early ingenious technique for the separate assessment of receptive and expressive skills, using identical linguistic content. Lerea, who originally devised the test, used the 'missing word' technique which is also found in the Grammatic Closure Test of the ITPA, and is intended to elicit specific grammatical constructions from the child, including regular and irregular nouns and verbs, different tenses, demonstratives, articles, pronouns, etc. The limitations of this method have been criticized elsewhere (Mittler 1970c), but it is now widely agreed that knowledge of morphological rules may provide a sensitive reflection of linguistic competence. Berko's (1958) original study of morphological skills has given rise to a number of psychometric instruments (*e.g.* Berry and Talbot 1966, Blake and Williams 1968, Berry 1969).

(d) *Sentence Repetition Tasks*. Elicited imitation has until quite recently been neglected as an assessment device, partly because imitation was thought to be a purely mechanical or perceptual-motor skill, and partly because such tasks were conventionally associated with memory testing. It is now becoming apparent that imitation involves the structuring and at least partial comprehension of the material, and that a detailed analysis of the imitation strategies used by the child and the exact type of errors made may provide a powerful assessment tool. Unfortunately, such assessment devices are still in their infancy. Menyuk (1969) studied the ability of preschool children to repeat sentences varying systematically in structure, and other workers have also paid particular attention to the exact nature of the linguistic material which the child is asked to imitate, and also stressed the need to keep the material within the child's short term memory span (Berry 1971a and b).

115

(e) *Tests of Syntactic Development.* In addition to the Sentence Comprehension Test developed by Hobsbaum and Mittler (described earlier), a number of other workers have described preliminary results of studies designed to assess the ability of pre-school children to understand sentences of gradually increasing complexity. Carrow (1968) presents a useful Table (reproduced in Berry 1969) showing the approximate ages at which 60 per cent of normal children understand specific grammatical categories, such as nouns, verbs, adjectives, adverbs, prepositions, tenses and genders.

The North West Syntax Screening Test (Lee 1969, 1970) consists of 20 sentence pairs to be identified receptively by picture selection, and 20 comparable sentence pairs to be produced in response to stimulus pictures. Useful norms for both receptive and expressive abilities are presented in percentile graphs, but, as the name implies, the test provides only a rapid screening measure yielding a global total score, and is not intended for detailed analysis of grammatical skills.

(f) *Tests of Speech Perception and Articulation.* A number of tests of speech perception are widely used by speech therapists. The Sound Discrimination Test originally developed by Templin (1957) requires the child to discriminate between pairs of words or sounds with a minimal contrast (*e.g.* keys-peas, chairs-stairs, etc.). In the Auditory Discrimination Test (Wepman 1958) the child has to indicate whether a pair of words is the same or different. Finally, the Picture Discrimination Test (Mecham and Jex 1962) uses a word-picture matching technique. The child is shown three pictures on a card, and then has to listen to three words, one of which is illustrated, while the other two are only acoustically similar to the other two pictures.

2. *Developmental Charts*

A number of scales are available which essentially consist of a more or less detailed check list of skills and abilities reached by normal children at specified ages. Most of these consist of items freely borrowed from the extensive literature on language development, reviewed at length by McCarthy (1954). They require a period of observation and assessment of the child's verbal behaviour in both natural and more formal test situations, and allow the examiner to structure his own observations, or direct the observations of others, such as teachers, nurses and above all parents. A recently completed project at the Hester Adrian Research Centre indicated that it was possible to train parents of pre-school mentally handicapped children to understand and use specially prepared developmental charts requiring no formal testing, but only the systematic observation of their own child at home.

Scales currently available may be no more than quick screening devices containing very few items, or longer and more detailed schedules with many items at each period of development. Among the shorter American scales are the Denver Developmental Screening Test (Frankenburg *et al.* 1967), the Utah Test of Language Development (Mecham *et al.* 1967) and the Houston Test of Language Development (Crabtree 1958). Relevant British scales that include, but are not exclusively concerned with, language development include the Sheridan scales (Sheridan 1958), the Progress Assessment Charts (Gunzburg 1963) and the charts recently prepared in the Hester Adrian Research Centre (Cunningham and Jeffree 1971).

Implications for Therapy

Spradlin (1968) criticises current language scales such as ITPA because they do not take sufficient account of the nature of language skills required in a particular community, or of the minimum language requirements regarded as necessary for adjustment in a particular society. The first step in any assessment or training programme must be the establishment of the goals of training: these in his view should relate to the minimum language requirements of the community and should, as far as possible, be based on an operational study of those requirements. The second phase should consist of the development of finely graded learning steps; the nature of these steps can only be inferred by a close study of both normal and deviant language acquisition. In general, Spradlin relies largely on principles of behaviour modification for the remedial programme, including immediate reinforcement of desired responses, careful grading of the learning steps, and the systematic use of prompting.

There is no doubt that behaviour modification techniques constitutes a powerful therapeutic weapon in the field of mental retardation. In the last decade, many reports have been published which testify to the effectiveness of these methods, and it is likely that they will be increasingly applied to the treatment of both language and behaviour disturbances. One of the advantages of these techniques is that they allow the psychologist to forge an organic link between assessment and treatment and to use behaviouristic as well as psychometric assessment techniques. In essence, the psychologist makes precise observations on a carefully specified piece of behaviour; this may refer to the amount of time spent vocalising, the exact nature of the vocalisations, the amount of time spent simply looking at the examiner, or at visual material. This functional assessment of behaviour involves a detailed study of the child, rather than a statistical comparison of his test scores with that of a normative population. Following the establishment of a baseline, a programme of systematic teaching can then be introduced which is designed to facilitate an increase in the frequency of the desired behaviour, or a decrease in the frequency of unwanted behaviour; this is done by means of a programme of carefully administered reinforcement (Bricker 1971).

It is possible that the use of principles of systematic assessment and teaching could release cognitive potential which has hitherto remained unexploited. There is every justification, therefore, for experimenting with new methods of assessment and teaching of language skills. Whatever the precise relationship between language and other cognitive processes, there can be little doubt that a teaching programme which sets out to enlarge language abilities would be of benefit to the child.

REFERENCES

Bateman, B. (1965) *The Illinois Test of Psycholonguistic Abilites in Current Research: Summaries of Studies.* Urbana, Ill.: University of Illinois Press.

—— (1968) *Interpretation of the 1961 Illinois Test of Psycholinguistic Abilities.* Seattle: Special Child Publications.

Berko, J. (1958) 'The child's learning of English morphology.' *Word,* **14,** 150.

Berry, M. F. (1969) *Language Disorders of Children.* New York: Appleton-Century-Crofts.

—— Talbott, R. (1966) *'Exploratory Test of Grammar.* (Cited by Berry, M. F. (1969).)

Berry, P. (1971*a*) 'Imitation of language in severe subnormality: a psycholinguistic assessment of technique.' Paper presented at the XVIIth International Congress of Applied Psychology, Liege, Belgium, July, 1971.

—— (1971*b*) *Imitation of Language in Subnormal Children.* University of Manchester, M.Ed. Thesis.

Binet, A. (1909) *Les Ideés Modernes sur les Enfant.* Paris: Flammarion.

Blake, K. A., Williams, C. L. (1968) *Use of English Morphemes by Retarded, Normal and Superior Children Equated for CA.* Athens, Georgia: University of Georgia.

Bricker, W. A. (1972) 'A systematic approach to language training.' *in* Schiefelbusch, R. L. (Ed.) *Language of the Mentally Retarded.* Baltimore: University Park.

Brimer, M. A., Dunn, L. H. (1962) *English Picture Vocabulary Test.* Bristol: Educational Evaluation Enterprises.

Carr, D. L., Brown, L. F., Rice, J. A. (1967) 'The PPVT in the assessment of language deficits.' *Amer. J. ment. Defic.,* **71,** 937.

Carrow, M. A. (1968) 'The development of auditory comprehension of language structure in children.' *J. speech Dis.,* **33,** 99.

Chomsky, N. (1965) *Aspects of the Theory of Syntax.* Cambridge, Mass.: M.I.T. Press.

Crabtree, M. (1958) *The Houston Test for Language Development.* Houston: Test Co.

Cunningham, C., Jeffree, D. (1971) Child Development Charts. Hester Adrian Research Centre, University of Manchester. (Unpublished.)

Dunn, L. (1959) *The Peabody Picture Vocabulary Test.* Minneapolis: American Guidance. Service.

Eisenson, J. (1966) 'Perceptual disturbances in children with central nervous system dysfunctions and implications for language development.' *Brit. J. Disord. Commun.,* **1,** 21.

Frostig, M., Lefever, D. W., Whittlesey, J. R. B. (1964) *Marianne Frostig Developmental Test of Visual Perception.* Palo Alto: Consulting Psychologists Press.

Frankenburg, W. K., Dobbs, J. B. (1967) *Denver Developmental Screening Scale.* Denver, Colorado: University of Colorado Medical Center.

Gunzburg, H. C. (1963) *Progress Assessment Charts.* London: National Association for Mental Health.

Hatch, E., French, J. L. (1971) 'The revised ITPA: its reliability and validity for use with EMRs.' *Journal of School Psychology,* **9,** 16.

Hobsbaum, A. (1970) Personal communication.

Kirk, S. A. (1968) 'The Illinois Test of Psycholinguistic Abilities: its origins, and implications.' *in* Hellmuth, V. (Ed.) *Learning Disorders,* Vol. 3. Seattle: Special Child Publications.

—— McCarthy, J. J., Kirk, W. (1968) *The Illinois Test of Psycholinguistic Abilities.* (Revised edn.) Urbana, Ill: University of Illinois, Institute for Research in Exceptional Children.

Lee, L. L. (1969) *The Northwestern Syntax Screening Test.* Evanston. Ill.: Northwestern University Press.

—— (1970) 'A screening test for syntax development.' *J. speech Dis.,* **35,** 103.

Lenneberg, E. H. (1967) *Biological Foundations of Language.* New York: John Wiley.

Lerea, L. (1958) 'Assessing language development.' *J. speech Res.,* **1,** 75.

McCarthy, D. (1954) 'Language development.' *in* Carmichael, L. (Ed.) *Manual of Child Psychology,* New York: John Wiley.

McCarthy, J. J., Kirk, S. A. (1961) *The Illinois Test of Psycholinguistic Abilities.* (Experimental edn.) Urbana, Ill.: University of Illinois, Institute for Research in Exceptional Children.

Marinosson, G. (1970*a*) 'A comparative study of normal, educationally subnormal and severely subnormal children on the revised Illinois Test of Psycholinguistic Abilities.' University of Manchester, M. A. Thesis.

—— (1970*b*) 'Language abilities of normal, ESN and SSN children: a comparative study.' *in* Mittler, P. (Ed.) *The Work of the Hester Adrian Research Centre: A Report for Teachers.* Monogr. Suppl. *Teaching & Training,* **8,** 17.

Mecham, M. J., Jex, J. L. (1962) *Picture Speech Discrimination Test.* Provo, Utah: Brigham Young University Press.

—— Jones, J. (1967) *Utah Test of Language Development.* Salt Lake City: Communication Research Associates.

Menyuk, P. (1969) *Sentences Children Use.* Cambridge, Mass.: M.I.T. Press.

Mittler, P. (1970*a*) 'Assessment of handicapped children: some common factors.' *in* Mittler, P. (Ed). *Psychological Assessment of Mental and Physical Handicaps.* London: Methuen.

—— (1970*b*) 'Language disorders.' *in* Mittler, P. (Ed.) *Psychological Assessment of Mental and Physical Handicaps.* London: Methuen.

118

—— (1970c) 'The use of morphological rules by four year old children.: an item analysis of the Auditory-Vocal Automatic subtest of the Illinois Test of Psycholinguistic Abilities.' *Brit. J. Disord. Common.*, **5**, 99.

—— Ward, J. (1970) 'The use of the Illinois Test of Psycholinguistic Abilities with English four-year-old children: a normative and factorial study.' *Brit. J. educ. Psychol.*, **40**, 43.

—— Wheldall, K. (1971) 'Language comprehension in the severely subnormal.' *Bulletin of the British Psychological Society*, **24**. (Abstract of paper delivered to the Annual Conference of the British Psychological Society, Exeter, April 1971.)

Osgood, C. E. (1957) 'A behavioristic analysis.' *in* Osgood, C. E. (Ed.) *Contemporary Approaches to Cognition*. Cambridge, Mass.: M.I.T. Press.

Paraskevopoulos, J. N., Kirk, S. A. (1969) *The Development and Psychometric Characteristics of the Revised Illinois Test of Psycholinguistic Abilities*. Urbana, Ill.: University of Illinois Press.

Phillips, C. J. (1968) 'The Illinois Test of Psycholinguistic Abilities: a report on its use with English children and a comment on the psychological sequeae of low birthweight.' *Brit. J. Disord. Commun*, **3**, 143.

Renfrew, C. E. (1971) *Renfrew Language Attainment Scales*. Churchill Hospital Oxford.

Reynell, J. K. (1969) *The Reynell Developmental Language Scales*. Slough, Bucks: N.F.E.R.

Rogers, M. G. H. (1971) *A Study of Language Development in Severe Subnormality*. Unpublished dissertation, Institute of Child Health, University of London.

Rosenberg, S. (1970) 'Problems of language development in the retarded: a discussion of Olson's review.' *in* Haywood, H. C. (Ed.) *Social-Cultural-Aspects of Mental Retardation*. New York: Appleton-Century-Crofts.

Shapiro, M. B. (1970) 'Intensive assessment of the single case: an inductive-deductive approach.' *in* Mittler, P. (Ed.) *Psychological Assessment of Mental and Physical Handicaps*. London: Methuen.

Shaw, D. J., Matthews, C. G., Kløve, H. (1966) 'The equivalence of WISC and PPVT IQs.' *Amer. J. ment. Defic.*, **70**, 601.

Sheridan, M. D. (1958) *Developmental Progress of Infants and Young Children*. London: H.M.S.O.

Smith, F. A., Miller, G. A. (1966) *The Genesis of Language: A Psycholinguistic Approach*. Cambridge, Mass.: M.I.T. Press.

Smith, P. A., Marx, R. W. (1971) 'The factor structure of the revised edition of the Illinois Test of Psycholinguistic Abilities.' *Psychology in the Schools*, **8**, 349.

Spradlin, J. E. (1968) 'Environmental factors and the language development of retarded children.' *in* Rosenberg, S., Koplin, J. H. (Eds.) *Developments in Applied Psycholinguistics Research*. New York: Macmillan.

Templin, M. C. (1957) *Certain Language Skills in Children*. Minneapolis: University of Minnesota Press.

Warburton, F. W., Fitzpatrick, T., Ward, J., Ritchie, M. (1970) 'Some problems in the construction of intelligence tests.' *in* Mittler, P. (Ed.) *Psychological Assessment of Mental and Physical Handicaps*. London: Methuen.

Ward, J. (1970) 'The factor structure of the Frostig Developmental Test of Visual Perception.' *Brit. J. educ. Psychol.*, **40**, 65.

Watts, A. F. (1944) *Language and Mental Development of Children*. London: Harrap.

Weener, P., Barrit, L. S., Semmel, M. I. (1967) 'A critical evaluation of the Illinois Test of Psycholinguistic Abilities.' *Except. Child.*, **33**, 373.

Wepman, J. (1958) *Auditory Discrimination Test*. Chicago: University of Chicago Press.

Wolski, W. (1962) *The Michigan Picture Language Inventory*. Ann Arbor, Mich.: University of Michigan.

119

CHAPTER 10

Cognitive Assessment in Young Children with Language Delay

M. BERGER and W. YULE

Psychological testing has a particularly important place in the assessment of the language retarded child. Language and cognition are closely interrelated (chapter 15) and a careful appraisal of cognitive abilities is necessary for an understanding of possible factors in the genesis and prognosis of language delay, of the nature of the language handicap, and of the child's educational needs. The purpose of this chapter is to provide the basis for a consideration of the rôle of cognitive assessment in the overall management of the language retarded child. In discussing this topic, we will be concerned with issues which specifically arise in children with this handicap. There are, however, other areas of knowledge essential to the effective use of psychological test findings with *any* children, *e.g.* what is meant by 'intelligence', how it is measured and what limitations attach to the use of scores such as intelligence quotients (IQs) and mental ages (MAs). For consideration of these and more general issues in cognitive testing see Anastasi (1963) and Butcher (1968).

The Need for Cognitive Assessment

Clinical observation and a careful history from the parents of the child can provide a useful guide to the child's general level of intellectual function (chapter 3). However, systematic and standardised psychological testing is necessary for any accurate estimate. This is particularly the case in the child presenting with language delay, when it is often difficult in clinical assessment to differentiate between *general* retardation and retardation in the development of *specific* skills. The purpose of psychometric testing can be summarised as follows:

1. In the differential diagnosis of speech delay one of the first questions is whether the delay is part of a general mental retardation, and if so to what extent, or is it more circumscribed in nature? Speech and language disorders are frequent in mentally retarded children (chapters 11 and 12), and before one can decide whether the child has a specific language disorder or a general developmental retardation, accurate estimates of both non-verbal intellectual skills and language performance must be available. Both require psychometric testing (see chapter 9 for language tests).

2. Treatment should be based on a reliable and objective description of the child's cognitive assets and deficits. Psychological testing can provide both a general measure of intellectual performance and measures of specific skills. The need to differentiate a child's abilities in the various aspects of language (*e.g.* understanding, production, imitation) has been argued in other chapters (3 and 6). The same need applies to non-verbal skills of perception, motor co-ordination, and perceptuo-motor function. Not only do test results indicate the general mental level to which educational programmes have to be geared, but they can also indicate those assets which may be developed and utilised to aid the child in overcoming his deficiencies (see below).

3. Given that a full and systematic description of intellectual skills has been obtained, this can be used as a baseline for comparing either spontaneous progress or progress resulting from treatment. In this connection, psychometric assessment, which can be standardised, has advantages over clinical judgement, which may vary between clinicians.

4. Within certain limits, test results can provide a basis for predictions about later language development, social progress, and educational achievement (Johnson 1963, Griffiths 1969, Lockyer and Rutter 1969, Rutter 1970a, Bartak and Rutter 1971) (see section below).

5. Knowledge of a child's overall level of intelligence is important in the interpretation of other test results. Scores on tests of specific skills, such as the Frostig test of per-ceptual-motor development (Frostig *et al.* 1964) or the Illinois Test of Psycholinguistic Abilities (McCarthy and Kirk 1961, Kirk *et al.* 1968), are much influenced by general intelligence (Olson 1968, Yule *et al.* 1969) and for their interpretation this must also be assessed.

6. Cognitive data also need to be collected with an eye to furthering our knowledge on children with language delay. Unless such children are routinely given a full cognitive assessment, we will never be in a position to know how far test results can be used to make judgements about the later development of language, educational progress, and the value of specific remedial programmes.

Choosing a Test of Intelligence

A very wide range of intelligence tests is available (see Anastasi 1963 and Buros 1965 for detailed descriptions and critiques). Here, only a few of those particularly useful for children with little or no speech will be described. Others are outlined in Berry (1969). The tests are divided according to the age for which they are most useful. Although the headings refer to chronological age (CA), with severely retarded children it may be better to choose tests according to expected mental age (MA).

Children under 2 Years

Infant tests often measure different aspects of development from those assessed by tests for older children. With the very young child, motor items predominate and these relate very poorly to later intellectual development. For this reason alone, it is difficult to make predictions from infant tests. However, social and adaptive functions have a somewhat better predictive power, and the best tests place greater emphasis on these items. Most tests derive from the Gesell scale (Gesell and Amatruda 1947, Gesell 1950) in which adaptive behaviour is assessed by items such as block building, cup and cube play, putting pellets in a bottle, 'posting' objects of different shapes into a box with special holes for each object, and putting pegs into a formboard. A detailed assessment is provided by the Griffiths scale (1954), but adequate screening assessments are obtainable from the simpler Denver scale (Frankenburg and Dodds 1968, Frankenburg *et al.* 1971) and the inventory developed by Knobloch and her colleagues (1966).

Evidence from longitudinal studies shows that it is not until after about two years of age that infant test scores relate significantly to later levels of intellectual

121

development. Whilst this general statement holds true, there is some evidence that very low scores on infant tests do predict later retardation in development (Hindley 1965, Thomas 1967, 1970, Werner *et al.* 1968, Rutter 1970*a*).

Children of 2 to 5 years

By the time the child reaches age 2 to 3 years, he can be assessed on a much wider range of cognitive functions. Probably the most generally useful test for language impaired children in this age group is the Merrill-Palmer Scale (Stutsman 1931). This covers the age-range 18 to 71 months and samples a variety of skills requiring different modes of response. Non-verbal items at the 24 to 29 month level, for example, include placing cubes in a box within a specified time, completing two peg-board items, and cutting with a pair of scissors. The test has the advantage of being interesting to most young children, of requiring the minimum of spoken instructions, and of having a wide range of items needing no speech from the child—all important characteristics of tests for the non-speaking child who may also have difficulties in understanding language (Lockyer and Rutter 1969). A further feature is that it has a procedure for dealing with items refused rather than failed—a not uncommon occurrence with young children.

The Arthur adaptation of the Leiter International Performance Scale (Leiter and Arthur 1955) requires no spoken instructions or responses and is particularly appropriate for deaf children or children with receptive language difficulties. The test has no time limit (an asset when testing young children not used to working against the clock) and can be modified to meet the needs of many types of handicapped children. It covers the age-range 2 to 18 years, but is of most value with young children. Children are required to match colours, shapes, blocks and pictures to examples presented individually by the tester. The chief disadvantage of the test is that it is somewhat cumbersome and time-consuming. While it is a 'performance' test, it would be wrong to regard it as an entirely 'non-language' test, particularly as scores on this test correlate highly (0.64 to 0.81, Anastasi 1963) with scores on the Binet. In practice, this seems to matter little with language retarded children as very high scores may be obtained by children with negligible language, spoken or otherwise.

The Columbia Mental Maturity Scale (1959) was designed for cerebral palsied children of 3 to 12 years of age and is often useful with language retarded children. It aims to assess form constancy and spatial relations in visual perception by the child picking which of a set of drawings 'does not belong with the others', the drawings being grouped on the basis of colour, size and form.

All of the tests mentioned suffer from defects in standardisation, so that scores at one age may not be exactly comparable with those of another. Both for this reason and because of the limited predictive power of IQ tests in children under 5 years of age, not too much attention should be paid to the precise MA or IQ obtained. On the other hand, the tests can provide a reasonably good estimate of whether the child is about average, below average, or markedly retarded.

The Binet test (in its various revisions) is also a heterogeneous item test which covers the age-range 2 to 16 years (Terman and Merrill 1961). Research has shown that this test is very dependent on verbal functions (Vernon 1961). This makes it particularly *un*suitable for use in testing children with language problems. Its most recent standardisation has also produced problems in interpreting scores derived from it, so that the test is of restricted value with the normal child (Berger 1970). It is unfortunate that in Britain, at least, it is still the test most often used among inadequately trained school medical officers who have the job of ascertaining children for special education. The great danger is that children with specific language handicaps may be misclassified because of inappropriate application and interpretation of this test—one of the dangers of mechanically interpreting IQ figures without regard to the content of the test employed.

School-age Children

For this age-group, the Wechsler Scales are the most generally useful. There are three Wechsler tests (1949, 1955, 1967) each following the same basic rationale and format but designed for different age groups. The Wechsler Pre-school and Primary Scale of Intelligence (WPPSI) covers the age range 4 to 6½ years; the Wechsler Intelligence Scale for Children (WISC) spans the years 5 to 16 (although it tends to be unreliable below the age of 6 because of the paucity of items); the Wechsler Adult Intelligence Scale (WAIS) covers the years from 16 onwards.

The Wechsler tests yield three IQs—Verbal Scale, Performance Scale and Full Scale IQs. Intelligent quotients on the WPPSI and WISC are computed on the basis of the child's score on 5 Verbal sub-tests, and 5 Performance sub-tests. The Full Scale IQ is derived from the score on all 10 sub-tests administered. Each sub-test consists of a set of items arranged in ascending order of difficulty. For example, on the Vocabulary sub-test of the Verbal Scale the child is required to give definitions ranging from words such as 'coat' and 'fork' to more abstract concepts such as 'litigation' and 'metamorphosis' (for obvious reasons, we cannot quote actual examples of test items). On the Block Design sub-test at the lower levels, the child has to construct copies of designs assembled by the examiner from four blocks, while the more difficult items require him to copy more complex two-dimensional pictures using nine blocks.

In developing his tests, Wechsler has introduced the somewhat arbitrary distinction between what he calls 'Verbal' and 'Performance' IQs: the major difference being that the Verbal Scale requires spoken answers to the questions, the Performance Scale does not. However, the high positive correlation between these scales contradicts the implied assumption that the two scales measure totally unrelated abilities. Thus, it is possible to obtain a rough estimate of general intelligence in handicapped children by giving the Verbal Scale to children with gross physical handicaps, and the Performance Scale to children with expressive handicaps. However, children with comprehension deficits may still be at some disadvantage on the Performance Scale because of the necessity to understand the spoken instructions.

As these tests usually take over an hour to administer, a number of shortened forms have been developed (Glasser and Zimmerman 1967). Obviously, IQs from these shortened tests will be less accurate than those obtained from the administration of the whole test.

A further useful test is Raven's Progressive Matrices (1956), which is appropriate for children of 6 years or older. There is also a version designed for younger children

(Raven 1960). The test consists of patterns and geometrical figures with one piece missing which the child has to chose from among a group of possible answers. It is interesting to most children, takes less than half an hour to administer, and provides a useful guide to intellectual level. However, it has only a modest correlation with scores on the WISC. It is designed to test reasoning skills not involving speech, but performance is also strongly dependent on visual perception, which may be deficient in some language retarded children.

The Vineland Social Maturity Scale

This is not a test in the formal sense (Doll 1947). It is described here because of its use in obtaining a rough estimate of a child's level of development in those cases where a combination of limited time and multiplicity of handicap preclude formal testing. The mother, or other caretaker who knows the child well, is taken through a formal interview to enquire about the child's accomplishments in various areas, such as dressing, feeding, and communication. For example, for a child who is 1 to 2 years old she will be asked whether the child marks with a pencil or crayon, eats with a spoon, unwraps sweets, or fetches familiar objects. It has been demonstrated that, at younger ages, scores on the Vineland Scale correlate moderately highly with IQ scores (Pringle 1966) and so yield a crude estimate of intellectual level.

Mecham (1958) has used a similar approach in deriving a scale for language development which is also administered by asking the mother a systematic series of questions on the child's use and understanding of speech, among other skills.

Testing of Specific Skills

If an accurate picture of a child's cognitive assets and deficits is to be obtained, it is necessary to use tests which tap specific functions and which do so in a way relatively independent of the child's general intellectual level. Unfortunately, such tests have proved extremely difficult to devise. Some progress has been made with tests of different language functions (chapter 9), but, even here, it has often been difficult to determine exactly which function is being assessed by each test. A beginning has also been made with visual perception through the Frostig tests (Frostig et al. 1964). However, these tests are complex, have a substantial correlation with measures of general intelligence (Yule et al. 1969), and it remains uncertain exactly what abilities are being measured.

Other tests have been devised to assess fine and gross motor co-ordination (Sloan 1955), motor impersistence (Garfield 1964), right-left differentiation (Williams and Jambor 1964), auditory discrimination (Wepman 1958), and audio-visual integration (Birch and Lefford 1963). These tests vary greatly in sophistication and standardisation, but they all represent attempts to introduce precision into the assessment of individual developmental characteristics. It has been argued elsewhere (Rutter et al. 1970) that the move away from global tests of 'intelligence' or 'brain damage' towards the development of specific diagnostic tests is most important and potentially of very considerable practical value. Already, psychologists can provide valuable information on a child's particular strengths and weaknesses in cognitive skills, but it has to be recognised that the tools currently at our disposal are deficient in many respects. Improvements will be necessary before this crucial aspect of cognitive assessment can take its proper place in diagnosis.

124

Diagnostic testing should also involve the application of research principles to the study of a single case, not only by the application of standard tests, but also by the design of experiments to investigate a specific problem in the individual (Shapiro 1951, 1961). Thus, experiments may be devised to determine whether a child's difficulties in learning to read are due to failure to learn, or failure to retain what he has learned (Shapiro 1957). This approach warrants further exploration.

Requirements of Tests for the Handicapped Child

Tests developed for use with non-handicapped children are likely to yield inappropriate conclusions when applied to handicapped children. It is therefore necessary in assessing such children to ensure that their particular disabilities do not place them at a disadvantage, and considerations over and above those which apply in testing the normal child must be borne in mind in selecting tests for use with language impaired children. It must also be appreciated that adapting procedures so that they accommodate the child's handicaps can place limitations on the validity of the measures.

Whilst no hard-and-fast rules can be put forward, clinical experience suggests that the following points should be given some weight in selecting assessment procedures. Motivation is important in all testing, and tests constructed for use with children generally incorporate items which will arouse and maintain their interest. This is especially necessary when testing handicapped children, who will often have experienced failure and may be unwilling to participate in, and persist with, items which they find difficult. It may be necessary to deviate somewhat from the prescribed testing procedures and to intersperse simpler items among those likely to tax the child. Beginning testing at a point very much below the level at which it is thought the child may be successful may encourage him to attempt more difficult items. Also, if the child appears to enjoy a particular task and is unwilling to attempt others, it is useful to allow him to work at what he likes on condition that he attempts other tasks later. If necessary, parents should be allowed to be present during the assessment. This is particularly useful in those circumstances where the parent can act as a translator of instructions and responses. Obviously, very young children are also more likely to be at ease if a parent is with them. It is, however, essential to ensure that parents do not directly or inadvertently help the child with the test items. Again, it must be remembered that the more the tester departs from standardised administration, the more he must qualify the results obtained.

Certain items on cognitive tests require the child to complete the task correctly within prescribed time limits. Some tests may also give bonus points for rapid solutions. Particular care needs to be exercised when these timed items are used in assessing handicapped children. Children with motor co-ordination problems, or children who are highly distractible, are most likely to be penalised if timed tests are used. Since many children with language problems can be multiply handicapped, this needs to be remembered.

Special considerations apply to the testing of children who lack speech, or whose understanding of speech is limited. It is essential to differentiate between items failed

125

because the child could not perform the task, and items 'failed' because the child did not know what task it was he was supposed to perform. When this is in doubt, instructions should be given in some form (such as mime or demonstration) which avoids the use of spoken language.

Reliable Assessment

A useful distinction can be made between a reliable assessment and a reliable test instrument. A reliable *instrument* is one which gives an accurate measure. By a reliable *assessment*, we mean that testing was undertaken under optimal circumstances. At the very least, this requires that the child co-operated fully in the testing, was not unduly anxious, and that the tester carried out testing in accordance with standardised instructions. A careful note should be made of any events which interfered with assessment: excessive distractibility, hyperactivity and poor persistence are among factors in the child's behaviour which can detract from the accuracy of the test results. If a systematic recording of the observations is made, then it becomes possible through discussion with parents and teachers, for example, to decide whether the behaviours shown are characteristic of the child or are situation-induced. Where test results are inconsistent with the reports of parents and teachers, and the tester is confident of the accuracy of his assessment, it becomes necessary to examine the observations of teachers and parents in detail, and it may also be necessary to re-administer the test after an interval of some weeks. This time lag is important in that it allows the child to 'settle' before being tested again.

Where there are possible inconsistencies between test findings and parental (or other) reports, two points need particular emphasis. (1) No psychological assessment is complete without a systematic account from the parents of what the child can do *outside* the test situations. (2) It is never acceptable to leave discrepancies between test findings and parental reports unexplained. The existence of a discrepancy is *always* an indication for a critical study of possible reasons for the discrepancy. The reasons may lie in the nature of the task (for example, the child may have more cues at home than in the controlled test situation), or in the interpretation of the child's behaviour, or in the cognitive abilities being assessed. If the parental report suggests marked skills or deficits on clinically important abilities which have not been assessed by the standardised tests, other tests should be used to sample the additional functions. Where the child seems able to perform a task at a higher level at home than he does in the clinic, and where no reasons in the nature of the task explain this discrepancy, the psychologist should attempt to repeat the observations in the home in order to determine the explanation for the discrepancy. Psychological assessment is complete only when this has been done.

Should it be the case that the child has reacted adversely to being tested and retesting is not possible, the results would need to be qualified accordingly. In any event, information about all attempts at testing, whether successful or not, should be noted in reports. It is also essential to include observations about the child's behaviour. If such information is incorporated in any report written on the child, it will enable the recipients of the report to gain an impression of the circumstances of testing and will be of help in their understanding of the results. It is to be noted that it takes some skill to be able to differentiate between observations and interpretations of behaviour. Unfortunately, this distinction is not always made, thus limiting the value of the information.

One facet of reliable assessment that is not often given sufficient consideration is the problem of deciding whether or not the child failed an item, as opposed to his being unwilling to do it. An aspect of this problem is the extent to which a child will persist on tasks irrespective of their difficulty. It is known that individuals differ on this temperamental attribute (Thomas *et al.* 1968) and it is likely that such a characteristic will interact with performance on tasks. If a child lacks persistence, then he may give up on tasks which are within his range of competence. Careful observation by the tester is necessary to differentiate between lack of persistence and lack of competence. Within the test situation, information about the degree of a child's persistence is best gained by close observation of his behaviour on all tasks. When considering the influence of poor persistence on test performance, it is useful to seek out other sources of information about the child's behaviour when confronted with difficult situations. Again, parents and teachers, suitably questioned, should be able to provide reliable information.

If it appears that the child is persistent, then it is probable that a failure is due to lack of competence. If the child lacks persistence, it is difficult to reach this conclusion, and this uncertainty should be commented upon in the report. Lack of competence is also more easily inferred when the child fails an item after having passed a sequence of similar items in a series that is graded in difficulty. If a pattern of random failures is observed in such a series, then it is possible that factors other than lack of competence are operating. Information of this type is very important for interpreting test results, especially in those circumstances where it is not possible to do a full assessment, as may occur when testing the language handicapped child.

Given that there are a variety of difficulties in differentiating 'true' failures from those which may arise as a consequence of the characteristics of the child and his reactions to being tested, it would appear to us that the most accurate assessments are obtained by concentrating on what the child can do and recognising that this may, under certain circumstances, underestimate his capabilities. This is particularly important when one is uncertain about the source of failure, a difficulty which often arises when testing handicapped children.

The 'Untestable' Child

Because psychological testing can be so very difficult in the young mute child, or in the child with a severe disorder of behaviour, clinicians have sometimes been led to disregard, or to deliberately avoid, obtaining psychological assessments. Psychologists, too, sometimes report that because of language difficulty, autistic withdrawal, or disruptive behaviour, the child is 'untestable'. This is simply a statement that the psychologist has failed in his endeavour and it says nothing about the child (except that he was difficult to test). In our experience, it is quite uncommon not to be able to provide some kind of systematic cognitive assessment of even the most difficult children, although of course it is not infrequent for this assessment to be incomplete in some respect. If testing is to be successful, it is necessary to use tests which interest the child and to establish a testing situation which is conducive to his best performance. A parental account may provide valuable leads to the best way of doing this, but with very young or very disturbed children, several sessions and several different tests may be needed.

When it proves impractical to assess the child in a test situation, it is still possible to obtain some estimate of his performance by means of the Vineland Social Maturity Scale (see above). This does not assess intelligence directly, but, in the absence of psychometric findings, it does provide a reasonable, though rough, guide to the child's general level of intellectual performance. An analysis of the social skills, where he is most advanced or most retarded, also provides a crude guide to the pattern of abilities. Finally, the psychologist should also make careful note of any particular skills which are reported outside those included in the social maturity scale. As far as possible, he should estimate the age level of these skills in terms of what is known about normal child development. It should *never* be necessary to come away without some assessment of the child's intellectual performance, and where estimates of abilities have to be based on reports rather than test findings, the psychologist should always specify precisely what reported behaviours have led him to make each part of his estimate.

The Problem of Score Interpretation

Perhaps the most important issue in the formal assessment of language and other handicapped children is the 'meaning', or validity, of the test results.

Test scores have meaning in the sense that they predict certain classes of behaviour in the non-handicapped population. High IQs generally imply that the child is capable of succeeding in the normal educational system, that the child can do cognitive tasks at levels above those of a major proportion of his age peers, and so on. Such predictions are based on the scores having been obtained through the administration of the full test in a standardised manner. One of the immediate practical implications of the research on the structure of abilities (Vernon 1961) is that any of a number of tests could be used to measure IQ. This would follow from the observation of positive correlation among cognitive tests when these have been given to the non-handicapped.

Unfortunately, we know very little about the structure of abilities in groups of handicapped individuals. However, we would argue that, rather than let this prevent us undertaking cognitive assessment of the handicapped, let us use whatever information we have at our disposal, but qualify our interpretations accordingly. The most useful assumption would be that, until proved otherwise, the meaning of test data is the same for handicapped and non-handicapped individuals.

But to what extent is it permissible to interpret scores from incomplete tests, as, for example, when a child completes only part of the Merrill-Palmer, or just 2 of the WISC sub-tests? When this happens, strict scoring and interpretation would result in an IQ which implied severe retardation. However, taking these scores on their own, it is psychometrically acceptable to regard these results as indices of the level at which the child can perform a class of cognitive tasks. In presenting an interpretation (*e.g.* that the child performs constructional tasks at a 5 year level), it is important to be constantly aware of the limitations which apply to such statements. These are, firstly, that the observations may be unreliable because they are based on a comparatively small number of items. Reliability would, however, be enhanced if other observations of the child were consistent with the obtained results. Secondly, interpretative statements should refer only to circumscribed areas of behaviour; namely, those sampled by the tests. Any attempt to generalise would need to be based on appropriate empirical evidence. Finally, test results should not be called 'IQs' unless it is made quite explicit that the 'IQ' is based on an incomplete or non-standard administration of the test. The reason for imposing this sanction is that 'IQ' has a particular meaning and special implications which may not hold if it is based on non-standard procedures, or if it is used to generalize about atypical individuals.

In the interpretation of psychological test scores, it is important to consider what it is that the test is measuring; put more formally, which abilities are being sampled by the particular tests being used? Answers to such questions are obtained through correlational analyses of batteries of tests. Cognitive tasks rarely, if ever, measure 'pure' or unitary functions: commonly, a number of abilities enter into task performance. To complete an item of the Block Design sub-test of the WISC requires, among other skills, the ability to discriminate colours, a degree of manual dexterity, pattern perception, and so on. These requirements can be inferred from an examination of the test items. From the positive correlation with the Vocabulary sub-test ($r - 0.54$ at age $10\frac{1}{2}$ years), it appears that verbal abilities may also enter into successful performance on the Block Design sub-test; or alternatively, that a common factor underlies success on both sub-tests. In the final analysis, the designation 'verbal' or 'non-verbal', or 'mixed' (the most likely designation), will depend on empirical studies demonstrating the presence or absence of correlation with other measures of verbal and non-verbal abilities.

Our knowledge of what functions are being tapped by cognitive tests derives primarily from studies involving non-handicapped individuals. We are as yet on uncertain ground when trying to elucidate which abilities are being sampled when these tests are applied to individuals with circumscribed or extensive handicaps. It is known that many autistic children can, for example, complete items on the Block Design sub-test (Lockyer and Rutter 1969, 1970). However, we do not know whether they can do this because they have intact verbal abilities, or because they have only those other abilities measured by this sub-test, or both. Until such time as the appropriate studies are undertaken, we will be unable to produce a solution to this problem. In the interim, it would be inappropriate to conclude that because autistic children can only be tested on performance tests they are deficient in all 'verbal' skills.

Stability of IQ

One of the criticisms levelled against cognitive test results is that these can change dramatically over time. How stable is the IQ? Bloom's (1965) survey of the literature showed that there is very high stability after about the age of 8, but less stability in early childhood. For example, at 4 to 5 years of age, the IQ correlates about 0.7 with IQ at age 17. As Jensen (1969) has stated, '....what these findings mean is that the IQ is not constant, but, like all other developmental characteristics, it is quite variable early in life and becomes increasingly stable throughout childhood'. The practical consequences of this can be more easily seen by considering mean changes in IQ during childhood and adolescence. On average, and disregarding direction of change, normal children change in IQ some 10 to 17 points (Bradway 1944, Sontag *et al.* 1958). This means of course that some children will change by more than this.

The implication is that the younger the child the less certain one can be in predicting later IQ scores. However, there is ample evidence that at the lower extreme of intelligence one can often make firmer predictions at earlier dates. In general, later subnormal functioning can be predicted from very low scores on infant tests. This has, however, to be qualified in light of the knowledge that low scores associated with extremes of deprivation (both psychological and material) may increase when such deprivation is alleviated (Skeels 1966).

It must be recognized, too, that predictions can be upset by major changes either in the child or in his environment as it impinges upon him. It is not unlikely that specific training can produce changes in test scores, although it is doubtful that such changes will be reflected in increased competence in more general areas of cognitive functioning. Unreliable assessments may also distort measurements sufficiently to lead to an impression that the test is producing misleading results. These and other factors need to be taken into consideration when the stability of the IQ is questioned.

Predictions from IQ Scores

The clear consequence of these findings is that it would be most unwise to place any child in some fixed category (such as 'ineducable') on the basis of an IQ test in early childhood. Nevertheless, a proper concern over the limitations of overall IQ scores (particularly in handicapped children with high scores on one sort of test and low scores on another) should not blind us to the very considerable predictions which can be based on cognitive testing.

For example, in autistic children an IQ score below 60 in early childhood has been found to be a good predictor of mental subnormality and poor social adjustment 12 to 20 years later (Rutter 1970*b*). Autistic children with an IQ below 60 were also much less likely to develop speech and were more likely than children of higher IQ to develop epileptic fits in adolescence. In this study, no autistic child with an IQ below 50 learned to read, and *within* the group of children with an IQ above that level there was a correlation of 0.52 between the initial IQ and the reading quotient (RQ) at follow-up in adolscence (Lockyer and Rutter 1969). Similar findings have emerged from a quite separate study of another group of autistic children who had much more intensive specialised schooling (Bartak and Rutter 1971). An IQ below 50 does *not* mean that progress will not occur, but it does imply that only very limited scholastic attainments are likely.

Less is known about predictions from early IQ scores in other groups of children with language delay, but what findings are available suggest that the results are similar. In the follow-up of the 'control' group of non-psychotic children attending the Maudsley Hospital (Rutter and Lockyer 1967), the correlation between initial IQ and later IQ was just as high (0.60) as in the previously mentioned autistic children studied by Lockyer and Rutter (1969). Most of this 'control' group had shown a considerable delay in language development. In her follow-up study of speech-disordered children who had attended John Horniman School, Miss Griffiths (1969) similarly found that reading backwardness was much greater in those children who had a low IQ as well as a delay in speech and language. The association between IQ and progress in language was less marked. Moreover, it should be noted that the association was due to the effect of very low IQ and it is doubtful whether IQ can be used to predict language development when IQ scores are within the normal range.

Rather more important than indicating which children may have a poor outlook, IQ scores can also indicate which children are likely to do well. As is widely recognised, the prognosis for autistic children is generally poor, with only a small minority achieving a good social adjustment. What is less widely appreciated is that the prognosis for the autistic child of normal intelligence is much better. In the Maudsley study, 42 per cent of those with an IQ of 70 or more were working or were in full time education when followed up (Rutter 1970*b*). Even better results have been found with receptive aphasic children (Moore House School 1970). These youngsters (all of whom had normal or above normal intelligence) continued to have very severe language impairment and some could not speak at all, but, in spite of this, the great majority held down a steady job (in some cases of a skilled nature) and showed a satisfactory level of social adjustment. In deaf children, too, good intelligence has been shown to be an important factor in a successful transfer from a special school for deaf children to an ordinary school (Johnson 1963).

Differences Between Test Scores

Special problems of interpretation arise in considering the significance of observed differences between two test scores obtained concurrently, whether these be components of a test such as the WISC or ITPA, or whether they are derived from two or more independent tests (*e.g.* comparing results on the EPVT with those on the WISC). With regard to the most commonly used within-test 'profile' or pattern analysis, one of the major problems encountered is that the number of items constituting each sub-test (or profile element) is small. It is known that tests with small numbers of items are less reliable than tests consisting of large numbers of items. The reliability of each sub-test is thus necessarily much lower than the reliability of the complete test. One must therefore be cautious in interpreting scores on short sub-tests, and it follows from this that the interpretation of differences between scores on sub-tests is a much more hazardous exercise.

A second problem concerns the frequency of occurrence of sub-test differences of a given magnitude in the general population. For example, the differences between IQs on the WISC Verbal and Performance Scales are frequently interpreted without regard to normative data. A difference of 9 IQ points in either direction occurs in over 50 per cent of the normal population at the age of $7\frac{1}{2}$. Differences as large as 22 points at the same age still occur in over 10 per cent of the population (Field 1960). For a difference to be statistically abnormal (infrequent), it has to be very large indeed, and the mere fact that a difference is *statistically* abnormal does not, in the absence of empirical evidence, imply any form of cognitive abnormality. Given that it is difficult to interpret huge differences between Verbal and Performances IQ scores, both of which are fairly reliable, it will be appreciated how much more difficult it is to interpret

131

differences between individual, short sub-tests. Although the WISC has been in existence since 1949, adequate data are still not available for making profile analysis a viable exercise. The position with relative newcomers to the psychologist's armamentarium, such as the Frostig Test or the ITPA, is infinitely worse. For these tests, there is no information on how large a difference between sub-tests there has to be for it to be of any clinical importance. Because scores based on a small number of items tend to be unstable, a fair amount of unreliability must be expected on profile or pattern analysis. Unless inter-test differences are quite large, one profile may be found today and another one tomorrow. Without information on the temporal stability of a difference, the clinical significance of the findings may be highly questionable.

There is, nevertheless, a very great need for this information. However limited the value of profile analysis today, it should be clear that the *potential* value of this type of diagnostic testing is very great. What is still required is the information on which to base this approach.

Prescriptive Teaching

Just as medical treatment should be based on an accurate diagnosis, so educational treatment (in this sense education would include speech therapy or psychological procedures) should be firmly based on a careful assessment of the child's assets and deficits. Various special remedial programmes based on ITPA or Frostig test profiles have been developed. Some of these programmes may be useful in themselves, but their rationale in profile analysis is weak, and many of the attempts to base educational programmes on patterns of psychological handicap have been quite naive (Mann 1970). Furthermore, although such programmes may lead to an increase in specific test scores (Rosen 1966), the hoped-for educational benefit frequently has not occurred (Allen *et al.* 1966, Bateman 1969).

Part of the reason for this rather disappointing state of affairs is the unsatisfactory state of profile analysis. If the pattern of scores was unstable, the programme may well have been based on a fiction. However, the basic difficulty may be more fundamental. If a child has good perceptual skills, but poor language skills, should teaching concentrate on the things he is best at or on those at which he is weakest? It is not immediately apparent which approach is superior and empirical data are lacking. The usual tendency is to concentrate on training the child on the most deficient skills, but this may be wrong. Thus, the old approach of insisting on purely spoken language in deaf children now seems to be mistaken. Language probably develops better if communication utilises at first those skills (namely gesture and mime) in which the child is most competent.

There can be no doubt that prescriptive teaching is here to stay, and rightly so. For too long it has been assumed that there is one approach which is appropriate for *all* children. Undoubtedly, it is a major step forward to try to tailor therapy to the assets and deficits of the individual child. Before we can do this with confidence, not only must better diagnostic testing occur, but also the link between diagnosis and treatment must be subjected to a fuller and more critical evaluation.

Conclusions

We have tried in this chapter to indicate that information about a child's level of cognitive development is important for both prognosis and treatment. In the case of language retarded children, particular difficulties are presented both in selecting and administering appropriate intelligence tests. We have tried to show the flexibility needed in testing such children, and to warn of the limitations that such departures from normal testing practices necessarily entail. Even when appropriate tests are selected, it is essential to ensure that a reliable assessment is obtained. We have also argued that, in our present state of knowledge, test results alone cannot prescribe specific educational treatment. Finally, we have noted that the interpretation of differences between scores on different tests remains problematical.

Cognitive testing is a complex matter. This does not mean that it is not worthwhile. On the contrary, in the hands of a skilled and knowledgeable psychologist, cognitive testing of language retarded children can be invaluable—invaluable, that is, both for the clinical management of the individual child and for increasing our understanding of disorders associated with language retardation.

Acknowledgements

We are grateful to Dr. Michael Rutter for helpful suggestions in the writing of this chapter.

REFERENCES

Allen, R. M., Dickman, I., Haupt, T. D. (1966) 'A pilot study of the immediate effectiveness of the Frostig-Horne training program with educable retardates.' *Except. Child.*, **33**, 41.

Anastasi, A. (1963) *Psychological Testing*. New York: Macmillan.

Bartak, L., Rutter, M. (1971) 'Educational treatment of autism.' *in* Rutter, M. (Ed.) *Infantile Autism, Concepts, Characteristics and Treatment*. London: Churchill Livingstone. p. 258.

Bateman, B. (1969) 'Reading: a controversial view. Research and rationale.' *in* Tarnapol, L. (Ed.) *Learning Disabilities. Introduction to Educational and Medical Management*. Springfield, Ill.: C. C. Thomas.

Berger, M. (1970) 'The third revision of the Stanford-Binet (Form L-M): some methodological limitations and their practical implications.' *Bull. Brit. Psychol. Soc.*, **23**, 17.

Berry, M. F. (1969) *Language Disorders of Children*. New York: Appleton-Century-Crofts.

Birch, H. G., Lefford, A. (1963) 'Insensory development in children.' *Mongr. Soc. Res. Child Develop.*, **28**, (5).

Bloom, B. S. (1965) *Stability and Change in Human Characteristics*. New York: Wiley.

Bradway, K. P. (1944) 'IQ constancy in the revised Stanford-Binet from the pre-school to the junior high school level.' *J. genet. Psychol.*, **65**, 197.

Buros, O. K. (Ed.) (1965) *The Sixth Mental Measurements Yearbook*. Highland Park, N. J.: Gryphon Press.

Butcher, H. J. (1968) *Human Intelligence: Its Nature and Assessment*. London: Methuen.

Columbia Mental Maturity Scale (1959) New York: Harcourt, Brace & World.

Doll, E. A. (1947) *The Vineland Social Maturity Scale. Manual of Directions*. Minneapolis: Educational Tests Bureau.

Field, J. G. (1960) 'Two types of tables for use with Wechsler's intelligence scales.' *J. clin. Psychol.*, **16**, 3.

Frankenburg, W. K., Dodds, J. B. (1968) *Denver Developmental Screening Test Manual*. Denver: University of Colorado Press.

—— Camp, B. W., van Natta, P. A. (1971) 'Validity of the Denver Developmental Screening Test.' *Child Develop.*, **42**, 475.

Frostig, M., Lefever, D. W., Whittlesey, J. R. B. (1964) *The Marianne Frostig Developmental Test of Visual Perception*. 3rd edn. Palo Alto, Calif.: Consulting Psychologists Press.

Garfield, J. G. (1964) 'Motor impersistence in normal and brain-damaged children.' *Neurology (Minncap.)*, **14**, 623.

Gesell, A. (1950) *The First Five Years of Life*. London: Methuen.

—— Amatruda, C. S. (1947) *Developmental Diagnosis: Normal and Abnormal Child Development.* New York: Hoeber.

Glasser, A. J., Zimmerman, I. L. (1967) *Clinical Interpretation of the Wechsler Intelligence Scale for Children.* New York: Grune & Stratton.

Griffiths, C. P. S. (1969) 'A follow-up study of children with disorders of speech.' *Brit. J. Disord. Commun.,* **4,** 46.

Griffiths, R. (1954) *The Abilities of Babies.* London: University of London Press.

Hindley, C. B. (1965) 'Stability and change in abilities up to five years: group trends.' *J. Child Psychol. Psychiat.,* **6,** 85.

Jensen, A. R. (1969) 'How much can we boost I.Q. and scholastic achievement?' *Harvard educ. Rev.,* **39,** 1.

Johnson, E. M. (1963) *A Report on a Survey of Deaf Children who have been Transferred from Special Schools or Units to Ordinary Schools.* London: H.M.S.O.

Kirk, S. A., McCarthy, J. J., Kirk, W. (1968) *The Illinois Test of Psycholoinguistic Abilities.* (Revised edn.) Urbana, Ill.: University of Illinois, Institute for Research in Exceptional Children.

Knobloch, H., Pasamanick, B., Sherard, E. S. (1966) 'A developmental screening inventory for infants.' *Pediatrics,* **38,** (Suppl.), 1095.

Leiter, R. G., Arthur, G. (1955) *Leiter International Performance Scale.* New York: C.H. Stoelting.

Lockyer, L., Rutter, M. (1969) 'A five to fifteen year follow-up study of infantile psychosis. III. Psychological aspects.' *Brit. J. Psychiat.,* **115,** 865.

—— —— (1970) 'A five to fifteen year follow-up study of infantile psychosis. IV. Patterns of cognitive ability.' *Brit. J. soc. clin. Psychol.,* **9,** 152.

MacAndrew, C., Edgerton, R. (1965) 'IQ and the social competence of the profoundly retarded.' *Amer. J. ment. Defic.,* **69,** 385.

Mann, L. (1970) 'Perceptual training: mis-directions and re-directions.' *Amer. J. Orthopsychiat.,* **40,** 30.

Mecham, M. (1958) *Verbal Language Development Scale.* Minneapolis: Educational Test Bureau.

McCarthy, J. J., Kirk, S. A. (1961) *Illinois Test of Psycholinguistic Abilities: Experimental Edition.* Urbana, Ill.: University of Illinois Press.

Moor House School (1970) *A Report on a Follow-up of Ten Receptive Aphasic Ex-pupils of Moor House School.* Private Publication.

Olson, A. V. (1968) 'Factor analytic studies of the Frostig Developmental Test of Visual Perception. *J. spec. Educ.,* **2,** 429.

Pringle, M. L. K. (1966) *Social Learning and its Measurement.* London: Longman Green.

Raven, J. C. (1956) *Progressive Matrices.* London: H. K. Lewis.

—— (1960) *Guide to Using the Coloured Progressive Matrices.* London: H. K. Lewis.

Rosen, C. L. (1966) 'An experimental study of visual perceptual training and reading achievement in first grade.' *Percept. mot. Skills,* **22,** 979.

Rutter, M. (1970*a*) 'Psychological development—predictions from infancy.' *J. Child Psychol. Psychiat.,* **11,** 49.

—— (1970*b*) 'Autistic children: infancy to adulthood.' *Semin. Psychiat.,* **2,** 435.

—— Lockyer, L. (1967) 'A five to fifteen year follow-up study of infantile psychosis. I. Description of sample.' *Brit. J. Psychiat.,* **113,** 1169.

—— Graham, P., Yule, W. (1970) *A Neuropsychiatric Study in Childhood.* Clinics in Developmental Medicine, No. 35/36. London: S.I.M.P.

Shapiro, M. B. (1951) 'An experimental approach to diagnostic psychological testing.' *J. ment. Sci.,* **97,** 748.

—— (1957) 'Experimental method in the psychological description of the individual psychiatric patient.' *Int. J. soc. Psychiat.,* **3,** 89.

—— (1961) 'The single case in fundamental clinical psychological research.' *Brit. J. med. Psychol.,* **34,** 255.

Skeels, H. M. (1966) 'Adult status of children with contrasting early life experiences.' *Monogr. Soc. Res. Child Develop.,* **31,** (3).

Sloan, W. (1955) 'The Lincoln-Oseretsky motor development scale.' *Genet. Psychol. Monogr.,* **51,** 183.

Sontag, L. W., Baker, C. T., Nelson, V. L. (1958) 'Mental growth and personality development; longitudinal study.' *Monogr. Soc. Res. Child Develop.,* **28,** (2).

Stutsman, R. (1931) *Merrill-Palmer Scale of Mental Tests.* New York: Harcourt, Brace and World.

Terman, L. M., Merrill, M. A. (1961) *Stanford-Binet Intelligence Scale: Manual for the Third Revision, Form L-M.* London: Harrap.

Thomas, A., Chess, S., Birch, H. G. (1968) *Temperament and Behaviour Disorders in Children.* New York: University of New York Press.

Thomas, H. (1967) 'Some problems of studies concerned with evaluating the predictive validity of infant tests.' *J. Child Psychol. Psychiat.,* **8,** 197.

—— (1970) 'Psychological assessment instruments for use with human infants.' *Merrill-Palmer Quart.,* **16,** 179.

Vernon, P. E. (1961) *The Structure of Human Abilities.* 2nd edn. London: Methuen.

134

Wechsler, D. (1949) *Wechsler Intelligence Scale for Children: Manual*. New York: Psychological Corporation.
—— (1955) *Wechsler Adult Intelligence Scale*. New York: Psychological Corporation.
—— (1958) *The Measurement and Appraisal of Adult Intelligence*. 4th edn. London: Balliere, Tindall & Cox.
—— (1967) *The Wechsler Pre-School and Primary Scale of Intelligence*. New York: Psychological Corporation.
Wepman, J. M. (1958) *Auditory Discrimination Test*. Chicago: Language Research Associates.
Werner, E. E., Honzik, M. P., Smith, R. S. (1968) 'Prediction of intelligence and achievement at ten years from twenty months pediatric and psychologic examinations.' *Child Develop.*, **39**, 1063.
Williams, M., Jambor, K. (1964) 'Disorders of topographical and right-left orientation compared with its acquisition in children.' *Neuropsychologia*, **2,** 55.
Yule, W., Berger, M., Butler, S., Newham, V., Tizard, J. (1969) 'The WPPSI: an empirical evaluation with a British sample.' *Brit. J. educ. Psychol.*, **39, 1**.

CHAPTER 11

Language Development and Mental Handicaps

PETER MITTLER

The ability to use language is obviously closely bound up with the development of intelligence, but the relationship between them is far from simple. That a child is mentally subnormal should not be regarded as a necessary or sufficient explanation for his inability to talk, nor should failure of language development be regarded as a sign of subnormal intelligence. Language is composed of a large number of skills and abilities, and some of these may be more directly affected by mental subnormality than others. In this chapter, some of the main problems that arise in considering the complex relationship between communication skills and intellectual functioning will be discussed, as will the question of whether the language difficulties shown by severely subnormal children can be regarded as a developmental disorder or as specific deficits. Finally, biological and social aspects of language development in the severely subnormal will be considered, with special reference to their complex inter-connection. The identification and assessment of specific language skills is more fully described in chapter 9.

Language and Intellectual Development

Many pre-school children are now being referred to paediatricians and other specialists because they are 'not yet talking', or because they have 'no intelligible speech'. In assessing such a child it is as essential to make a thorough study of all his language abilities as it is to try and consider possible causes of his failure to speak. For example, receptive language may be less impaired than productive skills, though it is no easy matter to assess how much language is understood by the child. On the other hand, the child may talk a good deal but be unable to use language for problem solving purposes, and may understand less of what is said to him than might at first appear.

Psychologists, speech therapists and educationalists in recent years have been developing techniques of investigating these problems, since there is no doubt that a detailed study of language behaviour is an essential aspect of the diagnostic process, whether the child is primarily subnormal, autistic, deaf, or suffering from a developmental language disorder. But current clinical practice is often limited to pin-pointing possible aetiologies. Psychologists, for example, are frequently asked to see children with delayed language development in order to 'exclude subnormality'; other specialists may also be seeing the child to exclude hearing loss, autism and other conditions. These investigations are usually necessary and worthwhile, but it is important to examine the assumptions behind them.

In the case of subnormality, we know too little about the relationship between general intelligence on the one hand and language development on the other to be in a position to 'explain' a child's failure to acquire language by reference to his mental subnormality alone. We have only to visit a subnormality hospital to observe many individuals whose level of language development is far below what might reasonably be expected from a knowledge of their intellectual level, as assessed by a standard intelligence test. It is not at all uncommon to encounter patients with a mental age of 5 or more, whose language abilities barely reach a 2 year level. The normal 2-year-old child has a vocabulary of one to two hundred words, and is rapidly mastering the more complex rules of grammar. By the age of 3-4 years, this process is thought to be virtually complete.

Few severely subnormal children can be expected to reach the level of linguistic competence acquired by the average 5-year-old. Unfortunately, doctors and others often assume that children are 'not suitable' for speech therapy until they are about 5 years old. In other cases, young children are not referred for speech therapy because it is assumed, rightly or wrongly, that the child's failure to speak is due to mental subnormality. Speech therapists would no doubt wish to take issue with the rather old-fashioned view of their work reflected in such an attitude; our aim here is to discuss the problem in terms of the complex relationship between the development of language and intelligence.

We do not precisely know the level of language development that can be expected at any particular stage of intellectual development. Clearly, there is cause for concern about a child whose mental and social development corresponds to a 4 or 5 year level but whose language development is well below a 2 year level. But what about a child with a mental age of 5 and a 'language age' of 4 years? Discrepancies as small as this may be of little real significance, and may be no more than measurement artefacts. Moreover, we have no basis for assuming that there should be a one-to-one relationship between intellectual development on the one hand and language development on the other. Even if the test results were reliable and accurate, we could not assume that a child with a mental age of 5 and a language age of only 4 was necessarily 'underfunctioning'. Similar problems occur at a later stage in considering the equally complex relationship between mental age and reading age (Burt 1967, cf. Graham 1967).

It is also difficult to separate verbal and non-verbal items in the intelligence tests with which the language tests are to be compared. The Binet test, for example, includes varying proportions of verbal and non-verbal items at different ages, thus causing contamination of criteria if a 'mental age' (MA) derived from a Binet is to be compared with a 'language age' derived from a test such as the Illinois Test of Psycholinguistic Abilities (ITPA) or the Reynell Scales.

Different problems are introduced by the use of non-verbal items, such as peg boards or form boards from the Merrill-Palmer or similar performance tests. In general, the correlation between verbal and non-verbal tests is rarely above 0.5, though correlations as high as 0.7 have been reported. Non-verbal tests, particularly those given to pre-school children, are often of doubtful reliability and validity, though they do have the advantage of being interesting to the child, and conveniently simple to administer (Mittler 1964). Unfortunately, they do not predict how the child will develop verbally or educationally, even though it is sometimes useful to be able to demonstrate that a child without language abilities can nevertheless function at a higher level on non-verbal tests. Evidence of this kind has often been used against decisions to declare children as 'unsuitable for education in school' on the basis of verbal tests alone. It is quite possible that performance on non-verbal tests is a better predictor of later development in children with language disorders than in normal children. This was shown to be the case in Rutter's (1970) follow-up studies of psychotic children for whom performance IQ was 'a remarkably good predictor of later intellectual and social performance'. Rutter argues on the basis of his follow-up studies that a low performance score 'strongly suggests that a child is unlikely to develop a useful level of language competence, that his social adjustment as an adult will be poor and that his IQ will remain at a low level as he grows older'. The implication is that performance tests are critical in cases where a child cannot speak. If the child scores poorly or not at all on performance tests, the prognosis for later intellectual development is poor; if he produces a good score, the prognosis may be more favourable. However, Rutter's studies refer only to psychotic children, and need to be validated on other language disordered populations before these conclusions can form the basis of generalisations relevant to other groups.

Discrepancies between verbal and non-verbal development are commonly found in the mentally subnormal. Children with Down's syndrome, for example, have been frequently shown to be more retarded in language skills than in perceptual or motor development (Lyle 1960, Carr 1970) though reasons for this are unclear, and there is no firm evidence to support the view that the language deficit might be directly related to the genetic abnormality. We do know, however, that children with Down's syndrome seem to be particularly susceptible to the adverse effects of institutionalisation on language development, as shown in Lyle's (1960) comparisons between children with Down's syndrome and those without brought up at home and in hospitals. But he also showed that much depended on the level of language development attained by the child prior to hospitalisation. Children who had acquired some language skills adjusted better to hospital than those who had failed to do so. In a recent longitudinal study of children with Down's syndrome living at home, Carr (1970) showed that 'motor' development was consistently ahead of 'mental' development (Bayley Scales).

Developmental Delays or Specific Deficits?
One of the unresolved questions in the field of mental handicap is concerned with the existence of specific cognitive deficits. A controversy has arisen between exponents of 'developmental' and 'defect' positions. On a developmental view the mentally handicapped are assumed to be going through the same stages of mental development as normal children, but at a slower rate and with a reduced likelihood of reaching the stages commonly reached by normal children around the age of 8 years or more. A defect theory on the other hand emphasises the probability of specific deficits being found in severely handicapped populations, because of the existence of genetic and neurological abnormalities. A defect position is supported if it can be shown that subnormals are inferior on a learning task to normal children matched for MA and, therefore, presumed to be at a comparable level of mental development. If subnormals perform at the same level as matched normals, this is taken as evidence in favour of a developmental theory.

138

Comparisons in terms of MA are artificial, partly because there are many different ways of reaching the same MA score, and because it may be unjustified to assume that two children or two groups are developmentally matched merely because they show identical MA scores. Moreover, the clinical and behavioural heterogeneity even within a small group of mentally handicapped children is so great that perfect matching on more than a small number of variables is impossible. These criticisms are more fully developed elsewhere (Baumeister 1967, Mittler 1972), but they are mentioned here in order to emphasise the artificiality of the 'developmental' versus 'defect' controversy. Nevertheless, a number of preliminary studies have provided evidence which is relevant, if not conclusive. Lenneberg *et al.* (1964) examined the language development of 61 children with Down's syndrome living at home, between 3 and 22 years of age, and with IQs ranging between the 20s and 70s. They reported a strong relationship between language development and motor development—especially age of walking, dressing and feeding independently. In general, language development was more strongly related to chronological age (CA) than to IQ. Children with Down's syndrome seemed to go through the same initial stages of language development as normal children in respect of babbling, and early one word utterances, although articulation defects were particularly marked. However, the language development of these children stopped far short of that reached by normal children. In other words, the rate of progress was slowed down at later ages, so that the children with Down's syndrome seemed to lag further behind the older they became. Although Lenneberg concluded that these findings were consistent with a 'maturational' or 'developmental' view of language development, it still remains true that the language development of mentally handicapped children is not merely slowed down but permanently handicapped, since most of them fail to reach levels of linguistic proficiency that would be characteristic of the average 5-year-old (*e.g.* Marshall 1967).

Many different skills and abilities must be involved in language development and some of these are the very abilities that have been shown to be severely impaired in the mentally subnormal. Experimental studies have consistently indicated that they have particular difficulties in dealing with incoming sensory information, and that many of their learning difficulties can be regarded as stemming from a disorder of attention. Information processing of auditory material is particularly difficult but is also seen in dealing with visual material (O'Connor and Hermelin 1963, Denny 1964). It is, therefore, important to try to differentiate between a large number of deficits, all of which could result in apparent language impairment, but some of which might be due to basic perceptual and attention disorders. It is not easy to make such a differentiation with the crude assessment techniques currently available, but an experimental analysis can often be suggestive. Needless to say, a programme of language therapy often needs to begin by teaching the child to attend, listen, discriminate and respond selectively to auditory and other material (Bricker and Bricker 1970).

The fact that mentally subnormal children appear to pass through the same sequential stages of development as normal children would be consistent with a developmental disorder, whereas their failure to progress beyond a low level of development represents a severe deficit. Thus, what begins as a developmental disorder may end as a defect when the individual reaches adulthood. It is also clear, however,

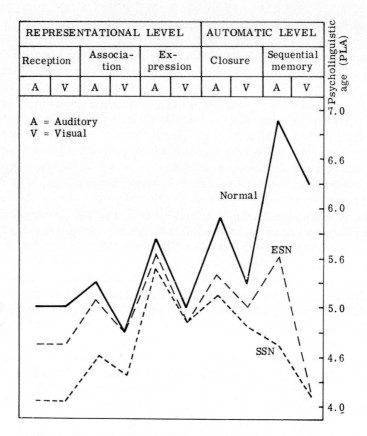

REPRESENTATIONAL LEVEL						AUTOMATIC LEVEL				
Reception		Associa-tion		Ex-pression		Closure		Sequential memory		
A	V	A	V	A	V	A	V	A	V	

A = Auditory
V = Visual

Normal

ESN

SSN

Psycholinguistic age (PLA)

7.0
6.6
6.0
5.6
5.0
4.6
4.0

Fig. Profiles representing performance of severely subnormal (SSN), educationally subnormal (ESN) and normal children, on 10 ITPA subtests as measured by Psycholinguistic Age (Marinosson 1970a).

that certain aspects of language functioning are so severely impaired from early childhood that it is more appropriate to consider them in terms of deficits from the beginning. The nature of these deficits will become more apparent once a larger number of specific linguistic abilities are identified, but several studies suggest that severely subnormal children have particular deficits in dealing with incoming auditory signals, and in particular in recalling sequences of auditory material such as digits or single words. The existence of both developmental disorders and deficits can be seen in the Fig. taken from a recent study by Marinosson (1970a and b) in which the revised edition of the Illinois Test of Psycholinguistic Abilities was administered to 30 normal, 30 ESN and 30 SSN children matched for overall verbal ability on the English Picture Vocabulary Scale (Brimer and Dunn 1962).

It is apparent from the Fig. showing psycholinguistic ages that even though the groups were matched on a crude measure of verbal ability, the normal controls were consistently superior, the ESN children intermediate and the SSNs lowest. The profiles are on the whole parallel and similar, suggesting that the pattern of linguistic

140

organisation is similar for the three groups, even though the SSN children are consistently at lower levels of development. On the other hand, the SSN children are significantly worse on the two sequential memory tests (auditory and visual), again suggesting the existence of specific deficits in this respect.

Another example of a possible specific deficit arises from work on the verbal regulation of behaviour. The nature of the relationship between language and thinking has pre-occupied philosophers and psychologists for centuries, but has not been the subject of a great deal of applied research in the field of subnormality. Perhaps the most ambitious attempt to explore this relationship is found in the work of Luria (1961) and other Soviet psychologists, who have developed Pavlov's later distinction between first and second signalling systems. Luria has described four stages in which behaviour comes under increasing control of the second signalling system. His experimental situation required the child to press (or not to press) a button on the appearance of a particular signal, usually a light or buzzer, though this basic paradigm has been extensively varied.

In stage 1, any utterance by the experimenter (E) causes the subject (S) to press, regardless of whether E says 'Press' or 'Don't press'. This is essentially the *orienting* phase, the words primarily serving to attract the child's attention. In stage 2, the child can inhibit pressing in response to E's 'Don't press'. This is described by Luria as the *releasing* or *impulsive* function of language which seems to cue the child to do what he was already going to do. In stage 3, the child tells himself aloud what to do, and can be heard quietly rehearsing 'Press', 'Don't press', or 'Yes', 'No'. At this stage, language has acquired a *selective* function. Stage 4 consists primarily of covert self-instruction (*preselection*) in which the child can respond appropriately to an instruction in the form 'Press if the red light comes on, but don't press if the green light comes on'. This stage is not normally reached until around 5 years. Even at this stage, the child may repeat the instructions to himself more or less verbatim, but later comes to condense them to telegraphic form. Luria (1963) particularly stresses the rôle of language in *inhibiting* behaviour, and argues that subnormals have a particular deficit in this respect. A small number of normative and experimental studies have been reported in recent years which suggest that Luria's model is potentially of therapeutic as well as theoretical significance (Burland 1969, Schubert 1969), though a recent study by Miller *et al.* (1970) failed to confirm the increasing use of verbal mediation with age.

O'Connor and Hermelin (1963) stress the need for the child to verbalise while carrying out a learning task, and Chalfant (1968) has published a preliminary report of a teaching programme along these lines. Work now in progress in Manchester suggests that the provision of verbal category cues facilitates conceptual organisation: a child is asked to remember a series of items (including, for example, a knife and a spoon) and is given either a verbal cue (for eating) or a manual cue (an eating gesture). Recall and organisation are significantly improved under these conditions (Herriot and Green 1971).

Some groups of children also seem to have particular difficulty in structuring incoming auditory material. Autistic children, for example, are in some respects at least quite different from SSN children. Although they show exceptionally good immediate rote memory, and do not show the characteristic deficits of sequencing found in the SSN, they seem to be extraordinarily unselective in what they remember, and perform equally well if they are asked to recall unstructured nonsense strings as they do when presented with structured and meaningful sentences (Hermelin and O'Connor 1970). They suggest specific deficiencies in coding and categorising processes which are relatively more marked in autistic than in matched subnormal or normal controls.

Biological and Environmental Aspects

Although we cannot in the present state of knowledge be as precise as we should like in differentiating between language and intelligence, or between deficits and developmental disorders, there is wide agreement that the mentally subnormal have particularly marked language difficulties, and that these tend to be more severe than might be expected from a knowledge of their skills and developmental maturity in other areas of behaviour, including non-verbal, motor and social spheres.

Reasons for such markedly skewed language development are highly complicated, and difficult to differentiate. In some cases, biological variables are implicated; there may be severe generalised or localised damage to the brain, or there may be peripheral anatomical defects, as in Down's Syndrome, where it is common to find structural abnormalities of the tongue, lips or palate (West *et al.* 1957, Fawcus 1965). In addition to their language deficits, the majority of severely subnormal children also show speech disorders, *e.g.* disorders of voice, articulation and rhythm. These may be related to various degrees of detected or undetected hearing loss, but also frequently occur in the presence of apparently normal hearing (for a recent brief review see Schiefelbusch *et al.* 1967, Webb and Kinde 1968). Articulation disorders are particularly common, while children with Down's syndrome have been frequently shown to have voice defects—*e.g.* huskiness and monotony.

Although biological factors play a crucial rôle in both speech and language disorders, they must be seen as interacting with environmental variables. A child with severe articulation difficulties is likely to suffer secondary language disorders in addition to primary speech disorders; his efforts at communication are often unsuccessful, he will be misunderstood or even ignored, and may come to regard his attempts at communication as inefficient and not worth-while. In this situation he will resort to non-verbal means of communication, such as gestures and mime, and hope that his needs will be understood without use of language. Furthermore, there is now ample evidence of the effect of environmental factors on language functioning. Children brought up in institutions tend to be more impaired in language development than those brought up at home; these differences are unlikely to be due to selection artefacts. The adverse effects of an institutional environment are by no means irreversible, as Tizard (1964) has shown in the Brooklands experiment, where the provision of a reasonably stimulating and more child-centred environment resulted in appreciable increases in verbal and social skills, compared with a matched control group who remained in the institution. No special language training programmes were provided in the Brooklands study, and use was made of a rather general programme of language stimulation in which children were treated as individuals rather than in groups, and many interesting activities were available which would be likely to encourage language. It is worth noting that no increases were recorded in non-verbal tests either between the experimental and control groups or within the experimental group as a result of treatment, despite the fact that much emphasis was placed on the practice of both gross and fine motor skills.

A number of studies have reported significantly lower levels of linguistic functioning in institutionalised children compared with children living at home. Muller and Weaver (1964) matched their groups on Binet IQ but found that the institutionalised children produced substantially lower scores on the Illinois Test of Psycholinguistic Abilities. Schlanger (1954) individually matched institutionalised and special class children on CA, MA, IQ and articulation skills, and reported that the former used shorter sentences and spoke fewer words per minute. The need to carry out a fine-grain analysis of environmental variables has been stressed in chapter 5; in the particular setting of the institution, it is probably the absence of consistent speech models that is most damaging. The institutionalised child is surrounded by peers who speak very little or very badly; moreover, the environment tends to reinforce non-verbal rather than verbal behaviour. As Spradlin (1968) put it; 'If the retarded child lines up and follows the other children, he may end up in the dining hall or in the picture show. If he imitates the verbal response of a peer, it is unlikely that anything very dramatic will occur'. Put in different terms, he has little opportunity to differentiate relevant foreground from irrelevant background. Indeed the constant background of radio during the day, and the tranquilising use of television in the afternoons and evenings also contributes to the difficulty of differentiating 'signal' from 'noise'. Adults rarely talk to him from close quarters, and he tends to hear language addressed to others rather than to him individually. Moreover, it is difficult to set up an institutional environment that reinforces language rather than discourages it. The constant existence of a set routine reduces the need for communication and the best way to gain adult attention is often non-verbal.

Although institutionalised children are at a strong disadvantage in respect of their opportunities for acquiring language, very little is known about the kind of linguistic stimulation available to handicapped children in their own homes. Studies of normal children have emphasised time and again the massive contribution of social class variables to language development (see chapter 5) but we do not know whether such variables are relatively as important and critical with mentally handicapped children. There are a number of case reports of patients with Down's syndrome with exceptionally advanced language abilities (Hunt 1968)—'islands of intelligence' perhaps—but it would be useful to compare the linguistic abilities of children with Down's syndrome from working class backgrounds to see whether the relative difference between the linguistic handicaps of children from different social classes is as great for patients with Down's syndrome as it is for normal children. So far the evidence does not suggest that social class factors are as critical for cognitive development in the SSN as they are for normal children. The study by Carr (1970) failed to demonstrate consistent social class differences in a sample of children with Down's syndrome.

Social class is obviously a crude index of environmental stimulation, and more refined measures of parental language behaviour are urgently needed. Bernstein's

(1965) work on differences between 'restricted' and 'elaborated' linguistic codes may eventually prove to be of some relevance in subnormality; some of his associates have developed interesting techniques of finding out what mothers say in response to their children's questions (Robinson and Rackstraw 1967), and it would be interesting to extend such techniques to the mothers of subnormal children. One recent study suggests that such mothers may lay undue emphasis on correct articulation rather than elaborate language production (Jeffree and Cashdan 1971).

It is a truism to emphasise that both biological and environmental factors are important in the development of language abilities in subnormal children; nevertheless, although we must obviously think in terms of an interaction between them, we know very little about the nature of such an interaction: nor have we progressed very far in refining terms as crude as 'biological' and 'environmental'. The former is concerned with a wide variety of variables, including broad maturational patterns, a hypothetical entity called a 'Language Acquisition Device' and pathological conditions of the central nervous system and peripheral speech organs. Environmental factors may include the availability of 'a good loving home', social class membership or something as specific as the type-token ratios used by the mother. In other words, both biological and environmental variables range from the molar to the molecular; no wonder that we have such difficulty in differentiating between them.

That environmental factors are of some importance is suggested by the possibility of helping severely subnormal children to develop language skills which were previously absent. Although many attempts to develop language abilities have been reported, many of the studies are poorly controlled, and it is not always easy to determine whether improvements were due to the teaching methods used and whether they were lasting in their effects (*see* Spradlin 1963 for a critical examination of earlier studies,). Some studies have taken the form of helping children to reach the labelling single word stage via a carefully designed programme of imitation training using systematic reward and shaping techniques (*e.g.* Lovaas 1966, Staats 1968); others have helped children to increase and diversify the use of linguistic skill already in their repertoire. In a recent study, for example, Jeffree (1971) has given examples of simple teaching techniques designed to facilitate an increase in sentence length, and also in the ratio of verbs to nouns.

Systematic attempts to improve language skills in the mentally subnormal have hardly begun, but seem to offer reasonably promising prospects. Although genetic and biological factors obviously set limits to the amount that can be achieved even by the best teaching methods, there is reason to believe that many severely subnormal children are 'underfunctioning' from the language point of view, and that their skills could be considerably extended. There is room for argument about the best methods needed to achieve this aim; for example, it may not be enough merely to provide a rich and stimulating environment in which mothers and teachers keep up a constant running commentary on their activities. More structured approaches may be needed in certain cases, including the use of 'systematic teaching' in which learning is graded into small steps, and successive approximations consistently rewarded.

Conclusions

There is no simple association between language and intellectual development, particularly in children with developmental disorders. The fact that a child appears to be mentally subnormal does not 'explain' his failure to speak, nor does late language development necessarily imply subnormality of intelligence. Nevertheless, mentally subnormal children usually show severe language impairments. These may be related to both biological and environmental factors. In cases of severe brain involvement, the same biological deficits may give rise both to severe subnormality and to failure to develop language, since both language and intelligence depend on at least a minimum level of cognitive development, particularly in respect of symbolisation and representational skills. Even in the milder disorders of language and intelligence, maturational factors play an important part; indeed, most children have to achieve certain physical milestones before they begin to acquire linguistic proficiency. Furthermore, genetic variables cannot be discounted in any consideration of language development or language disorder, since these set certain limits to the rate at which development proceeds and the point at which it reaches an asymptote. Environmental factors are also of great importance, though it is not easy to specify the nature of the processes involved, or how they interact with the biological variables.

Perhaps the most important of the environmental factors are those which can be mobilised in facilitating or accelerating language skills in mentally subnormal or language disordered children. While biological factors may set certain limits to the final achievements that may be expected of a child, skilled and systematic teaching of language has not yet been tried on any scale. It may therefore be premature to come to any firm conclusions about the ultimate level of language skill that a mentally subnormal child may be expected to reach at adulthood. It would also be unrealistic to exaggerate what could be achieved even if the best teaching methods were more widely available. It may be more appropriate to emphasise that many subnormal children are probably underfunctioning in respect of language skills, and that a properly designed teaching programme should at least aim for optimum levels of language skills of which they are potentially capable.

It is axiomatic, however, that any programme of language teaching must be based on a thorough assessment of a child's language abilities, and that any such analysis must consider language not as a global faculty or construct, but as a series of interdependent skills and abilities. The nature of these skills and their incorporation into an assessment programme will be discussed in the following chapter.

REFERENCES

Baumeister, A. A. (1967) 'Problems in comparative studies of mental retardates and normals.' *Amer. J. ment. Defic.*, **71,** 869.
Bernstein, B. (1965) 'A socio-linguistic approach to learning.' *in* Gould, J. (Ed.) *Penguin Survey of Social Sciences*. Harmondsworth, Middx.: Penguin Books. p. 144.
Bricker, W. A., Bricker, D. D. (1970) 'A program of language training for the severely language handicapped child.' *Except. Child.*, **37,** 101.
Brimer, M. A., Dunn, L. M. (1962) *English Picture Vocabulary Test*. Bristol: Educational Evaluation Enterprises.
Burland, R. (1969) 'The development of the verbal regulation of behaviour in cerebrally palsied (multiply handicapped) children.' *J. ment. Subnorm.*, **15,** 85.

Burt, C. (1967) 'Capacity and achievement.' *Education*, **130**, 198.
Carr, J. (1970) 'Mental and motor development in young mongol children.' *J. ment. Defic. Res.*, **14**, 205.
Chalfant, J. (1968) 'Systematic language instruction: an approach for teaching receptive language to young trainable children.' *Teaching except. Child.*, **1**, 1.
Denny, M. R. (1964) 'Research in learning and performance.' *in* Stevens, H. A., Heber, R. (Eds.) *Mental Retardation*. Chicago: University of Chicago Press. p. 100.
Fawcus, M. (1965) 'Speech disorders and therapy in mental subnormality.' *in* Clarke, A., Clarke, A. D. B. (Eds.) *Mental Deficiency: The Changing Outlook*. 2nd edn. London: Methuen. p. 447.
Graham, C. (1967) 'Ability and attainment tests.' *Education*, **129**, 902, 948, 1000.
Hermelin, B., O'Connor, N. (1970) *Psychological Experiments with Autistic Children*. Oxford: Pergamon.
Herriot, P., Green, J. (1971) 'Free recall in the severely subnormal.' *Bull. Brit. Psychol. Soc.*, **24**, 228A. (paper delivered to Annual Conference, British Psychological Society, Exeter, April, 1971.)
Hunt, N. (1968) *The World of Nigel Hunt*. London: Darwin Finlayson.
Jeffree, D. M. (1971) 'A language teaching programme for a mongol child.' *Forward Trends* (in press.)
—— Cashdan, A. (1971) 'Severely subnormal children and their parents: an experiment in language improvement.' *Brit. J. educ. Psychol*, **41**, 184.
Lenneberg, E. H., Nichols, I. E., Rosenberger, E. F. (1964) 'Primitive stages of language development in mongolism.' *Proc. Ass. Res. nerv. ment. Dis.*, **42**, 119.
Lovaas, I. (1966) 'A programme for the establishment of speech in psychotic children.' *in* Wing, J. K. (Ed.) *Early Childhood Autism: Clinical, Social and Educational Aspects*. Oxford: Pergamon. p. 115.
Luria, A. R. (1961) *The Role of Speech in the Regulation of Normal and Abnormal Behaviour*. Oxford: Pergamon.
—— (1963) *The Mentally Retarded Child*. Oxford: Pergamon.
Lyle, J. G. (1960) 'The effects of an institution environment upon the verbal development of institutionalised children. II. Speech and language.' *J. ment. Defic. Res.*, **4**, 1.
Marinosson, G. (1970*a*) 'A comparative study of normal, educationally subnormal and severely subnormal children on the revised Illinois Test of Psycholinguistic Abilities.' University of Manchester, M. A. Thesis.
—— (1970*b*) 'Language abilities of normal, ESN and SSN children: a comparative study.' *in* Mittler, P. (Ed.) *The Work of the Hester Adrian Research Centre: A Report for Teachers*. Monogr. Suppl., *Teaching & Training*, **8**, 17.
Marshall, A. (1967) *The Abilities and Attainments of Children Leaving Junior Training Centres*. London: National Association for Mental Health.
Miller, S. A., Shelton, J., Flavell, J. H. (1970) 'A test of Luria's hypotheses concerning the development of verbal self-regulation.' *Child Develop.*, **41**, 651.
Mittler, P. (1964) 'The use of form boards in developmental assessment.' *Develop. Med. Child. Neurol.*, **6**, 510.
—— (1972) 'New directions in the study of learning disorders.' *in* Clarke, A. D. B. (Ed.) *Learning Processes in the Mentally Subnormal*. London: Butterworths. (not yet published.)
Muller, M. W., Weaver, S. J. (1964) 'Psycholinguistic abilities of institutionalised and non-institutionalised trainable mental retardates.' *Amer. J. ment. Defic.*, **68**, 775.
O'Connor, N., Hermelin, B. (1963) *Speech and Thought in Severe Subnormality*. Oxford: Pergamon.
Robinson, W. P., Rackstraw, S. J. (1967) 'Variations in mothers' answers to children's questions as a function of social class, intelligence test scores and sex.' *Sociology*, **1**, 259.
Rutter, M. (1970) 'Autistic children: infancy to adulthood.' *Semin. Psychiat.*, **2**, 435.
Schiefelbusch, R. L., Copeland, R. H., Smith, J. O. (Eds.) (1967) *Language in Mental Retardation*. New York: Holt, Rinehart & Winston.
Schlanger, B. (1954) 'Environmental influences on the verbal output of mentally retarded children.' *J. speech hear Disord.*, **19**, 339.
Schubert, J. (1969) 'The V.R.B. apparatus: an experimental procedure for the investigation of the development of the verbal regulation of behavior.' *J. genet. Psychol.*, **114**, 237.
Spradlin, J. E. (1963) 'Language and communication in mental defectives.' *in* Ellis, N. R. (Ed.) *Handbook of Mental Deficiency*. New York: McGraw-Hill. p. 512.
—— (1968) 'Environmental factors and the language development of retarded children.' *in* Rosenberg, S., Koplin, J. H. (Eds.) *Developments in Applied Psycholonguistics Research*. New York: MacMillan.
Staats, A. W. (1968) *Language. Learning and Cognition*. New York: Holt, Rinehart & Winston.
Tizard, J. (1964) *Community Services for the Mentally Handicapped*. London: O.U.P.
Webb, C. E., Kinde, S. (1968) 'Speech, language and hearing of the mentally retarded.' *in* Baumeister, A. (Ed.) *Mental Retardation*. London: University of London Press. p. 86.
West, R., Ansberry, M., Carr, A. (1957) *The Rehabilitation of Speech*. 3rd edn. New York: Harper & Row.

CHAPTER 12

Psychiatric Causes of Language Retardation

MICHAEL RUTTER

There are many distortions of speech and language, both gross and subtle, associated with psychiatric disorder, particularly psychosis (Critchley 1964, Stengel 1964). However, there are only a very few psychiatric conditions associated with language retardation in the young child and it is these conditions which will be considered in this chapter.

Although the intellectual retardation and psychosocial causes of language delay are discussed elsewhere (see chapters 5 and 11), a note on them was felt to be appropriate here because they are, in fact, two of the most common causes why children with speech and language disorders are referred to the psychiatrist. The psychiatric aspects, therefore, are briefly discussed.

Intellectual Retardation

Much the commonest psychiatric disorder associated with a delay in the acquisition of language is intellectual retardation. Indeed, it is the most frequent disorder of any type associated with language delay (Ingram 1969).

Very few idiots (IQ 20 or less) use spoken language as a form of communication even when they reach adulthood, and language development is nearly always delayed in imbeciles (IQ 21 to 50). Among children with mild intellectual retardation (IQ 51 to 70), language delay is also common. Articulation defects, too, occur in about one in two children with any degree of mental subnormality (Spreen 1965, Jordan 1967). The strength of the association between IQ and language development is shown by the consistently positive correlations between the two, both in the normal range of intelligence (Spreen 1965, Moore 1967) and in the subnormal range (Matthews 1957, Spreen 1965). Most intellectually retarded individuals are limited in their use of spoken language throughout life.

Nevertheless, there are sufficient mentally subnormal individuals with fair language competence to make it clear that there is far from a one-to-one relationship between IQ and language (see chapter 11). Also, some children with mild intellectual retardation have a language handicap out of all proportion to their mental retardation (Morley 1965). As Mittler points out (see chapter 11), the diagnosis of mental subnormality should not be taken as a sufficient explanation for language delay. It is necessary to investigate fully in order to determine whether the language difficulties are due to organic brain disease, deafness, psychosocial deprivation, or other factors. Nearly all individuals with an IQ below 50 are known to have structural brain disease (Crome 1960). The gross language impairment associated with severe intellectual retardation is just as likely to be due to the brain disease causing the subnormality as to the low IQ directly. In this context, it should also be appreciated that language difficulties can impair intelligence (see chapter 15), just as low IQ can retard language development. Nevertheless, general intellectual retardation is probably the most common single factor in language delay, even if it is not usually the only factor (Fawcus 1965).

Whether or not the language development in subnormal children is deviant as well as delayed is not known. Mental subnormality is a term which covers a most heterogeneous group of conditions, and whether there are language differences between different types of subnormality has been surprisingly little investigated (Spreen 1965). In Down's syndrome, one of the few conditions systematically studied, language development follows much the same pattern as in normal children, with two exceptions: (a) that in Down's syndrome language ceases to develop at a time when behavioural development is still continuing (Lenneberg et al. 1964, Cornwell and Birch 1969) and (b) that the development of articulation is out of step with, and lags behind, language development (Lenneberg et al. 1964). Less is known about the process of language development in children with other types of mental subnormality but it seems that echolalia is sometimes a more prolonged and more pronounced feature than it is in normal children (Stengel 1964, Morley 1965).

The treatment and prognosis of language impairment in mentally subnormal children is discussed in chapter 11 and will not be considered here.

Psychosocial Retardation of Language

Psychosocial deprivation is a common cause of poor speech but, at least in the United Kingdom, it is a quite uncommon cause of a marked delay in speech development. There is an extensive literature documenting the fact that children reared in grossly deprived environments tend to be impaired in their language development (see chapter 5). However, for the most part these accounts are concerned with groups of speaking children whose use of spoken language is on average less mature than normal, rather than with individual children who show a marked delay in early language. Socially deprived children tend to have speech which is more appropriate to that of younger children in terms of articulation, vocabulary, sentence length, and use of grammar. They have a particular difficulty in using language as a means of problem-solving and of communicating ideas and concepts (Raph 1967).

However, it is less usual for children to be severely delayed in beginning to speak. Although most writers on language delay mention that it may be caused by psychosocial deprivation there is a surprising paucity of studies into the condition and its prevalence is not known. Nevertheless, psychosocial deprivation may lead to a delay in the onset of speech and in some circumstances it may even impair preverbal vocalisations and babble (Brodbeck and Irwin 1946, Provence and Lipton 1962). When speech develops there is usually a global impairment of both spoken language and word-sound production. Gesture is not much used in most cases. On the other hand, the comprehension of language is not usually retarded to the same extent (Provence and Lipton 1946, Klaus and Gray 1968). Speech is delayed but it probably follows a normal pattern of development. There are infantile consonant substitutions and omissions, poor vocabulary and immature grammar, as is usually seen in normal children just beginning to speak.

Diagnosis depends on the demonstration of environmental circumstances sufficiently severe to have caused language retardation. The quality of the language itself offers no clues except in so far as psychosocial language deprivation would be a doubtful diagnosis if language *comprehension* were markedly impaired. One feature which makes psychosocial retardation of language different from many other language disorders is that it probably occurs about as often in girls as in boys (Gerber and Hertel 1969), although this point requires further study. The behaviour and social responses of the deprived child follow no pathognomonic pattern but either extreme of social apathy or indiscriminately affectionate and demanding behaviour are fairly characteristic of many institutional children. Differential diagnosis is complicated by the fact that the children most vulnerable to deprivation are those already handicapped in intellect, personality or language.

The question of what sort of deprivation or what severity is required to cause a marked delay in early language development is clearly crucial with respect to diagnosis. Unfortunately no definite answer is yet available. Institutional upbringing is the best documented cause of deprivation leading to language retardation. Institutional environments tend to be deviant in many respects (Tizard 1970) and which particular feature is most important for language development is not known. However, the sheer lack of any form of contact with the child is one of the most striking features of many institutions (Rheingold 1960). There is very little communication or interaction between the staff and the child—a deficiency likely to impair language development. Yet, by no means all institutional children are seriously retarded in their language and in institutions where adequate stimulation is provided, severe developmental retardation is not found (Yarrow 1964). A further factor is the child's own temperamental attributes (Schaffer 1966). It seems that highly active children who demand attention thereby receive more stimulation and so are less likely to be deprived.

Circumstances in the home leading to speech delay are less well documented. Prince (1968) has described psychosocial language retardation in West Indian children. Poor quality child-minding arrangements in which a large number of children are left to their own devices in the care of one adult seem particularly likely to lead to language impairment. However, Moore (1968) found that regular placement in day nurseries for most of the second and third years of life was without effect on vocabulary. It seems that fairly gross deprivation must be present in order to cause significant speech delay in early childhood. On the other hand, lesser degrees of deprivation may have quite profound effects on language usage and on reading skills as the children grow older (Haywood 1965, Hess and Shipman 1967, Lawton 1968).

Similarly, subtle differences in family patterns of communication may have important consequences for children's later development, as Bernstein has pointed out (Lawton 1968, Bernstein and Henderson 1969, Bernstein 1970). The way children use language is likely to be influenced by the way language is used in the home—whether its use is limited to commands and requests or whether it is used to conceptualise ideas and explore the environment. These are important effects but they should not be confused with delays in early language development which are different in type and causation.

The prognosis of psychosocial language deprivation is uncertain. Probably, the outlook is usually fairly good provided the depriving circumstances can be remedied (Yarrow 1964, Taylor 1968). Where the deprivation cannot be remedied, the language handicap may be persistent. There is a case report showing that language development may begin even as late as 6 years and yet still be ultimately normal (Mason 1942, Davis 1947). This is unusual but the case does underline the error of assuming that it is 'too late' for recovery to take place merely because of the child's age. Treatment consists of remedying the depriving situation as far as possible and, where necessary, of providing language 'stimulation' and training.

Infantile Autism

Language retardation is almost an invariable feature of infantile autism (Rutter 1970a) and it is a failure to develop speech which often first leads to the autistic child being referred to hospital. It is a relatively rare condition, occurring in 2 to 4 children out of every 10,000 (Lotter 1966), but even so it is one of the more important causes of severe and persistent language retardation. Like the developmental language disorders, autism is much commoner in boys than girls—in a ratio of about 4 to 1.

Although autism is recognisable by the emotional and behavioural abnormalities characteristic of the conditions, autistic children show a distinctive pattern of language development which is of diagnostic importance (Pronovost 1961, Wolff and Chess 1965a, Cunningham 1966, 1968, Pronovost et al. 1966, Rutter 1966, Tubbs 1966, Rutter and Lockyer 1967).

Language and Speech Characteristics

In infancy, the most striking feature is often the autistic child's inconsistent response to sound. He fails to pay attention to his parent's voice, ignores most auditory stimuli and often fails to show a startle response to loud noises (Anthony 1958). Not surprisingly this frequently leads to the suspicion of deafness. The parents usually report that they do not believe he is deaf because sometimes he seems to turn in response to very quiet sounds. However, occasionally this may be quite difficult to confirm on audiometric testing and repeated examination is always advisable if there is the slightest suggestion that there may be a partial hearing loss. Nevertheless, in contrast to 'developmental receptive aphasia', autism is only rarely associated with a high tone hearing loss.

As the autistic child grows older it usually becomes apparent that his inconsistent response to sound is associated with a defect in the comprehension of language. As with other conditions, verbal understanding tends to improve with age, but in the pre-school child this difficulty is often one of the most handicapping of all manifestations of autism. The understanding of gestural communication is better than the understanding of spoken language but even the response to gesture may be impaired to some extent.

In early childhood, the comprehension defect is virtually always associated with a serious deficiency in 'inner language'. The intelligent autistic child is often highly skilled in the manipulation of shapes, performing at or above age level on constructional tasks or jig-saw puzzles. His failure to use toys for their appropriate function

150

and, in particular, his failure to use them in any imaginative way is, therefore, all the more striking. He may quickly discover how a toy car works but he will not use it to play 'races' or 'driving into the garage'. There will be no pretend games such as 'mother and father', 'cops and robbers', 'tea parties' or 'schools'. Usually, too, the autistic child is markedly retarded in his drawing in spite of good visuo-motor co-ordination—probably again a reflection of poverty of 'inner language'.

To date there are no published reports of systematic studies of the pre-verbal vocalisations and babble of autistic children. However, clinical observation, parental reports (Rutter *et al.* 1971) and Rick's (1972) systematic study, suggest that babble is usually delayed in development, and that, at least in some autistic children, it may be reduced in amount and deviant in quality.

Autistic children are almost always slow to produce meaningful words and even more delayed in their use of phrases. However, in a minority of cases (about a fifth) there seems to be a period of normal language development preceding regression at some point between 18 and 30 months, followed by impaired language development. At a time when spoken language is seriously impaired, much the most characteristic language feature of autism is the child's failure to use gesture or mime to communicate. He may point or take someone's hand to indicate his needs but there will very rarely be any other kind of gesture and certainly not a language of gesture.

When speech does develop it is abnormal both in quality and in use. Of the autistic children who acquire spoken language, and half do not (Eisenberg 1956, Rutter 1967, Rutter *et al.* 1967), three quarters have a prolonged period of echolalia in which they tend to repeat the last few words of whatever is said to them: this echoing is more rigid and lacking in meaning than that which occurs in normal children when they are learning to speak (Shapiro *et al.* 1970). Often, too, there is a frequent usage of stereotyped phrases copied from other people—'delayed echolalia'. As part of this same echoing tendency there is often pronominal reversal so that the child refers to himself as 'you' or 'he' instead of 'I'. That this is a result of echoing is suggested by the inflections used, *e.g.* interrogative when he says 'do you want chocolate?' (meaning 'I want chocolate') or neutral when he says 'he wants chocolate' to convey the same. Some mentally retarded children echo, but a marked echolalia together with pronominal reversal is much more characteristic of autism.

Sentences are grammatically incomplete, and many of the small connecting words are omitted. There may also be a particular tendency to omit pronouns of all types. A few autistic children produce neologisms and in a larger number much that is said appears inappropriate or purposeless.

The autistic child, even when he has a reasonable language competence, makes much less use of speech for communication than do other children. He may speak little, or if he does speak much, a lot of what he says is likely to consist of repetitive and seemingly 'obsessive' question and answer on his particular preoccupation at that time. Even the older autistic child who has considerable verbal fluency is unlikely to be able to 'chat' freely or join in a conversation between a group of people.

Most autistic children find difficulty following a story (*e.g.* at the theatre or on television), they miss nuances and tend to use words over-concretely. A difficulty with abstract concepts frequently persists long after speech has been well established. There is often a formality of language and a lack of ease in the use of words. Some older autistic children have pedantic ways of putting things—speaking in a kind of 'officialese'.

As language is developing, there may be some difficulties in word-sound produc_tion, usually in terms of the infantile consonant substitutions and omissions present in many normal young children who are just beginning to talk. In a few autistic children there may be more pronounced and persistent articulation defects. However, in most autistic children the language impairment far exceeds the articulation defect. In this respect, they contrast with some mentally subnormal children whose speech may be worse than their language.

In the older autistic child, abnormalities of speech delivery are not infrequently present. Some have a monotonous flat delivery with little lability, change of emphasis or emotional expression. In others, speech is staccato and lacking in cadence and inflection. In some cases the children use a special voice such as sing-song or whisper.

Emotional and Behavioural Characteristics

Apart from the language aspects, there are two other particularly characteristic features of autism—the quality of social relationships and the presence of ritualistic and compulsive phenomena (Wolff and Chess 1964*b*, Rutter 1966, Rutter and Lockyer 1967). In early life, the social abnormalities are shown by the autistic child's failure to engage in eye-to-eye contact, giving the appearance of aloofness and distance, and by his relative failure to become attached to his parents. He demonstrates little interest in people, tends to treat all adults in much the same way and shows little oɪ no separation anxiety. There is little variation in facial expression, a failure to cuddle or come for comfort and an apparent lack of warmth or affection.

About the age of 4 or 5 years, he may develop more social responsiveness and show some attachment to his parents. However, he will continue to be abnormal in his failure to join in group activities with other children and in his failure to develop personal friendships. Although most autistic children achieve normal eye-to-eye gaze as they grow older, they usually remain lacking in spontaneity and warmth. In adolescence, even those who have made the most progress are likely to be lacking in social 'know-how', deficient in empathy and without friends. By then they may be wanting to make friends but they lack the social skills to move from acquaintance to friendship. There are four types of ritualistic and compulsive phenomena:—abnormal attachments (to odd or unusual objects rather than a cuddly soft toy), abnormal preoccupations (varying in complexity from whirling a rag on a stick to complicated concerns with time or number), non-adaptability or resistance to change (often shown by distress when ornaments or furniture are moved in the home), and a variety of 'obsessive' activities which the child seems compelled to carry out repetitively regardless of the circumstances (many of the children have rigid and restricted eating habits and others have daily routines they have to perform).

Motor abnormalities (either hyper- or hypo-kinesis) are quite common in autism and stereotyped repetitive movements are a frequent occurrence. Charac-teristically, these take the form of hand and finger mannerisms (often done near the corner of the eye), or complicated whole body movements. Self-injury in the form of severe head-banging or wrist-biting may also be a problem, particularly in the child with a severe and persisting impairment in language comprehension.

The Nature of Autism

Autism is a descriptive and not an aetiological diagnosis, so that it is important to investigate possible pathogenic factors, biological, social and psychological. Not many autistic children show any abnormalities on neurological examination, but follow-up studies show that an organic brain disorder may nevertheless be present, Up to a quarter of autistic children followed into adulthood develop epileptic fits (Rutter 1970*b*). This is a much commoner occurrence in children who are intellectually retarded as well as autistic, but organic brain dysfunction is also demonstrable in a significant minority of intelligent autistic children.

Psychogenic theories had a vogue 10 to 20 years ago, but the evidence is rather against this explanation and few people now would suggest that autism is primarily a psychogenic disorder (Rutter 1968). However, it remains possible that environmental influences play a significant part in the development of *secondary* handicaps. Also, the curious finding that autism is commoner in children with professional or middle class parents (Lotter 1967) remains unexplained.

Possible genetic explanations for autism have not been adequately studied so far. The sibs of autistic children are usually normal and chromosome studies have been negative (Rutter 1967), but this does not rule out genetic influences.

At one time autism was regarded as a variety of schizophrenia but there is much against this view. Autism always begins before the age of 30 months, whereas schizophrenia rarely begins before middle childhood and usually not before pubescence. The two conditions also differ in many other respects including family history, social background, sex distribution, symptomatology, cognitive patterns and course of disorder (Rutter 1968, Kolvin 1971).

Others have classed autism as a sub-variety of mental retardation but this cannot be the case. Although three quarters of autistic children show some degree of intellectual retardation, a quarter are normally intelligent. Furthermore, to some extent the intellectual impairment is secondary to a language handicap (Lockyer and Rutter 1970). Low IQ is a severe handicap in many autistic children, but the autism cannot be due to low IQ alone.

Kanner (1943), who first described the condition, regarded autism as first and foremost a disorder of social relationships, but more recent evidence (Rutter 1968) suggests that the social abnormality is *not* the basic defect and certainly it cannot account for the language and intellectual characteristics of autistic children.

The cause of autism remains unknown but research findings suggest that in some cases (especially those with associated intellectual retardation), it is due to organic brain disease which causes a defect in the central processing of information, particularly in the coding and utilisation of information obtained through the modality of hearing. In other cases the social and behavioural abnormality may be secondary to a severe developmental disorder of language comprehension. As already noted, the language disorder in autism differs in some important respects from the ordinary

153

varieties of developmental language disorder. Autistic children, unlike children with a straightforward developmental disorder, rarely use gesture to communicate, there is a deficiency in the social utilisation of speech and echolalia is frequently persistent for long after speech develops. The meaning of these differences remains obscure but it seems likely that at least in part the differences are due to the autistic child's greater severity and greater persistence of the defect in the *comprehension* of language. It remains to be determined why children with so-called 'developmental receptive aphasia' are not also autistic. Preliminary findings from a comparative study now in progress have already made it clear that developmental receptive aphasia is a very rare condition (much rarer than autism) and that many children with 'aphasia' do go through a phase of autism (Rutter *et al.* 1971).

Prognosis

Autism is one of the gravest of all conditions associated with language retardation. Only one in two autistic children acquire spoken language. However, the poor prognosis is closely tied to the presence of intellectual retardation (see below). Follow-up studies have shown that the prognosis for the autistic child of normal intelligence (on performance tests) is better than once thought. For example, earlier reports suggested that five years was the watershed for language development—if the child was not speaking by then he never would. It is now known that this is not true. In the follow-up of 64 Maudsley Hospital autistic children, no less than 7 began to speak after the age of 5 years.

Altogether, almost two out of three autistic children are to be found in long-stay hospitals when they are adult (Rutter 1970*b*). About one in six attain a fair adjustment and a similar proportion achieve a good social adjustment and hold a steady job. But for those of normal intelligence (IQ 70+) the outlook is better. Thus, in the Maudsley study, 42 per cent of these children were working or still being educated when followed up in late adolescence or early adult life (Rutter 1970*b*) and only 16 per cent were in long-stay hospitals. Nevertheless, it should be added that, even of those with the best outcome, very few were completely normal. Most continued to have difficulties forming friendships.

The results given above were obtained for children most of whom had had little treatment by present-day standards. To what extent the outcome could be improved by effective early treatment is quite unknown. The pattern of findings at follow-up suggests that biological handicaps severely limit what is possible for many autistic children, but greater improvement may be possible for some.

As already suggested, the most important prognostic factor in autism is the level of measured intelligence. Where the child's IQ on performance tests is below 50 or 60, the outlook is very poor with the likelihood that he will eventually end up in a long-stay subnormality hospital. Above IQ 60, there is also some, but a lesser, association between IQ and prognosis. It has sometimes been thought that autistic children are only 'pseudo-retarded', but it is now clear that this is not the case (Lockyer and Rutter 1969, 1970).

Among autistic children of average intelligence the severity of language impairment is the next consideration. Those still without speech or still with severe difficulties in comprehension at age $4\frac{1}{2}$ to 5 years have a less good prognosis although their average intelligence is likely to ensure at least a fair level of adjustment ultimately. To some extent, too, the prognosis of autistic children is related to the overall severity of behavioural and emotional disturbance.

Lastly, the follow-up studies suggest that good schooling plays a part in ensuring a good level of adjustment in adolescence, emphasising the importance of providing a suitable school placement and also giving effective treatment in the pre-school period.

Treatment

Statements on treatment necessarily have to be rather tentative in the present state of knowledge. Nevertheless, in the last few years several independent groups in this country (Rutter and Sussenwein 1971), and in the United States (Schopler and Reichler 1971), have developed approaches which have much in common and which seem to offer promise.

In the pre-school period the emphasis is first of all on the development of communication and of social interaction. If the basic defect lies in the comprehension of spoken language it is necessary to communicate with the child through the use of gesture (which though impaired is usually less impaired than spoken language) and demonstration. That is, the child is contacted by *showing* him things rather than by *telling* him things. Similarly, people need to respond positively to any communication by the child—whatever the simplicity of the communication and whatever the modality used. As the aim is also to develop spoken language, demonstration and gesture need to be linked to words. However, because of the child's difficulties in comprehension and in processing information there is a danger of sensory over-load and initially it may be better to communicate and teach using only one sensory modality. For the same reason, the speech used to him needs to be simple in the first instance. Later on, a wide variety of language games may be useful. Of course, many are part of the usual repertoire of games played by parents and children—others have been developed for therapeutic purposes by speech therapists.

At least as important, however, is the development of *social* interaction and communication. Because the young autistic child does not spontaneously develop relationships, it is necessary at first to *intrude* on the child's activities. A policy of waiting until the child is ready to develop relationships has no place in the treatment of autism. The therapist must find ways of engaging himself in the child's interests and activities and, by doing things with the child, show the child that social interaction may be both useful to him and also fun. A task situation involving constructional elements is often best for this purpose, as the young autistic child's interests in objects predominate. By deliberately getting the child to participate in activities somewhat difficult for him, the adult can show his usefulness by aiding the child—in building blocks or completing puzzles or whatever it is. Throughout, the therapist needs to use his ingenuity to find ways of engaging the child's interest and then extending the activities in socially desirable directions.

Schopler, in particular, has shown the value of getting parents to carry out these activities. In a sense, parents are thereby used as co-therapists. It might be thought

155

that this gives rise to the danger of interfering with the normal parent-child relationship and transforming it into the more detached therapist-child relationship. However, it seems that this does not happen. By encouraging the parents to do things with their child and by giving them some gimmicks to help in this, parents find a renewal of interest and pleasure in their child.

Parents also need to be helped in their dealings with the child's deviant and disturbed behaviour. Parents of handicapped children—autistic and other—tend to be unduly protective and permissive and they need to realise that kindly firmness has an important place.

The way all this is done will vary with individual circumstances. Often it is useful to have someone see the child regularly for sessions designed to build up interaction —this may be a psychiatrist, psychologist, speech therapist or any other suitable person. In addition, the parents will have to be seen for guidance in their dealings with the child.

In some cases operant approaches to speech training or other types of behaviour modification may also be most useful (see chapter 17).

Most autistic children will require some form of special schooling and educational techniques have a major place in treatment.

Disintegrative Psychosis

Autism is associated with language development which is delayed from the outset (or occasionally from just after the outset). There is also a much less common disorder in which development appears normal on all counts up to age three or four years, at which time there is a profound regression and behavioural disintegration. This condition was first described by Heller and is sometimes known as Heller's disease. There may be a premonitory period of vague illness, the child then becomes restive, irritable, anxious and overactive. Over the course of a few months there is an impoverishment and then a loss of speech and language. Comprehension of language deteriorates and intelligence declines, although an intelligent facial expression is usually retained. There is a loss of social skills, impairment of inter-personal relationships, a general loss of interest in objects and the development of stereotypies and motor mannerisms (Heller 1930). There are no clinical signs of neurological damage but post-mortem studies have usually shown cortical degeneration, sometimes of a lipoid type (Kanner 1957, Malamud 1959, Ross 1959, Creak 1963). The prognosis is very poor, with the children usually remaining without speech and severely handicapped intellectually.

Schizophrenia

Schizophrenia is uncommon before pubescence and very rarely occurs before the age of 5 years. Although it is associated with marked distortions of thought and language, it is not usually associated with language retardation and therefore will not be considered here.

Elective Mutism

Elective mutism is a term coined by Tramer (1934) to describe children who are silent with all but a small group of intimates. It is a condition in which the children are able to talk but do not or cannot in certain circumstances or to certain people. In elective mutism there is no language retardation but rather a selectivity in the use of spoken language. It should properly be included with neurotic disorders but it is discussed here because of its possible confusion with language retardation.

Elective mutism occurs with approximately the same frequency in boys and girls or is slightly commoner in girls. It generally develops about age 3 to 5 years* after a period of normal speech development (Salfield 1950, Mora *et al.* 1962, Reed 1963, Pustrom and Speers 1964, Elson *et al.* 1965). The mutism then comes to attention after the child starts school. The usual pattern is that the child speaks normally fluently and freely at home but never speaks at school. The crucial point in diagnosis is the establishment that there is no abnormality in language comprehension or production but rather a motivational disorder with respect to speaking. Because of the initial difficulty in getting the child to talk at the clinic, this issue may have to be decided on the basis of the parental account and the confirmation by formal testing that language comprehension is normal.

Many 3 to 4 year olds, who can speak perfectly well at home, talk little or not at all in strange situations. When they do talk they often do so only in a whisper. This can easily be observed at the beginning of any new year at a nursery school or among young children in their first attendance at a hospital clinic. This is a reflection of the separation anxiety which is a normal feature of development at that age. However, as children become accustomed to the situation following repeated visits, anxiety diminishes and gradually normal talking follows. In some cases, elective mutism may be no more than an exaggeration of this pattern.

However, there are also cases of children remaining silent for many months or even several years and it is this condition which has more usually been referred to in the literature as elective mutism. In this chronic form it is a rare disorder, accounting for less than half a per cent of referrals to child psychiatric clinics (Reed 1963).

Neurological examination shows no abnormality, hearing is normal, and there is no family history of mutism. Intelligence is usually within the normal range and there is no verbal deficit on cognitive tasks. Developmental milestones are generally within normal limits. When the children do speak, their sentence structure, vocabulary and articulation are normal. The children vary in personality but most show temperamental features which are abnormal in some respect. Some of the children are apathetic, morose, unprepossessing and withdrawn. Others are timid, tense, anxious and fearful. Relationships with other children are usually poor. In some cases mutism is the only symptom but in most instances there are other neurotic manifestations. Usually there is an abnormally strong tie between the child and his mother, who is frequently anxious, dominating and overprotective. The children are often very dependent on their parents but frequently, too, the dependency is accompanied by ambivalence and hostility.

*There is also a condition of elective mutism occurring in adolescents which appears different and will not be considered here.

Reed (1963) has suggested that elective mutes may fall into a least two distinct sub-groups: (a) children who are immature and unresponsive and in whom the mutism is an attention-gaining and evasive form of behaviour and (b) tense, anxious, fearful children in whom the mutism is a fear-reducing mechanism.

Much of the psychiatric literature suggests that elective mutism is usually a 'pure' neurotic disorder. However, this is probably misleading and a more representative series of cases (Wright 1968) shows that in about a fifth of the children the mutism develops as a reaction to an underlying speech or language handicap. In some cases this is the main cause of the child being reluctant to speak (Smayling 1959). While an abnormal dependant relationship with the mother is the main pathogenic factor in most cases, some children avoid speech largely because of the teasing and mockery they receive on account of mispronunciations or other speech defect.

Treatment of elective mutism follows the lines used in other cases of neurotic disorder. Depending on the particular psychogenic mechanism present in each case, psychotherapy, social re-learning or reciprocal inhibition might be used. Direct approaches in which the child is systematically rewarded for speaking in social situations also have a place in treatment in some cases (Straughan *et al.* 1965, Reid *et al.* 1967). The ultimate prognosis is good, but in the more resistant chronic cases treatment may need to extend over several years (Reed 1963, Elson *et al.* 1965, Wright 1968).

Conclusion

The conditions discussed in this chapter constitute the most important psychiatric disorders associated with language retardation. However, there are other types of language delay in which psychological factors play a part. For example, twins are not infrequently slow to develop speech—a situation discussed in chapter 5 on environmental influences on language development. Also, it should not need stating that children with other language disorders, including developmental disorders, deafness, and neurological conditions, not infrequently get referred to psychiatric clinics. Child psychiatrists need to be familiar with the differential diagnosis of speech delay of all types.

REFERENCES

Anthony, E. J. (1958) 'An experimental approach to the psychopathology of childhood autism.' *Brit. J. med. Psychol.*, **31**, 211.
Bernstein, B. (1970) 'Education and society.' *New Society*, 26th Feb.
—— Henderson, D. (1969) 'Social class differences in the relevance of language to socialisation.' *Sociology*, **3**, 1.
Brodbeck, A. J., Irwin, O. C. (1946) 'The speech behaviour of infants without families.' *Child Develop.*, **17**, 145.
Cornwell, A. C., Birch, H. G. (1969) 'Psychological and social development in home-reared children with Down's syndrome (mongolism).' *Amer. J. ment. Defic.*, **74**, 341.
Creak, E. M. (1963) 'Childhood psychosis: a review of 100 cases.' *Brit. J. Psychiat.*, **109**, 84.
Critchley, M. (1964) 'The neurology of psychotic speech.' *Brit. J. Psychiat.*, **110**, 353.
Crome, L. (1960) 'The brain and mental retardation.' *Brit. med. J.*, **1**, 897.
Cunningham, M. A. (1966) 'A five-year-study of the language of an autistic child.' *J. Child Psychol. Psychiat.*, **7**, 143.
—— (1968) 'A comparison of the language of psychotic and non-psychotic children who are mentally retarded.' *J. Child Psychol. Psychiat.*, **9**, 229.
Davis, K. (1947) 'Final note on a case of extreme isolation.' *Amer. J. Sociol.*, **52**, 432.
Eisenberg, L. (1965) 'The autistic child in adolescence.' *Amer. J. Psychiat.*, **112**, 607.

Elson, A., Pearson, C., Jones, D., Schumacher, E. (1965) 'Follow-up study of childhood elective mutism.' *Arch. gen. Psychiat.*, **13**, 182.

Fawcus, M. (1965) 'Speech disorders and therapy in mental subnormality.' *in* Clarke, A., Clarke, A. D. B. (Eds.) *Mental Deficiency: The Changing Outlook*. 2nd edn. London: Methuen. p. 447.

Gerber, S. E., Hertel, C. G. (1969) 'Language deficiency of disadvantaged children.' *J. speech Res.*, **12**, 270.

Haywood, C. (1967) 'Experimental factors in intellectual development: the concept of dynamic intelligence.' *in* Zubin, J., Jervis, G. A. (Eds.) *Psychopathology of Mental Development*. New York: Grune & Stratton. p. 69.

Heller, T. (1969) 'Über dementia infantilis, 1930.' (Reprint of translated paper) *in* Howells, J. G. (Ed.) *Modern Perspectives in International Child Psychiatry—3*. Edinburgh: Oliver & Boyd. p. 610.

Hess, R. D., Shipman, V. C. (1965) 'Early experience and the socialisation of cognitive modes in children.' *Child Develop.*, **36**, 869.

Ingram, T. T. S. (1969) 'Developmental disorders of speech.' *in* Vinken, P. J., Bruyn, G. W. (Eds.) *Handbook of Clinical Neurology*, Vol. 4. Amsterdam: North Holland. p. 407.

Jordan, T. E. (1967) 'Language and mental retardation: a review of the literature.' *in* Schiefelbusch, R. L., Copeland, R. H., Smith, J. O. (Eds.) *Language and Mental Retardation: Empirical and Conceptual Considerations*. New York: Holt, Rinehart & Winston.

Kanner, L. (1943) 'Autistic disturbances of affective contact.' *Nerv. Child.*, **2**, 217.

—— (1957) *Child Psychiatry*, 2nd edn. Springfield, Ill.: C. C. Thomas.

Klaus, R. A., Gray, S. W. (1968) 'The early training project for disadvantaged children: a report after five years.' *Monogr. Soc. Res. Child. Develop.*, no. 120.

Kolvin, I. (1971) 'Psychosis in childhood—a comparative study.' *in* Rutter, M. (Ed.) *Infantile Autism: Concepts, Characteristics and Treatment*. London: Churchill Livingstone.

Lawton, D. (1968) *Social Class, Language and Education*. London: Routledge & Kegan Paul.

Lenneberg, E. H., Nichols, I. A., Rosenberger, E. T. (1964) 'Primitive stages of language development in mongolism.' *Proc. Ass. Res. nerv. ment. Dis.*, **42**, 119.

Lockyer, I., Rutter, M. (1969) 'A five to fifteen year follow-up study of infantile psychosis. III. Psychological aspects.' *Brit. J. Psychiat.*, **115**, 865.

—— —— (1970) 'A five to fifteen year follow-up study of infantile psychosis. IV. Patterns of ability.' *Brit. J. soc. clin. Psychol.*, **9**, 152.

Lotter, V. (1966) 'Epidemiology of autistic conditions in young children. I. Prevalence.' *Soc. Psychiat.*, **1**, 124.

—— (1967) 'Epidemiology of autistic conditions in young children. II. Some characteristics of parents and children.' *Soc. Psychiat.*, **1**, 163.

Mason, M. K. (1942) 'Learning to speak after years of silence.' *J. speech Disord.*, **7**, 295.

Matthews, J. (1957) 'Speech problems of the mentally retarded.' *in* Travis, L. E. (Ed.) *Handbook of Speech Pathology*.' New York: Appleton-Century-Crofts. p. 531.

Malamud, N. (1959) 'Heller's disease and childhood schizophrenia.' *Amer. J. Psychiat.*, **116**, 215.

Moore, T. (1967) 'Language and intelligence: a longitudinal study of the first eight years. I. Patterns of development in boys and girls.' *Hum. Develop.*, **10**, 88.

—— (1968) 'Language and intelligence: a longitudinal study of the first eight years. II. Environmental correlates of mental growth.' *Hum. Develop.*, **11**, 1.

Mora, G., Devault, S., Schopler, E. (1962) 'Dynamics and psychotherapy of identical twins in selective mutism.' *J. Child Psychol. Psychiat.*, **3**, 41.

Morley, M. E. (1965) *The Development and Disorders of Speech in Childhood*. 2nd edn. Edinburgh: E. & S. Livingstone.

Prince, C. S. (1968) 'Mental health problems in preschool West Indian children.' *Matern. Child Care*, 483.

Pronovost, W. (1961) 'The speech behaviour and language comprehension of autistic children.' *J. chron. Dis.*, **13**, 228.

—— Wakstein, N. P., Wakstein, D. J. (1966) 'A longitudinal study of the speech behavior and language comprehension of fourteen children diagnosed atypical or autistic.' *Except. Child.*, **33**, 19.

Provence, S. A., Lipton, R. (1962) *Infants in Institutions*. New York: International Universities Press.

Pustrom, E., Speers, R. W. (1964) 'Elective mutism in children.' *J. Amer. Acad. Child Psychiat.*, **3**, 287.

Raph, J. B. (1967) 'Language and speech deficits in culturally disadvantaged children: implications for the speech clinician.' *J. speech Disord.*, **32**, 203.

Reed, G. F. (1963) 'Elective mutism in children: a reappraisal.' *J. Child Psychol. Psychiat.*, **4**, 99.

Reid, J. B., Hawkins, N., Keutzer, C., McNeal, S. A., Phelps, R. E., Reid, K. M., Mees, H. L. (1967) 'A marathon behaviour modification of a selectively mute child.' *J. Child Psychol. Psychiat.*, **8**, 27.

Rheingold, H. L. (1960) 'The measurement of maternal care.' *Child Develop.*, **31**, 565.

Ricks, D. (1972) The Beginnings of Vocal Communication in Infants and Autistic Children. M.D. Thesis, University of London.

Ross, I. S. (1959) 'Presentation of clinical case: an autistic child.' *at* Pediatric Conference, The Babies Hospital Unit, United Hospital, Newark, N.J., Vol. II, no. 2.

Rutter, M. (1966) 'Behavioural and cognitive characteristics of a series of psychotic children.' *in* Wing, J. K. (Ed.) *Childhood Autism: Clinical, Educational and Social Aspects.* Oxford: Pergamon. p. 51.

—— (1967) 'Psychotic disorders in early childhood.' *in* Coppen, A., Walk, A. (Eds.) *Recent Developments in Schizophrenia.* British Journal of Psychiatry Special Publication, No. 1. London: R.M.P.A.

—— (1968) 'Concepts of autism: a review of research.' *J. Child Psychol. Psychiat.*, **9**, 1.

—— (1970a) 'The description and classification of infantile autism.' *in* Churchill, D· W., Alpen, G. D., De Meyer, M· K. (Eds.) *Infantile Autism.* Springfield, Ill.: C. C. Thomas.

—— (1970b) 'Autistic Children—infancy to adulthood.' *Semin. Psychiat.*, **2**, 435.

—— Lockyer, L. (1967) 'A five to fifteen year follow-up study of infantile psychosis. I. Description of sample.' *Brit. J. Psychiat.*, **113**, 1169.

—— Sussenwein, F. (1971) 'A developmental and behavioural approach to the treatment of pre-school autistic children.' *J. Autism Childhd Schiz.*, **I**, 376

—— Bartak, L., Newman, S. (1971) 'Autism—a central disorder of cognition and language?' *in* Rutter, M. (Ed.) *Infantile Autism: Concepts, Characteristics and Treatment.* London: Churchill. Livingstone.

—— Greenfield, D., Lockyer, L. (1967) 'A five to fifteen year follow-up study of infantile psychosis. II. Social and behavioural outcome.' *Brit. J. Psychiat.*, **113**, 1183.

Salfield, D. J. (1950) 'Observations on elective mutism in children.' *J. ment. Sci.*, **96**, 1024.

Schaffer, H. R. (1966) 'Activity level as a determinant of infantile reaction to deprivation.' *Child Develop.*, **37**, 595.

Schopler, E., Reichler, R. J. (1971) 'Developmental therapy by parents with their own autistic child.' *in* Rutter, M. (Ed.) *Infantile Autism: Concepts, Characteristics and Treatment.* London: Churchill Livingstone.

Shapiro, R., Roberts, A., Fish, B. (1970) 'Imitation and echoing in young schizophrenic children.' *J. Amer. Acad. Child Psychiat.*, **9**, 548.

Smayling, L. M. (1959) 'Analysis of six cases of voluntary mutism.' *J. speech. Disord.*, **24**, 55.

Spreen, O. (1965) 'Language functions in mental retardation: a review: I. Language development, types of retardation and intelligence level.' *Amer. J. ment. Defic.*, **69**, 482.

Straughan, J. H., Potter, W. K., Hamilton, S. H. (1965) 'The behavioural treatment of an elective mute.' *J. Child Psychol. Psychiat.*, **6**, 125.

Stengel, E. (1964) 'Speech disorders and mental disorders.' *in* de Reuck, A. V. S., O'Connor, N. (Eds.) *Disorders of Language.* Ciba Foundation Symposium. London: Churchill. p. 285.

Taylor, A. (1968) 'Deprived infants: potential for affective adjustment.' *Amer. J. Orthopsychiat.*, **38**, 835.

Tizard, J. (1969) 'The role of social institutions in the causation, prevention and alleviation of mental retardation.' *in* Haywood, H. C. (Ed.) *Social-Cultural Aspects of Mental Retardation.* New York: Appleton-Century-Crofts. p.281.

Tramer, M. (1934) 'Electiver Mutismus bei Kindern.' *Z. Kinderpsychiat.*, **1**, 30.

Tubbs, V. K. (1966) 'Types of linguistic disability in psychotic children.' *J. ment. Defic. Res.*, **10**, 230.

Wolff, S., Chess, S. (1965a) 'An analysis of the language of fourteen psychotic children.' *J. Child Psychol. Psychiat.*, **6**, 29.

—— —— (1965b) 'A behavioural study of schizophrenic children.' *Acta psychiat. scand.*, **40**, 438.

Wright, H. L. (1968) 'A clinical study of children who refuse to talk in school.' *J. Amer. Acad. Child Psychiat.*, **7**, 603.

Yarrow, L. J. (1964) 'Separation from parents during early childhood.' *in* Hoffman, M. L., Hoffman, L. W. (Eds.) *Review of Child Development Research*, I. New York: Russel Sage Foundation. p.89.

CHAPTER 13

Deviant Language Acquisition: The Phonological Aspect

R. BERESFORD

The purpose of this chapter is to show how phonological studies of spoken language may help us to understand both normal language development and deviant language acquisition. The acquisition of speech occurs, on average, over a period of three years, rapidly at times, in the normal child, but with some children this development seems slower. Some such children subsequently are intelligible in English while others of this group remain deviant.

Phonological and Phonetic Elements

A *phonetic* description of speech, which is usually made in auditory and articulatory terms, refers to the production of speech sounds as physical events and *not* as signals or meaningful sounds. Phonetic elements of speech can be studied by seeing what sounds the child can produce or is able to imitate. In contrast, a *phonological* description aims to describe what sounds the child is using meaningfully in his speech. Phonological components are stated as rules of contrast (sound system) and rules of sequence (sound structure). If we are to be intelligible in our speech, we must signal such contrasts and signal them by an agreed sound in permitted sequence. In addition to phonetic and phonological components of spoken language, there are two other pieces of information we require if we are to account adequately for the generation of utterances (meaningful strings of noise): these are the *semantic* and the *syntactic* components. The syntactical level refers to the meaningful organisation of linguistic units, such as words, phrases and sentences. The semantic level relates to the interrelation between the items of the utterance and the context and situation in which they occur. In this chapter I shall principally be concerned with the phonological component.

To illustrate the importance of the study of phonological development, I am going to describe two children. These are essentially normal children with no evidence of neurological dysfunction and both are thought to have intelligence within the normal range. Neither has a hearing loss and both presented with unintelligible speech.

The spoken language of these children has some features in common.

1. There appears to be no significant deviation at the syntactic and semantic level.
2. There are no significant rhythmic or intonational deviations.
3. The deviations are principally at the phonological level and mainly involve the consonantal sounds rather than the vowels.
4. (*a*) A restricted number of the consonantal sounds of English are used meaningfully (24 consonants are usually recognised as the normal requirement).

(*b*) Some of the meaningful consonantal sounds are different in certain phonetic features from the consonantal sounds of English.

(*c*) Some sounds outside the sound system of English are used meaningfully.

5. (*a*) There is a failure to signal certain meaningful sound differences which English requires, e.g. the words *bin, fin, pin, thin*, are all signalled [bin] ('bin')

(*b*) Meaningful differences are being signalled but in a way different from English, *e.g. thin* is signalled as [bin] ('bin'), or [ɸin] ('fin').

6. There are restrictions on the number of consonant clusters used.

7. However, it must be remembered that such spoken language is consistently meaningful and consistently signalled; that is, an integrated and organised individual language (*i.e.* an idiolect).

Table 1 gives the consonantal sound system and structure of the spoken language of a boy (Kenneth) at the age of 4 years and 2 months. Of the 24 consonantal sounds of English, two are not used [/θ/and/ʒ/] and [ts] is used as a distinctive sound. Many necessary meaningful sound differences which English requires are not being signalled. Column 3 (Table 1) shows many syllable initial contrasts are not signalled and even more syllable final contrasts [t/d/k/n/y/v/θ/s/z/ʃ/ʤ] would not be signalled at all; *bat, bad, back* and *bang* would all be signalled as [ba]. Many meaningful sound contrasts are signalled deviantly.

A feature not shown in the Table is the occurrence of variants, *i.e.* meaningful utterances occurring in more than one form, *e.g. bin* realised as [bin] or [pin]. Sometimes such 'variants' are both deviant; *thin* realised as [bin] or [ɸin], *fin* realised as [bin] or [pin]. Such examples, along with a number of others, suggest linguistic changes reflecting a process of 'monitoring'. A further important feature, only indirectly shown in Table 1, is the fact that the phonetic features of even the deviations are those of English. Thus, the voicing and manner of articulation are not deviant and, although there are deviations in the placing of articulation, only two [ɸ] and [ts], fall outside the range of normal English. These features suggested to us that what we were observing was an essential normal stage in language acquisition with a very much slower rate of change than is normal. This inference is supported by observation of the boy's speech eight months later (Table II).

Over this eight month period, a number of significant changes will be seen to have occurred, many more meaningful differences are signalled as is required in English, and there are many fewer deviant differences. Not only are many more non-deviant meaningful differences being signalled, but also [ʒ] now occurs, and phonetic deviants such as [ɸ] and [ts] do not occur. In short, the change has been in the direction of English, or, more correctly, the English of his speech community (playmates, family) and away from his 'individual language'. This would seem to be a consequence of a 'natural' process, albeit slower (or later) than his developmental peers.

Deviant Development

Kenneth's 'slow' acquisition of speech is manifest at the phonological rather than at the phonetic level and his problems are distinct from those of children who have articulation difficulties. Table III phonologically summarises findings on another boy, Stanley, aged 4 years and 3 months, who is similarly of normal intelligence with no apparent hearing loss or neurological dysfunction, and who is able to comprehend language and imitate speech sounds. However, the phonological analysis shows that the number of sounds used is fewer even than Kenneth's, a large number of meaning-

162

ful contrasts required by English are not signalled. Further, there is less evidence of any process of change that is 'self corrective' towards an approximation of the phonological rules of English.

Five months later (Table IV), the changes which have occurred are fewer than they were with Kenneth. A large number of meaningful contrasts of English are still not being signalled, a large number of deviant differences are still being signalled, and the system, although enlarged, is still very restricted and phonetic deviants now occur. There have been some changes, but not in the direction of an approximation to English. These differences between Kenneth and Stanley mean we must classify Stanley as a child with deviant acquisition of speech. He is developing his own individual speech.

Some Remarks on Phonological Acquisition

I feel that children do not just learn speech sounds but rather they learn patterns of articulatory movement correlated with perceived sounds. This is a process which is active rather than passive and there seems to be what could be called a 'matching' process which might be hypothesised on an analysis-synthesis model: a process which might be labelled one of progressive differentiation, but a differentiation of distinctive features rather than specific sounds; a recognition of sound differences correlatable with meaningful differences.

Two phonological features which might seem to be distinguished at an early age are stress and tone—the intonational markers of an utterance (in terms of a meaningful unit) we call a 'sentence', within which 'coarser' distinctive feature differences are distinguished, e.g. voicing and nasality, friction and duration, place and quality. It is relevant here that the sequence of such contrasts might be dependent upon ease of perception, i.e. voiced/voiceless and oral/nasal differences appear to be easier to recognise than differences of place of articulation. This suggests that there will be a sequence of acquisition, but precisely what this is may well be an individual matter because of perceptual and cognitive differences. Thus, marked and unmarked items in the set of meaningful sounds may not necessarily correlate with the same distinctive feature in the spoken language of different children, yet such sound systems will be complete at all times, even though restricted.

From this it follows that language is predominantly learned auditorily and that learning is dependent upon ease of perception. Here, of course, an inability to 'imitate', and any restriction upon the length of a perceived unit, would clearly interfere with such a learning process. It could well be, therefore, that the children whose language we have labelled 'deviant' have a learning problem but one which presents more at a cognitive level.

Linguistic studies of the type described form the basis of assessment of language and it is possible to isolate the level of communicatory breakdown and to show what changes may be taking place. Inferences from such a linguistic statement provide a basis for decision about management and a possible remedial approach. Such an approach needs to be made in individual terms relative to individual deviations and related to any apparent changes in acquisition. Any supervision or remedial help must take into account the fact of an on-going process and individual differences.

TABLE I
Consonantal sound system and structure of Kenneth's speech at 4 years 2 months

Sounds meaningfully used	Permitted place of occurrence in the syllable		Meaningful sound contrasts not signalled	
	Initial	Final	Initial	Final
p	p	p		
b	b	b		
t	t			t
d	d			d/g
k	k			k
g	g			
m	m	m		m/ŋ
n	n	n		n/ŋ
ŋ	-	ŋ		ŋ
f	f	f	f/θ/s	θ
v	v			f/v
ð	ð			
s		s	s/ʃ	s/ʃ
z	z			z
ʃ	ʃ			ʃ/tʃ
h	h	-		
tʃ	tʃ			
dʒ	dʒ			dʒ
l	l	l	l/j	
r	r	-		
w	w	-		
j	j	-	j/ð	
ts		ts		ts/tʃ

TABLE II
Kenneth's speech at age 4 years 10 months

Sounds meaningfully used	Permitted place of occurrence in the syllable		Meaningful sound contrasts not signalled	
	Initial	Final	Initial	Final
p	p	p		
b	b	b		
t	t	t		t
d	d	d	d/ð	
k	k	k		
g	g	g		
m	m	m		
n	n	n		
ŋ	-	ŋ		
f	f	f	f/θ	f/θ
v	v	v		
ð	ð	/		
s	s	s		
z	z	z		
ʃ	ʃ	ʃ		
ʒ	-	/		
h	h	-		
tʃ	tʃ	tʃ		
dʒ	dʒ	dʒ		
l	l	l	l/j	l
r	r	-		
w	w	-		

TABLE III
Consonantal sound system and structure of Stanley's speech at 4 years 3 months

Sounds meaningfully used	Permitted place of occurrence in the syllable		Meaningful sound contrasts not signalled	
	Initial	Final	Initial	Final
b	b		b/p,f,v, θ	b
d	d		d/t,k,g,s,ʃ, tʃ, dʒ	d
m	m	m		m/n
n	n	n		n/ ŋ
ŋ	-	ŋ		ŋ/m
h	h	-		
r	r	-		
w	w	-		
			l/j	p/t/d/k/g/ f/v/s/ʃ/ tʃ/dʒ/l

TABLE IV
TABLE IV
Stanley's speech at age 4 years 8 months

Sounds meaningfully used	Permitted place of occurrence in the syllable		Meaningful sound contrasts not signalled	
	Initial	Final	Initial	Final
p	p		p/b, f	p
b	b		b/p, f, v, θ	b
t	t		t/d, k,ʃ,tʃ	
d	d		d/t, g, s, tʃ	
m	m	m		m/n
n	n	n		
ŋ	-	ŋ		
l	l			
r	r	-		
ʊ	ʊ			
ɸ	ɸ			
			z 1/h/j	p/b/t/d/k/ f/v/θ/s/z/ dʒ/1

CHAPTER 14

The Paediatric Rôle in the Study of Children with Communication Disorders

MARTIN BAX and R. C. MAC KEITH

The paediatrician, and any other doctor who has the task of seeing children regularly, seeks to identify as early as possible any child with a communication disorder. When such a child is identified, as with any other handicapped child, one physician assumes the responsibility for the overall care and management of the child and this physician is usually the paediatrician. The paediatrician specialises in helping children with health problems rather than in disease entities and has special skills in understanding the approach and management of these young people.

Early identification of handicap, of whatever aspect of function, can only be achieved by periodic developmental assessment of all children at suitable ages throughout the pre-school period. This assessment cannot be a once-and-for-all process for several reasons. Even if gross handicap has been excluded at 6 weeks or 6 months or later, a mild one will be evident later and handicap can be acquired. Secondly, it is impossible to screen at 6 or 10 months for language or speech disorders, or at 2 to 3 years for cognitive functions which do not emerge until the age of 4 or later. One scheme for carrying out developmental assessment has been suggested (Egan *et al.* 1969) and here we shall only comment on aspects of the examination which relate to identification of communication disorders.

Developmental Assessment

In the neonatal period the physician will observe certain responses to sound, although, as these are not always easy to obtain consistently, he may find it difficult to spend enough time with each neonate to observe these responses himself. To a loud noise the awake neonate (Prechtl's State III) will give a startle response and he may 'still' to a low-pitched sound. Eye movements towards the sound may be identified and it may be possible to see the baby turning towards the mother's voice at a very early age. The physician will also have the opportunity to hear the child crying and from his knowledge of normal and abnormal cries (Wasz-Höckert *et al.* 1968) he will think about the quality of the cry and if concerned about it will study it further. It is wise to pay particular attention to the comments of experienced attendants at this time. Nurses who have worked in nurseries are particularly alert at noting a child who has a strange cry, and the response to sound of the hyper-excitable child (who tends to give a startle response to the slightest noise) may also alert the physician to studying the particular baby more carefully. The mother's comments on the responsiveness of the child are also extremely important.

Observation is more useful at 6 weeks when, if time is taken, it is usually relatively easy to see an awake child make a response to his mother's voice. Again, however, in a quick examination where the child is not in the ideal state for the examination, it may be impossible to carry out this test and the physician can merely note the startle response, perhaps the stilling of a cry to a loud noise, and be content with the mother's report that the child seems to look and listen to her and her own feeling that these responses are normal. It is important already at this age to note the intergration of the different senses. The child looks at the mother's face, the mother smiles, the child smiles then laughs or coos and as the weeks go by this develops into tuneful babble. Any disorganization of this pattern of response is cause for concern.

By 5 to 6 months the child may make this sort of response to a stranger. He will invariably smile back at a smiling stranger and commonly babble back if the stranger makes the appropriate noises. The doctor should, therefore, be able to listen to a tuneful babble from a 5-to 6-month-old child and its normal tone and quality is reassuring. Perhaps the most important single aspect of the screening examination of the child of 6 months is the test of lateral turning to both high-pitched and low-pitched sound. The response is usually swift and automatic at this age, but the child may become visually involved and for a period be difficult to distract. The response may show some difference of quality on the two sides and if there is any doubt about the quality of the response the examiner should see the child again in a fortnight. It is difficult at this age for the mother to describe the sounds her child is making and the examiner may have to suggest to her the type of noises which he expects from a 6-month-old child (see chapter 1). But it is often easier to get a 5-or 6-month-old to babble in the clinic than it is to get a 10-month-old to vocalize.

We usually see the child again between the ages of 10 and 12 months and between 15 and 18 months for a developmental assessment, and on each occasion the child's hearing is rechecked. At these examinations the child is observed turning to high and low-pitched sounds. It is often more difficult to test the hearing of a 15-month-old child than it is a child of 6 months. He becomes more sophisticated and will not turn to a repeated signal. The examiner may, however, be fortunate and see him turn when somebody moves or speaks in the room, but he should stand away from the child and make soft pitched sounds of varying qualities and hopefully see him turn to these noises. Where unequivocal responses are obtained in the limited time that is often all that is available, it is most important to record this so that at the next visit the examiner can make certain he obtains the child's hearing responses, omitting, perhaps, to be quite so detailed in his examination of the vision on this occasion. From the age of 3 years onwards, Reed and STYCAR tests are possible providing the examiner forms a good contact with the child, and this problem is discussed in the third section of this paper.

The speech of the 10-and 15-month-old child is discussed in chapter 1. During a quick assessment, however, it is not often possible to elicit very much vocalization and the examiner depends very much on historical information from the mother. At the 2 year examination, it is often possible to get the child to talk, but if he is shy and good speech is not heard he should be referred for six months and seen again at $2\frac{1}{2}$ years. Statements made by mothers should be treated with the utmost respect and they usually give accurate information about their children's performance. However, this is not invariably so and the mothers can sometimes describe as talking in sentences children who do not and alternatively say they do not when they do.

Sometime between the ages of 2 and 3 the examiner must himself hear the child talk. At the pre-school or first school examination the doctor should make a thorough assessment of the child's speech and language. He should listen to single words and we make a point of recording the following 6 consonants: s, l, k, sh, th and r (see Rutter and Bax for the time at which the child normally acquires these consonants). The child should repeat a sentence after the examiner and the examiner should hear several spontaneous sentences. These are not usually difficult to elicit. If the child is very shy difficulties may be encountered, but the use of pictures during the tests of single words will usually elicit some conversation. Faced with total failure it is worth recalling that the child will probably start to talk to his mother when he leaves the room and if the examiner follows him to the door he may very quickly hear sentences which were not previously forthcoming.

Language is always difficult to assess quickly in an objective way. The examiner should have some knowledge of the sorts of words children usually know and the range of play material they habitually use. He should also be aware that the knowledge of words can vary sharply within a culture of a boy's school cap. A few years ago any child from three onwards could identify this, but in the part of London where we work the children do not wear caps and many children between the ages of 3 and 5 not only fail to identify it by its name, 'cap', but they do not even identify it as a hat. Again, at 3 years, in the area of Southwark at least, the drawing of the tree on the Reed card is frequently described as 'flowers'. Usually by $4\frac{1}{2}$-5 years this identification is made correctly. It is particularly important to be aware of the normal variation of a cultural sub-group who may be living in the community but not yet sharing the same form of child-rearing practice which is used by the indigenous population. Not all the immigrant groups of the United Kingdom provide their children with the sorts of toys that the average U.K. child is exposed to. If a child fails to play with toy dolls or to identify them, find out if he has ever seen them at home. If not, choose other objects with which he may be more familiar to see what sort of language skills he possesses.

The management and treatment of language and speech disorders is the subject of other chapters of this book. Here we just wish to discuss the problem of when and where to refer the young child who seems to be slow in developing speech and language but who has no other abnormalities. It is essential first of all to reassess the child and confirm that no other abnormalities are present. His whole development is reassessed and particular at tention should be given to his hearing responses and his understanding of the world around him. Ask the mother about behaviour at home. Check that he is playing meaningfully with toys such as cars, dolls, tea-sets, and not just treating them as objects. Find out if he helps his mother with household tasks. Will he ever point at objects she names? Hopefully, one will observe him indulging in this sort of play and hear him vocalize even though sounds are not yet meaningful. Nevertheless, there are children who at 2-$2\frac{1}{2}$ years of age are still only saying a bare dozen words and not making sentences at all. Services in our area are not such that all children with this problem can be assessed in the manner outlined below.

What about the child who has no other developmental delays or abnormalities but who is simply slow at developing speech? Our own practise at the moment is to observe this child during the year from 2-3 and to encourage the mother and others in his home to talk to him in a one-to-one relation. Inarticulate people, particularly when they are worried and nervous in a doctor's consulting room, may not clearly remember instructions and may learn better from a demonstration. The child is sat on the doctor's knee and together they look at a picture book and discuss the pictures. One must also be certain that toys and picture books are available in the child's home if not they should be 'prescribed'. Poor families may be reluctant to admit to the poverty of their homes and the doctor or health visitor or social worker should visit their homes to see whether such material is available. If the child's speech is not developing well at 3 years we invite our speech therapy colleagues to assist us and if there is any doubt at all about the child's overall development he is referred for a fuller assessment. Many people encourage the parents of 3 + children with speech difficulties to place them in nursery schools in the hope that this will help their speech development. As we believe that speech is mainly learnt from an adult we don't feel on theoretical grounds that this will help the child's speech development and our uncontrolled clinical impression is that the nursery school has little influence in the child's speech development *per se*, but will of course affect his social competence. Although, in general, we believe that the nursery school education is helpful to young children, one should be aware of the shy, socially immature 3-year-old who is not able to cope in a day nursery and who may in consequence become even more withdrawn and less accessible to the speech therapist who might work with his speech problem. The child must be socially accessible if his language and speech development is to be helped.

The Handicapped Child with a Communication Problem

Sheridan has outlined the eight needs of the handicapped and they are: (1) early identification (which we have already discussed); (2) full assessment; (3) immediate appropriate treatment and education; (4) support for the parents; (5) periodic reassessment and review of the care; (6) continuing treatment and education and support of parent; (7) vocational training; and (8) placement in employment or long-term care. Ingram and Henderson describe (see chapter 6) the assessment of the child with a speech disorder, we discuss more generally the paediatrician's rôle.

The child is referred from the child health clinic or the general practice for assessment because the doctor has identified or suspects developmental delay, because he has found or suspects handicap, or because the mother is worried that all is not well: (the person who responds to such a mother with 'don't worry, he's all right' usually concentrates at least two errors into these five words; she cannot stop worrying and there is usually something wrong.)

Assessment, whether done by the paediatrician in his ordinary outpatient clinic, in a district assessment centre or in a Regional Assessment Centre, has four parts: (a) screening, so that developmental delay is confirmed (or sometimes excluded); (b) comprehensive assessment by history and examination by which the disorders or handicaps underlying the delay are discovered; (c) immediate action; (d) preparation of a diagnostic profile on which the care of the handicapped child is planned for further investigation and for treatment without delay.

The assessment must be comprehensive for two reasons. The first is that any delay in development is a symptom and like all other symptoms can be due to a variety of underlying disorders *or* to various combinations of underlying disorders, *e.g.* poor response to sound stimuli may be due to deafness, but it may be due to disorder in another area of function. Every child with any developmental delay must have an assessment of function. We use the following headings:

motor, visual, auditory, language,
learning, 'drive', emotional, social.

'Drive' is difficult to define, but it describes the use the individual makes of his abilities. We find it a very useful category in practice.

The second reason why the handicapped child must have a comprehensive assessment is that if there is one handicap there is likely to be another. Thus, we know that children with congenital heart disorder are at a high risk for important errors of refraction or for deafness.

Where there is a chronic neurological disorder such as cerebral palsy, other disorders, including those of hearing and language, are usual. Having assessed the child comprehensively and identified disorders, the paediatrician attempts to *diagnose the cause of the handicap(s)*. This is partly because it may, very rarely, indicate a need for specific treatment, partly because it may lead on to genetic advice to the parents and partly because prevention can only come from a knowledge of causes.

The next step is to prepare a *diagnostic profile*. Diagnosis is a tricky word. It is sometimes restricted to naming the underlying cause of the handicaps, *e.g.* pre-, peri- or post-natal insult of the brain. But any diagnostic summary to be complete must include four statements:

(a) a statement about function—*i.e.* of the ability or disability in everyday functions, *e.g.* he does not talk;

(b) a statement about physiology—*e.g.* he has articulatory dyspraxia *or* loss of hearing of high pitch sound;

(c) a statement about anatomy—*e.g.* the ears are normal;

(d) a statement about cause—*e.g.* perinatal hyperbilirubinaemia.

The diagnostic profile is best illustrated by an example:—

John Smith is a 4-year-old boy in good general physical health (a statement about his general health).

He has a chronic neurodevelopmental disorder; the cause of this was perinatal hyperbilirubinaemia (a statement putting the child both into a general class and into a special compartment in this class. Once in this particular class you know, for example, that he is at risk for high-tone deafness).

Then follows a review of the child in eight aspects, in each of which physiological and functional statements are made.

Motor function: mild choreoathetosis; slight motor delay and clumsiness.

Visual function: normal.

Auditory function: moderate high tone deafness; impaired hearing.

Language function: appears normal.

Learning: at level for age.

'Drive' and powers of concentration: appear good.
Emotional state: a happy responsive child.
Social health: physical environment; good housing community facilities; good relationship with others in his family; accepting parents, with warm relations with child.

Planning and initiating the overall care of the child derives from going through the diagnostic profile and considering whether any help can be proffered in any of these various fields. The plan is discussed in full with the parents and we try to think of some practical way in which they can help their child at this particular time. We also discuss with them others who may be involved in further diagnostic work or therapy. The work of individuals—other than the paediatrician—involved with children with communication difficulties are reviewed elsewhere in this book.

The paediatrician will often have a rôle in helping the parents understand the advice they are getting from another expert. Thus, after seeing the orthopaedic surgeon the parents of a child with cerebral palsy may well want to discuss the operation he suggests with the paediatrician. Sometimes the paediatrician may have to help the parents in another way and the following case is an example.

The parents of I.E., a blind disturbed 4-year-old child, were worried about his failure to speak and took him to a speech-hearing clinic at another hospital. The child was reported as being profoundly deaf and in need of a teacher of the deaf. According to the parents, when ear-phones had been placed on the child he had become disturbed and had only responded to a drum-beat. Their own paediatrician commented that he had sat in their home and had often watched the child responding to soft sounds: he wondered whether they could not confirm this themselves. Later the parents rang him back to say that they had done so: the child would come to the whispered word 'Sweet' and when sweet papers were rustled. The parents agreed with the paediatrician that the child was not profoundly deaf. In this particular instance the paediatrician was unable to exclude some deafness as the child was hard to test formally, but we still do not believe that deafness plays a major part in this child's problem.

Approach to the Child

The paediatrician, with his skill in getting the child to respond rather rapidly in a clinical situation, may be able to help the specialist who sees few children. If the child's communication abilities, his response to sounds and his own speech and language are to be studied, the child must co-operate with the examining doctor and his own. The examining doctor must therefore know how to get young children to carry out certain tasks for him. At 6 months the child is not usually frightened of strangers and will smile and laugh at the doctor, but by 8-10 months jany children are more sophisticated and if the examiner unwisely bends down towards the child and thrusts his large, adult face at him, the child may begin to cry. Throughout the rest of of the child's life (both childhood and adulthood), his social responsiveness towards the friendly approaches of strangers varies in relation to his experience of them and the development of his own 'personality'. It is very common for children to go through a period sometime between the ages of 15 months and 3 years when they are

173

very shy of strangers but if the examiner sees them again after six months they have often moved out of this stage. It is useful to remember, however, some of the things which put children off. They do not like being stared at by adults (the more adults present the more uneasy a shy child will feel). They do not like people talking down at them from a great height. They do not like being poked or prodded or even having strange objects placed on their bodies, *e.g.* stethoscopes and tape measures. They usually dislike lying on their backs with somebody strange bending over them. They like to become accustomed to a new physical environment and new people. All these features of children's social responsiveness are against the physician who wants to examine the child as rapidly as possible and pass on to his next case.

There are certain characteristics of children which will help him. Two and 3-year-olds are very conscious of adults who are within 5 or 6 feet of them, but if the adult moves 10 feet away the child seems to become less aware of him and will play quite happily. If the doctor watches the child from the other side of the room he may be able to observe a whole range of activities which the child will not perform if the examiner is standing too close to him, or, if the child does not wish to take objects from the doctor or communicate with him, he may well communicate through his mother even if he has heard the doctor giving the mother instructions. (Thus, if you ask the child to give you an object from the table in order to test his comprehension, he may take no notice of you: when the mother asks him to get her something he may do it. The doctor has to see that the mother does not add clues that will help the child carry out the intended action. If the mother says 'get me a cup from the table' and at the same time points to the cup, the examiner cannot be certain that the child comprehended the statement or merely followed the mother's guiding finger and picked up the object pointed to.)

With older children at school, the shyness or social difficulty may take the form of total refusal to do anything. It is often possible to trick the child into carrying out some action at the examiner's request after which the child may continue to respond. Thus, you can lift the child's hands up in the air at the same time telling him to lift his hands and put them down. Usually the child will automatically lower his hands and then you can point out to him that he has in fact obeyed one of your instructions. After a little of this simple sort of play he may suddenly start to co-operate. If the child refuses to perform a relatively difficult task, another trick in this situation is to move back to a simpler task suitable to a younger child. For example, the 5-year-old child who refuses to draw will often agree to play with one inch cubes (suitable in the examination of 2-to 3-year-olds) and then slowly start to carry out tests appropriate to his age. Again, where speech cannot be elicited in the clinic, the ideal situation is to observe the child in his own classroom with an adult familiar to him, such as his teacher, who will usually be able to get him to talk without too much difficulty.

The other main group of school children who are difficult to examine are the uninhibited, highly active ones who will not co-operate with the doctor. At this age, although the child is apparently so uninhibited in his strange surroundings, he will be less happy in the absence of a familiar adult and if he is briefly taken to another clinic room without his parents, may well quieten down quickly and even strike a bargain to behave if he is allowed to return to his mother. Although all these points may seem very simple and naive, we have frequently seen doctors fail to elicit speech and language from children because they do not pay attention to the social relationship with the child. The doctor may talk to the mother perhaps when the family first enter the room, but he should have his eyes on the child all the time and be quick to take the opportunity to make social contact, such as observing that the child is looking interestedly at a toy and making a gesture to him that he may handle it. Avoid confrontation at all times. Look at a book with the child from behind. Don't ask him directly to do something that he has already indicated he does not want to do, but ask him to do another task which seems quite different but which involves the same skills. If he begins to be anxious during the course of the examination, get up and talk casually to another person, appearing for the moment to have lost interest in the child. This will give him a period in which to relax and (although you *are* interested) perhaps he will gain the impression that you don't really mind whether he does the task you have allotted him or not.

The doctor is still something of a mythical figure in our society and children will often have been impressed by the importance which their parents attach to the consultation. An articulate 5-year-old recently commented to the doctor, 'I'm sweating because of coming to see you'. He asked to rest at one point in the examination because he was exhausted, but his parents and teachers reassured the doctor that with other adults he was a relaxed and happy child. It is the doctor's task to impress on the child that although he thinks it is important to see his 'guest' there is no alarming ritual to be gone through, he merely wishes the child to play and talk to him in the way the child would to a friend of the same age. The doctor has to alter his behaviour to accommodate his guest and not the other way round.

REFERENCES

Egan, D. F., Illingworth, R. S., Mac Keith, R. C. (1969) *Developmental Screening at 0-5 years.* Clinics in Developmental Medicine, No. 30. London: S.I.M.P. with Heinemann.
Wasz-Höckert, O., Lind, J., Vuorenski, V., Partanen, T., Valenne, E. (1968) *The Infant Cry: A Spectographic and Auditory Analysis.* Clinics in Developmental Medicine, No. 29. London: S.I.M.P. with Heinemann.

CHAPTER 15

The Effects of Language Delay on Development

MICHAEL RUTTER

The possession of a complex code of language symbols used for communication marks man as different from other species. If language can be regarded as one of the main features which constitutes what it means to be human, then it might be expected that a retardation in the development of language would have far-reaching consequences in terms of its effects on other aspects of development.

Language and Thinking

As a large proportion of what is generally regarded as intelligence involves the use of language, it may be appropriate to start by examining the effects of language on intellectual growth.

Thinking has been regarded as nothing but subaudible speech—that is, you had to have words in order to think. That is now seen as a nonsensical suggestion. There are ample studies, such as those of the deaf, which clearly indicate that thinking does not require words (Furth 1966). However, it may still be that words to some extent shape our thoughts. For example, Whorf (1956) suggested that the language of a particular society influences the thinking of individual members of that society. Thus, Eskimos have many words for different types of snow and they think of snow in terms of subtle distinctions (essential for their way of life) which never enter our thinking at all. We have just one word for snow. Similar connections can be seen in the way that different cultures name colours or shapes. There is evidence that, to a minor extent, the way in which we conceptualise and think about our environment and experiences is influenced by the words we have available (Carroll and Casagrande 1958, Stefflie et al. 1966, Lenneberg 1967), This is relevant to the deaf child who may have difficulty in certain sorts of abstraction and conceptualisation (especially in thinking about emotions and feelings) because of the relative poverty of gestural language as a medium of communicating subtle ideas (Lewis 1963, 1968, Fry 1964). Language skills undoubtedly influence the ease with which concepts are formed (Carroll 1964) but concepts may certainly be achieved in the absence of relevant words.

Russian psychologists, especially Vygotsky (1962) and Luria (1957, 1961), have urged the importance of spoken language in the organisation of experience and the formation of thought processes, and hence in the regulation of behaviour. The existence of spoken language allows the establishment of internal mechanisms of thinking which make humans more than a reflex organism. They have carried out a series of experiments which show that learning a task may be facilitated by the child speaking aloud what he has to do. For example, children more rapidly learn to press a button to a red light when they say as they do so, 'I have to press for a red light and not for a green' (Luria 1961).

However, it is not just the word that matters but rather the multiple thought connections that language provides. Thus, in another experiment, toddlers had to learn to select a doll from an array of toys (Razran 1961). One group were given sentences which merely labelled the object, *e.g.* 'Here's a doll'. In contrast, the second group were given sentences which referred to the doll in terms of what could be done with it, *e.g.* 'Rock the doll', 'Dress the doll'. This group who had been given a variety of attributes of the doll were better in learning which object in the array of toys was a doll, presumably because their language experience had enabled them to build up a *concept* of what is a doll rather than having to rely on rote memory of the object to which the label 'doll' had been applied.

American experimenters have been concerned also with the rôle of language as a mediator in the learning of concepts and in the solution of conceptual problems (Bruner 1964, Bruner *et al.* 1966, Blank 1968). It has been found that language is frequently an aid in the learning of generalised ideas, such as the concept of 'the bigger one', and furthermore that language may make it easier to shift from one concept to the opposite one, *e.g.* from 'biggest' to 'smallest' (Kuenne 1946, Kendler and Kendler 1962). However, language is not essential for this type of learning as it can be found in animals (Paul 1965). Furthermore, language may occasionally be a hindrance by encouraging the child to stick with an idea which no longer applies (O'Connor and Hermelin 1959).

Language is only one element in the development of logical thought (Piaget 1950) but it is an important element (Inhelder and Piaget 1964). We may take it as established that language is an aid to many, but not all, sorts of learning. However, the mechanisms involved remain obscure (Herriott 1970) and so far most of the studies have not differentiated between language competence and the ability to produce spoken language. To make this distinction we have to turn to investigation of two particular handicaps—deafness and infantile autism.

Language and Thinking in Deaf Children

Most severely deaf children are greatly handicapped in both the understanding and production of spoken language. On the other hand, their potential at birth for language competence should be normal when no brain defect is involved. In fact, as they grow older their language competence falls somewhat below normal because gestural language is so much more limited in scope than spoken language. The development of any form of intelligence, including language competence, requires *experience* as well as biological potential for its development and in this respect deaf children are handicapped. Because of the discrepancy in deaf children between their language competence (which is fairly good) and their spoken language (which is very poor), they provide a useful opportunity to see which faculty is necessary for intelligence.

In general, deaf children perform as well as normal children on puzzle-type tasks and slightly below normal on tests involving concepts (Lenneberg 1967, Furth 1964, 1966). It seems also that where deaf children perform poorly it is sometimes partly due to their lack of experience rather than their lack of ability. In other words, spoken language is important not so much in its own right but rather because its use greatly enlarges a person's experience and hence his opportunities for learning. In identical twin pairs in which one twin is deaf and the other hearing, the deaf twin usually lags slightly behind the hearing twin in intellectual development (Rainer *et al.* 1963). However, Furth (1966) quotes one case where this was not so and attributes the good intellectual development of the deaf twin to the fact that deaf parents provided ample communication in early childhood by means of manual signs including finger spelling. This is just one case, but other studies also suggest that in deaf children it is most important to provide rich *communication* in early childhood (see below). At this stage, gesture frequently offers more than speech. It is often thought by teachers of the deaf that the use of gesture will inhibit the development of spoken language but there is no evidence that this is the case. Communication should be encouraged in whatever medium seems most appropriate at the time. *Language* is what is needed and although spoken language is certainly the richest of the language media it is a disservice to the deaf child to rely on it exclusively.

Language and Thinking in Autistic Children

Studies of autistic children also throw light on the rôle of language in thinking. Autism is usually thought of as a disorder of social relationships but research over the last 5 or 10 years has shown that it is more reasonable to consider autism primarily as a disorder of language and thinking (Rutter 1968, Rutter *et al.* 1971). Hermelin and O'Connor (1970) found that autistic children have a serious and widespread cognitive deficit in relation to language processes. They lack language competence or 'inner language'. If 'inner language' is required for conceptual thought, autistic children should be seriously deficient in this respect. So far, only a limited range of cognitive tasks have been examined but the results are quite consistent. Autistic children may perform at a normal level on puzzle-type tasks but, if the task involves even the simplest sort of concept, the children do very badly in spite of the tests requiring *no speech whatsoever* (Lockyer and Rutter 1970). Thus they are usually unable to put a short series of pictures into an order which tells a story. It seems that although language *production* is not necessary for conceptual thought, a language *capacity is* needed. Unfortunately there have been scarcely any psychological studies of children with developmental language disorders—a glaring gap in our knowledge which urgently needs to be filled. From the very meagre findings available it appears that children with a developmental language disorder show a rather similar cognitive performance to deaf children—that is to say on conceptual tasks they perform a little, but not much, below normal (O'Connor and Hermelin 1965, Blank and Bridger 1966, Eisenson 1968, Weiner 1969). However, the studies have not differentiated receptive and executive language disorders so that it would be extremely hazardous to draw any firm conclusions.

Children with autism and children with a severe developmental language disorder have recently been compared using detailed observations and testing of the children together with an extensive parental interview (Rutter *et al.* 1971). It was found that the non-autistic children even, when there was *receptive* disorder, did *not* have a global language deficit. Unlike the autistic child who did have a global language impairment, the child with a developmental receptive language disorder usually had fair skills in gestural communication and his play activities and test performance suggested the availability of 'inner language'.

178

Many of the facts are still not available, but it seems reasonable to suppose that the intellectual development of children with a purely *executive* language disorder should be near-normal, whereas that of children with a *receptive* language disorder should show some impairment in conceptual thought, but far less than that of autistic children who are grossly handicapped in this respect.

Much further research is required, particularly with regard to the psychological development of children with a developmental language disorder. Nevertheless, it is evident that spoken language is of very little *direct* importance in the development of thought and intelligence. On the other hand, the understanding of language and the availability of 'inner language' are important because they facilitate the development of concepts, and concepts aid the organisation of our thoughts. In addition, language usage in some medium (be it written, gestured or spoken) is of great importance *indirectly* though its rôle in widening experience. Intelligence requires experience if it is to develop, just as the body requires food for growth (Eisenberg 1967). In our care of children with language disorders, we need to make sure from infancy that we do all we can to aid the development of language in all media and that we provide the opportunities for learning that might otherwise be lost because of the language handicap.

Language and Play Activities

In turning next to the effects of language retardation on play activities, the distinction between language comprehension and language usage is again important. If, as the evidence indicates, 'inner language' is needed for the normal development of thought processes, we might expect to see a similar effect on imaginative play activities which are the outward sign of a child's inner thought. And we do.

Luria and Yudovich (1959) have described a most interesting study concerning a pair of 5-year-old identical twin boys who had limited language comprehension and were able to say only a few words. Their play was primitive and monotonous, there were no constructive activities, no pretend games and their drawings were without recognisable meaning. As their language improved over the next 10 months their play activities changed. Constructional play, pretend games, and modelling with plasticine began, and their following of rules in group games improved. Furthermore, these imaginative play activities were said to improve most in the twin who received language therapy and whose language improved earlier.

If it was speaking as such which led to the development of imaginative play, the play of young deaf children should be markedly concrete and lacking in dramatic qualities, but, in fact, this is not the case. Pre-school deaf children love make-believe games and constructional play and their drawings are as good as those of other children (Lenneberg 1967), although as they grow older their play may remain somewhat more restricted than that of others (Heider and Heider 1941).

Mentally retarded children and children with a developmental language disorder do not show any marked differences from normal children in their overall play patterns, but children with impaired language do engage somewhat less in *symbolic* play (Hulme and Lunzer 1966, Lovell *et al*. 1968). Furthermore, there is a relationship between the complexity of language and the amount of symbolic play (Lovell *et al*. 1968).

Children with *receptive* language disorders are often delayed in their development of imaginative play activities, but the one group who are *very* severely handicapped in make-believe play are autistic children (Bartak and Rutter, in preparation). The comparative study of autistic children and children with a severe developmental language disorder, showed that even in autistic children of normal non-verbal intelligence, creative and imaginative play was grossly impaired. Autistic children, at least when young, do not engage in make-believe games, their drawings and models are primitive and lack imagination and they are unable to participate in group games or follow the rules of games.

More than anyone else, Sheridan (1969) has emphasised the importance of assessing a child's imitative skills and play activities when evaluating language development. She has recently constructed a 'common objects' and 'miniature toy' test which is used to determine whether a child comprehends the function of objects and whether he can use them to develop make-believe games. Such play activities probably offer a most useful guide to a child's 'inner language' and basic language competence and hence may provide an item of some predictive value with respect to later language development. Also, it may be that treatment which encourages the development of imitation and of imaginative play activities actually aids the child's skills in language production (Sheridan 1969).

Of course, any improvement in play activities is worthwhile in its own right. The language retarded child who is impaired in his symbolic play is likely to be handicapped in his relationships with other children. Group games involving make-believe (playing families, schools, shops and hospitals) are a very important part of social relationships at age 4 to 6 years and the child who cannot participate is at a considerable disadvantage in making social contacts. Make-believe play serves many functions, as a means of exploring feelings, lessening fears, increasing excitement, understanding an event by re-enacting it, confirming a memory, altering a stressful happening to make it pleasant in fantasy, and as a method of rehearsing and so developing social skills (Adams 1967, Millar 1968).

Language and Reading

There are several different language media, one of which is written language. It is important to recognise that reading is both a perceptual skill (a child must be able to recognise the difference between 'b' and 'd' and between 'm' and 'n' in order to read) and a language skill. Words constitute a system of symbols and that is one of the hallmarks of language. To understand the *meaning* of what he reads (and without meaning reading is an empty useless activity), a child must have language skills.

Thus, children who are delayed in talking are likely also to be delayed in reading, because both reflect language impairment. Ingram and his colleagues in Edinburgh have followed a group of speech retarded youngsters into ordinary primary schools and have found that the majority have difficulties in learning to read (Ingram 1963, Mason 1967). Children with more severe language handicaps at special schools have also been found to have pronounced reading difficulties (Canning and Davies-Eysenck 1966, Griffiths 1969).

Looked at from the other end, the results are similar. Numerous studies have shown that older children with severe reading difficulties frequently have a history of speech delay and many still show language impairment and verbal deficiencies in abstract thinking (Blank *et al*. 1968, Rutter *et al*. 1970*a*). Furthermore, there is some evidence that within a group of children with reading disability those with language impairment may have a worse prognosis (Lytton 1968).

Children who have difficulties solely in speech (that is in the articulation of words) also often have difficulties in learning to read (Crookes and Green 1963). However, in their case the difficulties probably stem from problems in perception (learning which letter is which) rather than from problems in learning a written *language*. Preliminary findings suggest that their educational difficulties are less persistent and widespread than those of children with language retardation (Crookes and Greene 1963, Griffiths 1969).

Because most children who are late in talking ultimately speak normally, there is a tendency to assume that speech delay is of no consequence in most cases. These findings emphasise how mistaken this view is. Although most children catch-up in their speaking, many are left with subtle language handicaps which may continue to impede their educational progress. The association between speech delay and later reading retardation is quite strong.

This association is the strongest of all the psychological effects of speech delay and perhaps the most important. The educational implications of reading failure need no emphasis. As Burt (1950) pointed out, most teaching in schools is by the blackboard or the textbook and the child who cannot read is thereby severely handicapped. If he cannot understand what is written on the broad or printed in his books he is likely to fall increasingly behind in other subjects as well.

One point of concern with regard to the education of children with language handicaps is that several studies have suggested that some children who have made good progress in special schools fall behind after transfer to ordinary schools (Ministry of Education 1963, Griffiths 1969). This is a point returned to later in the chapter after considering social, emotional and behavioural development.

Social, Emotional and Behavioural Development

The frequency with which speech disordered children show abnormalities in emotional development has been commented on by many writers. Ingram (1959), in his important study of young children with developmental speech disorders, noted that out of a group of 80 children, 10 were having psychiatric treatment. The commonest complaint was of withdrawn and solitary behaviour but also the children were often found to be dependent and immature. They resented being left alone and reacted to frustration by temper tantrums or tears. Among those with severe comprehension difficulties an unawareness of the environment and an inability to make relationships sometimes closely resembled the behaviour of autistic children. Myklebust (1954) has made similar observations.

Deaf children are often described as socially immature, lacking in self-confidence and initiative, together with a poor toleration of frustration and a poor control of their feelings (Lewis 1968). In a study of children attending schools for the deaf (Ministry of

181

Education 1964) it was found that 12 per cent were maladjusted (a rate probably above that in the general population).

In order to find out how language retardation affects personality development, we need systematic comparisons between language retarded children and children in the general population. The effects of different types of language handicap must then be studied separately. Unfortunately such comparisons are very few and far between (Goodstein 1958, Lewis 1968).

Sociometric studies of children with speech impediments show that those with a mild defect are only slightly less popular than other children (Perrin 1954, Freeman and Sonnega 1956, Marge 1966). On the other hand, mothers' reports suggest that speech defective children are more often maladjusted than controls and in particular are fearful, tense, anxious and do not make friends easily (Solomon 1961). The issue can also be examined the other way round by seeing how often psychiatrically ill children show speech defects. In an investigation of 10-and 11-year-old boys, those with psychiatric disorders had twice as many speech difficulties as boys in the general population (as judged by parental and teachers' reports). The difference for girls was less (Rutter *et al.* 1970*a*).

These findings refer to children with a *speech* disorder. With respect to *language* impairment, information is again very limited but some data are available from the Isle of Wight studies. In a very small group of language retarded children, 4 out of 9 had a neurotic disorder and in the small number of partially deaf children studied the rate of psychiatric disorder was nearly twice that in the general population (Rutter *et al.* 1970*b*).

For findings on children with a more severe language impairment, it is necessary to turn to a similar study of neuro-epileptic children (Rutter *et al.* 1970*b*). Within a group of children all of whom had epilepsy, cerebral palsy or some similar condition, emotional and behavioural abnormalities were twice as common in those who were markedly impaired in their use of spoken language.

Wing (1969) used a detailed parental questionnaire to determine the occurrence of autistic features in children with various other handicaps. She found that impaired social relationships (of an autistic type) had been present at some time in most children with 'developmental receptive aphasia' but in only a few of those with purely executive problems.

Rutter *et al.* (1971) showed that most children with receptive language disorders showed *few* autistic manifestations at age 5 to 7 years. But an appreciable minority had shown impaired personal relationships when younger and in some cases the children had shown a syndrome indistinguishable from infantile autism. Similar cases have been reported by others (*e.g.* Berg 1961). Obviously, the important question is what distinguishes this subgroup of children with a receptive language disorder who appear indubitably autistic at 3 to 4 years of age but who show little evidence of autism some 3 years later. The number of carefully studied children is much too small for any confident answer to be given, but it would seem that this phenomenon is usually seen in children who show a severe global impairment in both 'inner language' and language comprehension from which they recover (at least in part) as they grow older. Thus, when young they do not play imaginatively or use gesture but as they

182

approach school-age these skills develop and the autistic traits diminish or disappear. This most interesting subgroup of children undoubtedly merits further study.

In both autism and developmental receptive language disorder there is a serious delay in language, but in autism, unlike developmental disorders, there are also serious social and behavioural abnormalities. Although no final answer is yet available, the reason probably lies in differences in the *extent* and *severity* of language impairment. The child with a receptive language disorder has a defect in both the understanding and production of spoken language but he has a reasonable proficiency in gestural language and his 'inner language' capacity is near-normal. The autistic child, however, is handicapped in *all* aspects of language and because of this in many cognitive functions as well. Note that there are areas (particularly motor development) in which the child with a developmental receptive language disorder is more handicapped, so that the nature of the handicap is important in the development of autism. The parental characteristics of the two groups of children are generally similar with the one curious exception that autistic children more often come from middle-class and professional families. Autism probably develops in relation to a severe defect in all aspects of language functions. Transient autistic features are seen in some children with a developmental language disorder, usually when there is a particularly severe defect in language comprehension together with some impairment of 'inner language'.

To summarise what has been said so far on language retardation and emotional development, children with speech defects show a slight excess of social and emotional problems compared with the general population. These problems are rather more common where there is also language impairment, and autistic-type difficulties are probably only seen where there is a severe defect in language comprehension.

To understand better the *reasons* for these emotional and social difficulties, we require evidence on the circumstances of their association with language retardation. The first point to note is that studies of deaf, retarded and normal children all show that there is only a very weak relationship between the severity of language disorder and the frequency of emotional problems (Lewis 1968, Graham 1970). This emphasises that the psychological ill-effects of language impairment are indirect rather than direct.

This conclusion is also supported by Miss Johnson's study of 33 deaf children transferred from special schools to ordinary schools (Ministry of Education 1963) which showed that in about half the cases transfers were followed by serious problems. Most of the children found the change of school bewildering and unsettling. Their speech defects had sometimes led to teasing and unhappiness. Difficulty in following classroom teaching caused falling standards in school work in some children, especially those with poor reading skills. Worry and discouragement then followed. But perhaps most striking was the children's loneliness and social isolation. Because of their deficiencies in spoken language and in their understanding of conversations, few had joined in school club activities. It was noteworthy that these difficulties tended to be most marked in secondary schools.

It is important not to get these findings out of balance. In some cases the transfer worked well—particularly where there was good intelligence, a useful degree of hearing, reasonable competence in spoken language and well-developed reading skills. The child's personality characteristics were also important: not surprisingly children adjusted most easily when they were confident, self-sufficient and determined to succeed.

Another relevant study is Meadow's (1968) comparison of deaf children reared by hearing parents, and deaf children reared by deaf parents. In almost all respects the deaf children brought up by deaf parents were better adjusted in terms of sociability, popularity, emotional responses, willingness to communicate with strangers and lack of communicative frustration. They wrote better English compositions and their achievements in school work were greater. Only in speech and lip-reading ability were there no differences.

This is an important finding—the more so because at first sight one might expect the opposite. It demonstrates that the personality difficulties shown by some deaf children are not a *necessary* consequence of deafness. Why it was better for the deaf children to have deaf parents is not known with certainty but probably the important reasons were: (a) deaf parents were more accepting of a deaf child, and (b) they communicated better and earlier with the child by means of signs and gestures. Early *oral* training is most important for the emergence of speech, but manual communication does not discourage speech development. On the contrary, communication skills in one medium probably facilitate the development of skills in any other language medium.

The last study to be mentioned in this connection is Griffith's (1969) study of language retarded children who had attended John Horniman school. She found that children who had appeared happy, confident and well adjusted at the residential school for children with language impairment sometimes showed serious maladjustment after they left, especially in secondary school. Where they went on to another special school, however, this occurred less often in spite of the fact that these children were more handicapped in language.

What can be learnt from these three studies in each of which language handicapped children made better progress in 'abnormal' environments, namely special schools, and families where the parents were deaf? Obviously, it would be foolish in the extreme to conclude that all language retarded children should remain in specialised environments where they encounter only children with similar handicaps. This is foolish because our ultimate aim is to enable the children to live among ordinary people when they leave school, so that the transition has to be made sometime. A few children may always require a sheltered setting but for most the question is not *whether* to transfer to an ordinary environment but rather *how* and *when*? We do not yet know if it is better earlier or later in childhood, but merely postponing the transfer provides no solution.

Conclusions

In considering how psychological difficulties might be reduced, it is necessary to briefly review some of the possible reasons why language retarded children have a higher rate of these than do other children.

The first point is to get the perspective right: most children with language difficulties do *not* show abnormalities in social and emotional development. Although the rate of emotional difficulties is higher than in the general population, only a minority of the children are affected. Secondly, although the psychological problems tend to be more frequent in children with the most severe language handicaps, this is not a very strong relationship and it is clear that language retardation does not *directly* lead to emotional problems.

There are at least five different ways in which language retardation *indirectly* leads to emotional and behavioural difficulties: through educational failure, through the effects of communication difficulties in social relationships, through lack of social integration, through the effects of teasing and rejection by other children and through associated brain dysfunction.

Some types of language retardation are due to abnormalities in brain function which may be associated with temperamental differences making the child less resilient and more susceptible to the usual stresses of growing up (Rutter *et al.* 1970b). In this case, the language impairment is important only through its association with a more general defect in brain functioning. This mechanism probably accounts for no more than a small minority of the psychological difficulties.

Children with oddities of any kind tend to be particularly prone to teasing, and handicapped children are generally less popular than other children. As unpopularity is associated with emotional difficulties (Rutter *et al.* 1970b) this may be one partial explanation for the problems of language retarded children. Incidently, it may also be one reason why some children are better adjusted in special schools where they do not stand out as different from others.

A lack of social integration may be important in several different ways. Children's behaviour is much influenced by their self-image. When they see themselves as capable, self-sufficient, interesting and attractive people they are more likely to behave in ways which fulfil that self-expectation. Where parents are distressed, bewildered and un-certain about their child's handicap, the child himself is likely to sense this and view himself negatively. Similarly, where parents are unduly over-protective, the child may not learn to be confident and able to look after himself. All parents need help in adjusting to the birth of a handicapped child and need knowledge on what is realistic to expect of him and what things to do to help him. In the absence of such help and instruction, early diagnosis may even be positively disadvantageous by increasing parental distress (Williams 1968, 1970).

Later on, the difficulties posed by lack of social integration may be seen with the language retarded child in the ordinary school. Teachers frequently have not been taught or told how to help a child with language problems or hearing impairment. They may have inappropriate expectations of him, and may assume that he can fend for himself socially when in fact he needs help to do so. Social isolation is not inevitable, but its prevention does require greater knowledge of ordinary teachers than they usually possess. This is *not* a plea for putting children with mild handicaps into special schools—that is undesirable for many reasons, and certainly uneconomic. What is necessary is that the skills of the special school be transmitted to the ordinary school, perhaps by greater use of specialised peripatetic teachers.

Children need to communicate in order to make friends as has already been mentioned. The two groups who most need special help in this connection are deaf

185

children and autistic children. The severity of the language handicap in the autistic child means that enormous ingenuity and persistence are needed if ways of communicating with him are to be found.

Lastly, there is the importance of educational difficulties which constitute the one handicap *directly* related to language retardation. There is a strong association between reading retardation and anti-social behaviour (Clark 1970, Rutter *et al.* 1970*a*). The nature of the association suggests that in some cases the educational failure may be a contributory factor in the causation of anti-social disorders (Rutter *et al.* 1970*a*). For children with the most severe language handicaps special education is needed and it is not necessary to comment further on the appalling shortage of such schools. Undoubtedly, more are needed. However, most children with language disorders will need to be educated in ordinary schools. The studies already discussed make it clear that if this is to be a success there must be better arrangements there for teaching language retarded children. It is not just a question of a difficulty in speaking but also it is a disorder of language which is likely to make the acquisition of reading skills more difficult than for normal children.

The psychological difficulties of language retarded children are in part intrinsic, but in larger part secondary, to the way in which they are dealt with by society, and are therefore potentially preventable. The two most important implications are the need for early communication by whatever medium seems appropriate and the need for adequate educational provision in both ordinary and special schools.

REFERENCES

Adams, D. K. (1967) 'The development of social behavior.' *in* Brackbill, Y. (Ed.) *Infancy and Early Childhood.* New York: The Free Press. p. 397.

Berg, I. S. (1961) 'A case study of developmental auditory imperception: some theoretical implications.' *J. Child Psychol. Psychiat.*, **2**, 86.

Blank, M. (1968) 'Experimental approaches to concept development in young children.' *in* Lunzer E. A., Morris, J. F. (Eds.) *Development in Human Learning.* London: Staples Press. p. 68.

—— Bridger, W. H. (1966) 'Conceptual cross-modal transfer in deaf and hearing children.' *Child Develop.*, **37**, 29.

—— Weider, S., Bridger, W. H. (1968) 'Verbal deficiencies in abstract thinking in early reading retardation.' *Amer. J. Orthopsychiat.*, **38**, 823.

Bruner, J. S. (1964) 'The course of cognitive growth.' *Amer. Psychol.*, **19**, 1.

—— Oliver, R. R., Greenfield, P. M. (1966) *Studies in Cognitive Growth.* New York: Wiley.

Burt, C. (1950) *The Backward Child (3rd Edition).* London: University of London Press.

Canning, A., Davies-Eysenck, M. (1966) 'An attempt at analysis of developmental disorders of language and articulation.' *De Therapia Vocis et Loquelae*, **1**, 35.

Carroll, J. B. (1964) *Language and Thought.* Englewood Cliffs, N. J.: Prentice-Hall.

—— Casagrande, J. B. (1958) 'The function of language classifications in behavior.' *in* Maccoby, E. E., Newcomb, T. M., Hartle, E. L. (Eds.) *Readings in Social Psychology.* London: Methuen. p. 18.

Clark, M. M. (1970) *Reading Difficulties in Schools.* London: Penguin Books.

Crookes, T. G., Green, M. C. L. (1963) 'Some characteristics of children with two types of speech disorder.' *Brit. J. educ. Psychol.*, **33**, 31.

Eisenson, J. (1968) 'Developmental aphasia (dyslogia). A postulation of a unitary concept of the disorder.' *Cortex*, **4**, 184.

Eisenberg, L. (1967) 'Clinical consideration in the psychiatric evaluation of intelligence.' *in* Zubin, J., Jervis, G. A. (Eds.) *Psychopathology of Mental Development.* New York: Grune & Stratton. p. 502.

Freeman, G. G., Sonnega, J. A. (1956) 'Peer evaluation of children in speech correction class.' *J. speech Disord.*, **21**, 179.

Fry, C. (1964) 'Language problems in profoundly deaf children.' *in* Renfrew, C., Murphy, K. (Eds.) *The Child who does not Talk.* Clinics in Developmental Medicine, No. 13. London: S.I.M.P. with Heinemann. p. 117.

Furth, H. G. (1964) 'Research with the deaf: implications for language and cognition.' *Psychol.*, *Bull.*, **62**, 154.
—— (1966) *Thinking without Language*. London: Collier-Macmillan.
Goodstein, L. D. (1958) 'Functional speech disorders and personality: a survey of the research.' *J. speech Res.*, **1**, 359.
Graham, N. C. (1970) *The Language of Educationally Subnormal Children*. Final Report to the Department of Education and Science.
Griffiths, C. P. S. (1969) 'A follow-up study of children with disorders of speech.' *Brit. J. Disord. Commun.*, **4**, 46.
Heider, F., Heider, G. M. (1941) 'Studies in the psychology of the deaf: the language and social behaviour of young deaf children.' *Psychol. Monogr.*, no. 242.
Hermelin, B., O'Connor, N. (1970) *Psychological Experiments with Autistic Children*. Oxford: Pergamon.
Herriott, P. (1970) *An Introduction to the Psychology of Language*. London: Methuen.
Hulme, I., Lunzer, E. A. (1966) 'Play, language and reasoning in subnormal children.' *J. child Psychol. Psychiat.*, **7**, 107.
Ingram, T. T. S. (1959) 'Specific developmental disorders of speech in childhood.' *Brain*, **82**, 450.
—— (1963) 'Delayed development of speech with special reference to dyslexia.' *Proc. roy. Soc. Med.*, **56**, 199.
Inhelder, B., Piaget, J. (1964) *The Early Growth of Logic in the Child*. London: Routledge & Kegan Paul.
Kendler, H. H., Kendler, T. S. (1962) 'Vertical and horizontal processes in problem solving.' *Psychol. Rev.*, **69**, 1.
Kuenne, M. R. (1946) 'Experimental investigation of the relation of language to transposition behavior in young children.' *J. exp. Psychol.*, **36**, 471.
Lenneberg, E. H. (1967) *Biological Foundations of Language*. New York: Wiley.
Lewis, M. M. (1963) *Language, Thought and Personality in Infancy and Childhood*. London: Harrap.
——(1968) *Language and Personality in Deaf Children*. Slough: N.F.E.R.
Lockyer, L., Rutter, M. (1970) 'A five to fifteen year follow-up study of infantile psychosis. IV. Patterns of cognitive ability.' *Brit. J. soc. clin. Psychol.*, **9**, 152.
Lovell, K., Hoyle, H. W., Siddall, M. Q. (1968) 'A study of some aspects of the play and language of young children with delayed speech.' *J. Child. Psychol. Psychiat.*, **9**, 41.
Luria, A. R. (1957) 'The role of language in the formation of temporary connections. *in* Simon, B.. (Ed.) *Psychology in the Soviet Union*. London: Routledge & Kegan Paul. p. 115.
—— (1961) *The Role of Speech in the Regulation of Normal and Abnormal Behaviour*. Oxford: Pergamon.
—— Yudovich, F. (1959) *Speech and the Development of Mental Processes in the Child*. London: Staples Press.
Lytton, H. (1968) 'Some psychological and sociological characteristics of "good" and "poor" achievers (boys) in remedial reading groups: clinical case studies.' *Hum. Develop.*, **11**, 260.
Marge, D. K. (1966) 'The social status of speech handicapped children.' *J. speech Res.*, **9**, 165.
Mason, A. W. (1967) 'Specific (developmental) dyslexia.' *Develop. Med. Child. Neurol*, **9**, 183.
Meadow, K. P. (1968) 'Toward a developmental understanding of deafness.' *J. Rehab. Deaf*, **2**, 1.
Millar, S. (1968) *The Psychology of Play*. London: Penguin Books.
Ministry of Education (1963) *Report on a Survey of Deaf Children who have been Transferred from Special Schools or Units to Ordinary Schools*. London: H.M.S.O.
—— (1964) 'Survey of children born in 1947 who were in schools for the deaf in 1962-63,' *in The Health of the School Child: Report of the Chief Medical Officer of the Department of Education and Science for the years 1962 and 1963*. London: H.M.S.O. p. 60
Myklebust, H. (1954) *Auditory Disorders in Children*. New York: Grune & Stratton.
O'Connor, N., Hermelin, B. (1959) 'Discrimination and reversal learning in imbeciles.' *J. abnorm. soc. Psychol.*, **59**, 409.
—— —— (1965) 'Visual analogies of verbal operations.' *Lang. Speech*, **8**, 197.
Paul, C. (1965) 'Effects of overlearning upon single habit reversal in rats.' *Psychol. Bull.*, **63**, 65.
Perrin, E. W. (1954) 'The social position of the speech defective child.' *J. speech. Disord.*, **19**, 250.
Piaget, J. (1950) *The Psychology of Intelligence*. London: Routledge & Kegan Paul.
Rainer, J. D., Altshuler, K. Z., Kallman, F. J., Deming, W. E. (1963) *Family and Mental Health Problems in a Deaf Population*. New York: New York State Psychiatric Institute.
Razran, G. (1961) 'The observable unconscious and the inferable conscious in current Soviet psychophysiology; interoceptive conditioning, semantic conditioning, and the orienting reflex.' *Psychol. Rev.*, **68**, 81.
Rutter, M. (1968) 'Concepts of autism: a review of research.' *J. Child Psychol. Psychiat.*, **9**, 1.
—— Tizard, J., Whitmore, K. (1970a) *Education, Health and Behaviour*, London: Longmans.
—— Graham, P., Yule, M. (1970b) *A Neuropsychiatric Study in Childhood*. Clinics in Developmental Medicine, No. 35/36. London: S.I.M.P. with Heinemann.

—— Bartak, L., Newman, S. (1971) 'Autism—a central disorder of cognition and language.' *in* Rutter, M. (Ed.) *Infantile Autism: Concepts, Characteristics and Treatment.* London: Churchill Livingstone.

Sheridan, M. (1969) 'Playthings in the development of language.' *Hlth Trends*, **1**, 7.

Stefflie, V., Vales, V. C., Morley, L. (1966) 'Language and cognition in Yucutan: a cross-cultural replication.' *J. Personal. soc. Psychol.*, **4**, 112.

Solomon, A. L. (1961) 'Personality and behaviour patterns of children with functional defects of articulation.' *Child Develop.*, **32**, 731.

Vygotsky, L. S. (1962) *Thought and Language.* Cambridge, Mass.: M.I.T. Press.

Weiner, P. S. (1969) 'The perceptual level functioning of dysphasic children.' *Cortex*, **5**, 440.

Whorf, B. (1956) *in* Carroll, J. B. (Ed.) *Language, Thought and Reality.* New York: Wiley.

Williams, C. E. (1968) 'Behaviour disorders in handicapped children.' *Develop. Med. Child. Neurol.*, **10**, 736.

—— (1970) 'Some psychiatric observations on a group of maladjusted deaf children.' *J. Child Psychol. Psychiat.*, **11**, 1.

Wing, L. (1969) 'The handicaps of autistic children—a comparative study.' *J. Child Psychol. Psychiat.*, **10**, 1.

CHAPTER 16

The Child's Acquisition of Codes for Personal and Interpersonal Communication

MARY D. SHERIDAN

For some years I have been studying the spontaneous behaviour of normal and handicapped infants and young children in free field and in loosely structured situations, with special reference to the early development of general understanding, codes of communication and social adaptation. This has involved direct observation of children's everyday activities, manipulations and explorations and the way in which they relate to the people and happenings in the world around them (Sheridan 1960, 1969).

My studies have been carried out at home and in day and residential nurseries, schools, clinics and hospital wards. They have led me to a number of conclusions regarding the child's inborn urge and developing capacity to represent his experiences, needs and emotional states and also his self-awareness and his notions of space and time, using various language codes. These codes he uses to communicate with himself, *i.e.* to think, and with other people, *i.e.* to receive their various messages and express his own thoughts and sentiments in exchange. Although my tentative and entirely personal conclusions may not be generally acceptable, I can claim that they are founded on watching and listening to hundreds of babies and young children and recording their spontaneous activities, utterances and behaviour as objectively as possible. The result of my observations are offered in the hope that they may throw further light on the baffling problems of differential diagnosis, day-to-day management and prognosis of children showing delay or failure in ability to communicate in the ordinary way.

Terminology

Existing terminology regarding human communication remains so confused and confusing that it tends to prevent rather than assist communication between the various groups of workers caring for or teaching normal and handicapped children. Paediatricians, otologists, neurologists, psychiatrists, phoneticians, linguists, psychologists, speech therapists and teachers continue to use their own professional jargon (Sheridan 1964 *a*). It is axiomatic that a commonly accepted semantic reference, as well as a common coding system, is a pre-requisite for effective communication within any social group. This should also apply to professional workers, but does not.

Having found it essential for my own deliberations to distinguish as precisely as I could between physiological and psychological processes, and since my own self-communications are conducted in basic English, I must begin by defining my own terminology (Sheridan 1964 *a* and *b*). Of course, all psychological processes are basically physiological, but at present we are unable to express psychological activity in terms of neuro-physiology.

189

Hearing is the reception of sound by the ear and its transmission to the central nervous system. I am not prepared to particularise the pathways and cortical areas involved but, in my view, the process of hearing is mainly a physiological one.

Listening is paying attention to the sounds heard with the object of interpreting their meaning; in other words this is mainly a psychological process.

Speech is the use of systemised vocalisations to express verbal symbols or words. This is probably mainly a physiological process.

Language is the symbolisation or codification of concepts (ideas) for the purpose of *self-communication* regarding the present, past and future, also for the purpose of *interpersonal communication* in reception and expression; in other words this is mainly a psychological process.

The word 'language', however, is also commonly used to denote that repository of concept-in-code upon which the de-coding of incoming messages and the encoding of outgoing communications depend. This strictly personal repository is usually referred to as the possessor's 'inner-language'. For convenience I retain this term, but, in order to distinguish between the code and the repository, I always use the qualifying term 'inner-language ' when referring to the repository. (The word 'language' is also commonly used with reference to grammatical structure but I never employ the term in this sense in regard to young children).

My present discussions are chiefly concerned with the child's *primary or biological learning* in relation to the registration of experiences in his memory-bank, and his development of one or more language codes wherewith to represent and recall these memories of the past and manipulate them in relation to present deliberations and future planning.

Without entering into age-old controversies regarding the relationship of brain and mind, we can all agree that somewhere within the living brain are situated the magnificent neurological structures which originate and regulate the dynamic processes of physical, intellectual and emotional activity. Here every function of human existence is initiated, processed, maintained or inhibited but never fully arrested until death.

In everyday circumstances, *sensation* is never restricted to a single modality although one modality may be dominant, particularly in handicapped children. Hence, *stimulations* are always multi-sensorial and the memories they produce are correspondingly multiplex. Similarly, all *learning situations* have affective as well as cognitive elements which are stored in the memory-bank in permanent association. These combined sensory, mental and emotional processes stimulate the child's intellect and personality to develop each in his own fashion and at his own rate.

Communication Codes

The codes in which any individual human being represents his concepts to himself or to other people, are uniquely personal and exceedingly complicated. It will be obvious that the child's memoranda regarding his everyday experiences are being continually formed, assimilated, re-inforced and amalgamated. At first, while these memoranda are few and simple, the child's memories are usually recalled (or re-activated) mainly in situations identical with, or very similar to, those in which they were originally acquired. Soon, however, the number and complexity of his memoranda, and the concepts he evolves from them, increase so rapidly that it becomes essential to categorise his ideas and compress them, without loss of substance, before storing them in his memory-bank. He must then employ some coding system to facilitate rapid and effective recognition (de-coding), cross-reference (interpretation) and evokation (encoding). Codes may be constructed in at least four different ways, *i.e.* in words, pictures, gestures or three-dimensional models. These are discussed in more detail later.

Primitive identification of the self, as separate from other people and objects in the environment, is an essential preliminary to the construction of any form of communication code. Realisation of 'me' and 'not me' depends upon the integration of *body awareness* (which might be formulated as follows)—'I respond to various sensory stimulations and engage in numerous motor activities without reference to other people and things. Therefore I have separate existence'; *cognitive awareness*— 'I think my own thoughts, therefore I have separate existence'; and *affective awareness* —'I experience my own emotions, therefore I have separate existence'.

Within this organisation of the self, in order to prevent personal confusion and social chaos, cognition or reasoning must eventually assume, and maintain, control over physical activity and emotional impulse.

The Acquisition of Codes

Prolonged observation confirms the ancient truth that given functional motor, visual and auditory equipment together with adequate cognitive and affective potential, the most favourable opportunities for learning are provided by mother-teaching at mother-distance, in other words from consistent, affectionate and unhurried every-day care and experience in an ordinary family home. The child's experiences are localised at first within the small, physically enclosed world of his mother's arms, close to her face, voice and warmth of person and feeling. This world gradually expands as he grows in size and independence. Watching, listening and touching, he begins to imitate what he sees, hears and feels occuring in organised *movement* which, in everyday circumstances, is equivalent to *function*. The child's imitations of the simple activities and vocal utterances which occur in his small world usually precede his comprehension. He babbles and imitates, at first, without understanding the meaning of these activities. *Comprehension*, however, eventually follows imitation and must do so in order to produce *spontaneous meaningful expression* whether in motor praxis or in language code. In young children, it is sometimes difficult to distinguish between delayed imitation and primitive expression.

Communication with the self, *i.e.* to think in coded form, which involves the ability to scan one's past experiences, to relate them to the present, judging their signifi-cance in the light of intellect and the warmth of emotion, and then to plan the future, appears to be conducted in another code. This is usually a highly sophisticated and abbreviated version of the code in common use within one's social group. It is a 'code of codes' designed for purely personal and internal use and not amenable to expression. Hence the self understands the self's ideas better than anyone else can, but often has to admit 'I find it difficult to put into words'. The self-code in which thought is conducted, however, can only be evolved after the common code, from which it is derived, has been mastered. This perhaps accounts for the young child's addiction to self-talk, which is really thinking aloud, until he has learned how to keep his thoughts to himself—and why.

Interpersonal communication, upon which most of human happiness and all social competence depend, necessitates a slower and more conventional use of the common code. In everyday situations, the child's familiars, adults and older children, are constantly talking to each other and also to him, encouraging, forbidding or explaining. He listens to and assimilates what he can of the vocal cadences, words and phrases and their various associations and implications.

In the course of my own manipulations of ideas and introspections and many subsequent discussions with friendly colleagues, I have found it desirable to invent two new, but I trust, simple words, 'memord' and 'codeme'. Although I have consulted numerous authorities, I have not been able in either case to discover any generally accepted term which carries the same basic, unambiguous meaning.

A *'memord'* (a portmanteau word from 'memory-record') may be defined as *a* memory which is recorded in *the* memory, or more elaborately, as a unit or molecule of memory which is recorded in connection with a single perceptual event or conceptual insight. Like other molecules, a memord may be simple or highly complex, deriving from motor, sensory, emotional or intellectual experience, or from a combination of all these.

I discarded the term 'memory trace' (which in any case, seems latterly to have fallen into disuse) because for many of my respondents it carried inprecise, attenuated or vaguely two-dimensional implications and sometimes even a suggestion of un-wanted residue or waste. For most people, too, the word 'trace' seemed to deprive the term of auditory or affective attributes. The other possible term 'mental image' was unsatisfactory because of visually overloaded implications.

The word *'codeme'* (analogous to 'phoneme') is used to designate a unit of code, whether the code is verbal, pictorial, mimed or other. Again I have found it desirable to discard the words 'signal', 'sign' and 'symbol' because all these carry too many differing semantic implications. (In this connection I should perhaps note, since later I must refer to the play of young children, that long ago I found it desirable to discard the highly ambiguous terms 'dramatic', 'symbolic', 'imaginative' and 'fantasy' in connection with the situational and rôle-play of very young children, preferring the plainer terms 'imitative', 'pretend' or 'make-believe' as more appropriate to my purpose.)

Before he learns to use language codes of any sort, however, the infant employs a pre-linguistic form of communication which is singularly affective at its own level.

Pre-linguistic (or Non-codemic) Communication

Pre-linguistic communication deserves closer study than it has yet received, since the child who is unable to use a codemic system has to resort to this primitive form of communication in order to maintain any sort of contact with his fellow beings.

Pre-linguistic communication *normally* exists between infants and their familiars until it is replaced by spoken language. It manifests itself in welcoming or resistive body movements, visual engagement, facial expressions, emotionally-charged utterances, laughter, sobbing, panicking, or tantrums. Amongst its later manifestations are purposeful touching, pulling, pushing, pointing or moving another's hand to carry out an activity which is physically beyond the child's own capacity. It begins soon after birth, reaches a peak between 16 and 20 months and then gradually declines as the child's spoken language becomes more firmly established. It *abnormally* persists when the acquisition of the language-coding system is delayed, fails to occur, or is lost as a result of physical or mental illness.

This form of communication, the pre-linguistic child shares with the higher mammals, which also use it effectively, although they cannot progress, as can the normal $1\frac{1}{2}$ to 2 year human child, into the possession of a language code. Pre-linguistic communication is employed to draw another's attention to a pressing need, happening or object or to express a pervasive physical or emotional state. Its use is necessarily restricted to the 'here and now'. It may produce satisfactory response, but it cannot represent what is past or to come.

Communication in Language Codes

There are four main varieties of language code, *i.e.* using words, pictures, mime or three-dimensional models.

1. The Verbal Code

This is man's principal codemic system. The process of communication in verbal language, whether in speaking, writing, finger-spelling, Braille or Morse, is usually described as threefold: reception, interpretation and expression.

Reception (decoding) depends upon the child's capacity to see and hear and also upon his willingness and/or ability to watch and listen to spoken or written words. Some children with cerebral palsy, for example, may be willing to listen but lack the ability to control their excessive distractability so that they cannot pay full attention to what they hear. Some mentally ill children, on the other hand, appear to lack the necessary capacity for making the decision to listen.

Interpretation (association) depends upon the adequacy of the child's personal 'inner language' verbally coded. This, in turn, depends upon the orderly maturation of the child's neurological structures and inborn drives, with simultaneous favourable opportunity to build up his stock of memords and related concepts-in-code.

Expression (encoding) involves first the marshalling of ideas from the memory-store of concepts, then the appropriate representation of these ideas in verbal codemes and finally putting into action the necessary motor processes to speak, write, or finger-spell the selected words.

Recognition of codemes, *i.e.* matching received codemes against those previously stored in the 'inner-language' repository, is presumably a less complicated psychological activity than *retrieval* which is the evokation of codemes from the same repository. The normal child is able to echo and understand words said to him several months before he can spontaneously speak them. This fact must always be taken into consideration in relation to auditory training and speech therapy. In young children with language disorders, the time-lag between ability to interpret the spoken word and ability to reply may be very prolonged.

2. Communication in pictorial form

This involves the ability to receive, interpret and express ideas through the medium of two-dimensional representations, *e.g.* drawings, diagrams and maps. These pictorial codemes may be static or moving. The code has unrestricted use since it can represent the past, the present and the future.

3. Communication in mime

This employs two forms of representation, *i.e.* improvised pantomime and the conventional sign-language. Improvised mime consists of orderly serial actions used to describe past events, ask a question or indicate a future plan. It requires the minimum amount of instruction, but intelligent selection and precise execution. It has unrestricted use.

Sign language is the conventionalised action-code or 'shorthand mime' and is used extensively by the deaf amongst themselves. It possesses wide possibility as a coding system. Interpretation and execution depend upon prolonged individual instruction and constant practice. Its use, therefore, is restricted to a special group. Both forms are codemic.

4. Communication using objects or models

The codemes of this system consist of three-dimensional objects. They may be of ordinary size or enormously magnified (for instance those used in micro-biology) or miniaturised as scale models. This system has wide representative possibilities.

The Acquisition of Language Codes

Speech may be mere parrot-like echolalia of other people's vocal utterances and without meaning for the speaker, but *spoken language* must be founded on verbal understanding. Similarly, a baby's manipulation of everyday objects, *e.g.* cup, spoon, hairbrush, comb, or mirror, may be mere immediate or delayed imitation and certainly begins as such. About the age of 12 months, however, a child usually begins to show unmistakable, spontaneous, meaningful self-directed definition-by-use in his manipulation of familiar or real-life sized objects. This, in my opinion, marks his comprehension that there is a consistency of association between the familiar object itself and its purpose. This realisation is quickly followed by another that there is an indivisible relationship between an object and its name because, at this stage, he can often hand over an object or correctly indicate it in some other way, such as visual regard, on spoken request. The infant's earliest comprehension of the function of any person or object is entirely ego-centrated but has usually appeared by 11 to 12 months.

The next step in definition-by-use is demonstrated by the child's application of real-life sized common objects to other people and larger dolls or pets. This appears some weeks or months later than his self-directed definitions but has usually appeared by 18 months, by which time the child is normally able not only to hand the object on request but also to speak its name. Transfer of similar definition-by-use play to miniature (*i.e.* doll's-house sized) toys appears a month or two later, but is normally well-established by 2 years. Before 18 to 20 months, the child usually treats these miniature toys like other small objects, scattering them about, piling them in heaps, putting them in and out of containers, or occasionally lining them up in tidy but meaningless rows. In my view, this transfer to representative play with miniatures indicates the child's newly acquired ability to externalise (*i.e.* express) his already internally memorised and coded experiences. He has begun mentally to detach people, things and happenings from sole reference to himself (as the hub of the universe) and categorise them, showing primitive realisation not only of 'me' and 'not me' and of the separate existence of and between people and things in his environment, but also something of the rules of space and time.

The difficult realisation that he must conform to certain accepted patterns of everyday social behaviour, whether he likes it or not, slowly follows. All this time the child still only has a limited command over words, phrases and selective mime and no ability whatever for graphic representation. It is little wonder that he sometimes explodes into a tantrum of anguished frustration (see Figs. 1-8).

Differential Diagnosis

The child's use of common objects and, later, of miniature toys, single words, mime, drawing and of rôle and make-believe play, therefore, in my view, gives valuable information concerning the possession or non-possession of a codemic system. His manipulations, demonstration of general understanding regarding the world around him, social behaviour and, most particularly, his ability to use codemes in his social communications, provide clues wherewith we may assess the nature and development of his 'inner language'. The object of all paediatric diagnosis is not only immediate treatment for relief of distress but also the discovery of aetiological factors and the application of reliable preventive measures. In young children between 18 months and 4 years, the differential diagnosis of delayed language development is one of the most baffling problems in paediatric practice. There is no necessity to stress the need to take a careful medical and social history and to eliminate the possibility of lack of adequate opportunity to learn, auditory impairment, neurological disorder, global mental retardation or the rare cases of elective mutism in non-talking children who otherwise appear to be normal. Without entering into speculations regarding the vexed question of aetiology, the remaining non-speaking children may be said to fall into four groups according to the clinical manifestations presented (Sheridan 1964*b*).

Group I

Children who *hear* and *comprehend* spoken language adequately but cannot use oral expression to the expected level for their age. They can, however, express themselves effectively in other ways, such as sign-language, mime, models, drawings, or sometimes even verbally through finger-spelling or writing. They engage in make-believe play with other children of their age and are usually well accepted by them. In other words they possess adequate 'inner language' The majority of these children develop spoken language by the age of 5 or 6 years, although they may need expert help. A small minority remain mute although they have the potential capacity to develop a useful alternative codemic system and should be encouraged in every way to do so.

Group II

Children who *hear* and *comprehend* very simple spoken language when they are addressed close by, in short sentences, at slow rate and in familiar situations. They are very dependent upon the constant presence of familiar, understanding adults and helpful older children. They usually have a limited spoken vocabulary which they eke out with gestures. They engage in very simple rôle-play alone or with one or two younger children; in other words, they possess a primitive 'inner language' which is largely restricted to the concrete and to the present. Although they are often, but not always, globally retarded in their development, given help, they have potential capacity for limited but definite improvement.

Group III

Children who *hear* and may *repeat* words or even long phrases in parrot-like fashion but do *not comprehend* the meaning of what they say. They may recall musical themes and enjoy playing with sound-making instruments. They manifest varying degrees of awareness of their environment and show willingness and sometimes urgent desire to communicate with other people in pre-linguistic fashion by pulling, pointing, clinging, screaming, or weeping. These children appear to possess memords which are capable of reactivation in appropriate situations but to have no codemes. Their capacity to develop an 'inner-language' is doubtful but should be actively encouraged, particularly in children under 7 years.

Group IV

Children who *hear* but seem unable to pay attention either to spoken utterances or to other meaningful environmental sounds. Even their prelinguistic communications are notably reduced. They appear to be unable to relate to other people in any positive way. It is doubtful if they possess memords. They may be hyperkinetic and obtrusively noisy, or silent, inactive and wholly withdrawn. In either case, they appear to be depersonalised, or perhaps more accurately 'unpersonalised' and virtually inaccessible to any form of human communication (see Figs. 9-17).

Immediate imitation at one end of his language developmental scale and full spontaneous *codemic expression* at the other, are readily distinguished, but the transition stages of delayed imitation and partial codification are not so clearly defined. Without entering into controversial discussion regarding short, medium or long-term memory storage, I must restate my conviction that a child needs to watch, listen to and manipulate common objects of *ordinary size* which are repeatedly employed by his familiars in everyday situations in close connection with individualised sensory-tied experience before he can comprehend the conventional usage and separate properties of these objects and, still later, attach names to them. Infants demonstrate the stages of this gradual learning when they apply common objects functionally, first to themselves, and then to other people or pets and later in the earliest fragmentary 'pretend' play with their dolls. It is still later before they can externalise their accumulating concepts and codemes in meaningful play-activities with miniature models. In this connection the stages of doll's-house play, from the bringing of single objects to mother, through grouped floor-assembly to more elaborate play inside the house, briefly described elsewhere (Sheridan 1969), can be very revealing (see Figs. 18-24).

In spite of their often grossly aberrant behaviour, therefore, the majority of non-speaking children under 7 years give the impression of possessing a functional memory-bank although it may contain only a meagre store of memords. They also usually indicate at least potential capacity to use a communication code of some sort even though this may not be composed of verbal codemes. Although the effective use of spoken language should always be aimed at, in my view therapy should never be restricted to this single codemic input channel. The child should be encouraged to communicate in any code or mixture of codes which he can learn to imitate, comprehend and put into practice.

Lacking a language, the child is denied the dignity of human status which is his birthright. He is condemned to a half-life of emotional solitude and intellectual silence. If, in the present state of our ignorance, we are unable to help him acquire even the most rudimentary stock of codemes, we must allow him to communicate with us in pre-linguistic fashion and gently but firmly train him to use this form of expression within socially acceptable limits. Meanwhile, we must give him assurance of our concern by our facial expressions, affectionate vocal tones and compassionate physical contacts. Then we shall at least have the consolation of knowing that we have done our best to help him.

Note: The paper was illustrated by 50 coloured slides, from which the black and white pictures given overleaf are a selection.

REFERENCES

Sheridan, M. D. (1960) *Developmental Progress of Infants and Young Children*. London: H.M.S.O. (Also 2nd edn, 1968)
—— (1964*a*) 'Development of auditory attention and the use of language symbols'. *in* Renfrew, C., Murphy, K. (Eds.) *The Child who does not Talk*. Clinics in Developmental Medicine, No. 13. London: S.I.M.P. with Heinemann Medical. p. 1.
—— (1964*b*) 'Disorders of communication in young children.' *Mth. Bull. Minist. Hlth. Lab. Serv.*, **23**, 20.
—— (1969) 'Playthings in the development of language.' *Hlth Trends*, **1**, 7.

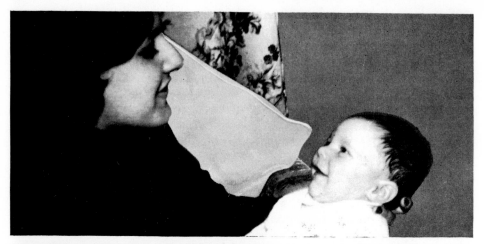

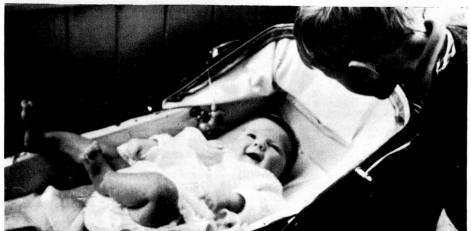

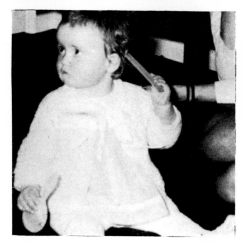
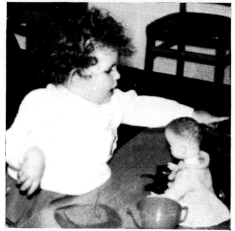

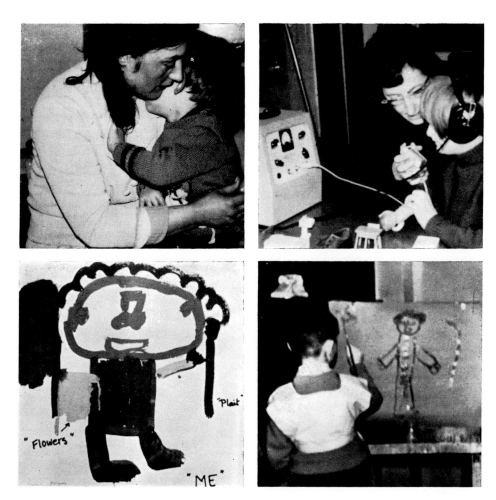

Facing page:

Fig. 1 (*top*). Normal boy, 6 weeks. Note visual engagement and broad social smile. The baby responded with 'cooing' sounds to his mother's voice.
Fig. 2 (*centre*). Normal girl, 19 weeks. Delighted response to face and voice of 6-year-old brother.
Fig. 3 (*lower left*). Normal girl, 12 months, demonstrating spontaneous self-directed definition-by-use of a familiar real-life object.
Fig. 4 (*lower right*). Severely deaf girl (maternal rubella), 16 months. A natural verbaliser who responded well to auditory training. She is pointing at her ball, while saying the word 'ball'.

This page:

Fig. 5 (*top left*). Severely deaf boy, 3½ years. Not a natural verbaliser. He worked willingly during auditory training session, but became tired and sought comfort from mother. (Compare this affectionate interchange with the impersonal lapsitting in Fig. 15.)
Fig. 6 (*top right*). Blind-deaf girl, 10 years. Congenital absence of eyeballs and severe auditory impairment, but some useable hearing. Limited, well-articulated vocabulary. Related life-size shoe to those on own feet, but it was doubtful if she understood that miniature toys represented everyday objects.
Fig. 7 (*lower left*). Self-portrait by normal (coloured) girl, 6½ years. She realised that she had 'black' hands and feet, but thought her face was pink.
Fig. 8 (*lower right*). Deaf boy, 7 years. Originally diagnosed as mentally handicapped. Not a natural verbaliser, but used drawings and signs effectively as means of communication.

199

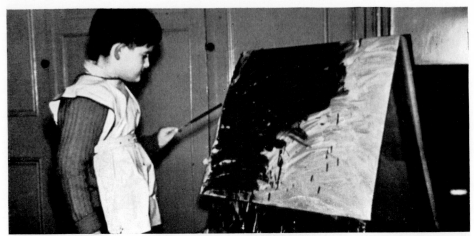

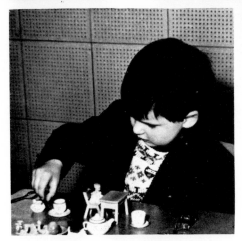

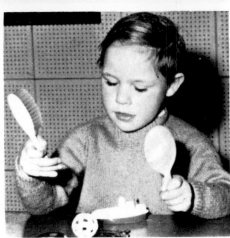

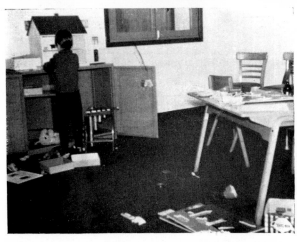

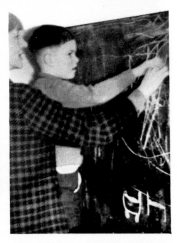

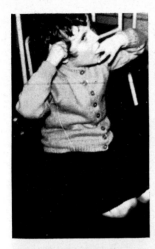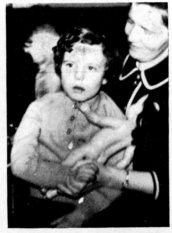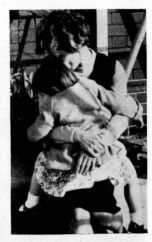

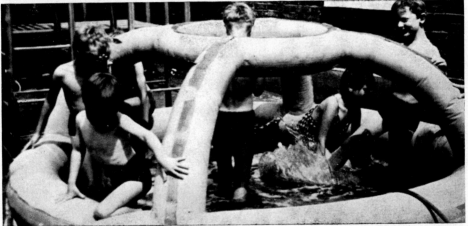

Facing page:

Fig. 9 (*top*). Non-speaking boy, 7 years. No evidence of possessing any system of codemes. Painting was meaningless brushwork. (Compare with Fig. 8.)

Fig. 10 (*centre left*). Non-speaking boy, 4 years. Normal hearing and good verbal comprehension. Meaningful assembly of miniature toys.

Fig. 11 (*centre right*). Non-speaking boy, 4 years. Hearing normal but very limited verbal understanding. Numerous signs of minor neurological dysfunction. Immature manipulation of common objects with doubtful indication of definition-by-use.

Fig. 12 (*lower left*). Non-speaking boy, 4½ years. Hearing normal but no verbal comprehension. No indication of possessing any system of codemes. Over-active behaviour rapidly produced environmental chaos.

Fig. 13 (*lower right*). Non-speaking boy, 8 years. Normal hearing but no verbal or other codemic understanding. Made friendly overtures, and guided adult's hand to perform activity beyond own capacity.

This page:

Fig. 14 (*top left*). Non-speaking girl, 7½ years. Typical autistic behaviour. Normal hearing but no verbal understanding.

Fig. 15 (*top centre*). Same child, sitting on lap with no attempt to make personalised relationship.

Fig. 16 (*top right*). Non-speaking girl, 3½ years. Hearing normal but no verbal understanding. Sought physical contact and clung to anyone who could tolerate her need for this type of re-assurance.

Fig. 17 (*lower*). Playtime on a summer afternoon in a school for intelligent autistic children. There was no attempt at conversation between the children, or to engage in any form of group activity. Boy kicking water made no attempt to splash another child.

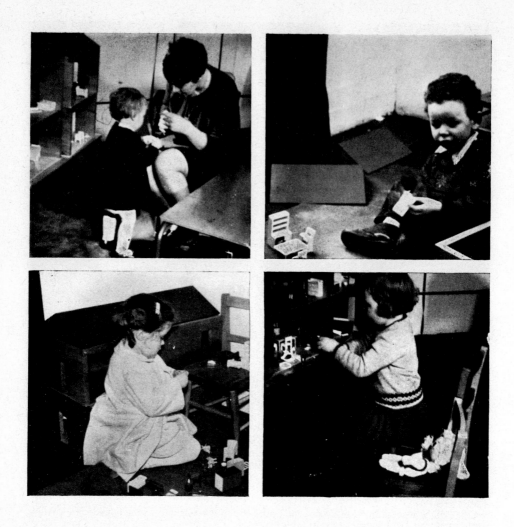

Figs. 18-24: *stages in doll's-house play*

Fig. 18 (*top left*). Girl, 18 months, bringing single objects to mother, naming one or two, and vocalising continually to draw mother's attention.
Fig. 19 (*top right*). Boy, 2¼ years. Assembly of a few related pieces of furniture on floor near mother's chair, talking intermittently to self and to mother.
Fig. 20 (*lower left*). Girl, 2¾ years. Assembly of related pieces on chair near doll's house, talking mainly to self.
Fig. 21 (*lower right*). Girl, 3 years. Play in one room of doll's house, talking to self and occasionally to large doll on chair.

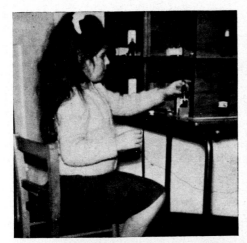
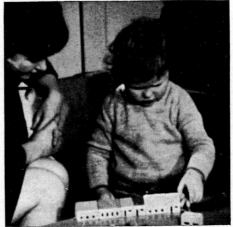
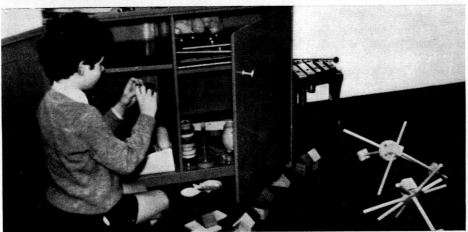

Fig. 22 (*top left*). Girl, 4½ years. Organised play all over doll's house. No audible self-talk.

Fig. 23 (*top right*). Girl, 3 years, playing with toy village. Assembly of similar objects in tidy rows is typical of this age. She talked continuously and sensibly to her mother as she built. (Compare with Fig. 24).

Fig. 24 (*lower*). Late-speaking boy, 8 years. First choice of play material was wooden construction on the right; he jargoned softly to himself in the making. Second choice was the blocks, used to build the 'street' by the cupboard door, saying more loudly to himself 'Houses..houses..houses'. He then built square structure at the near end of the street and said 'garage'. Finally went to cupboard searching for small toys, saying 'Cars..cars..cars'. None of the talk was directed at adults present, although he seemed pleased when his street was admired. (Compare with Fig. 23.)

CHAPTER 17

Behaviour Modification Principles and Speech Delay

W. YULE and M. BERGER

Introduction

Over recent years there has been a rapid expansion in the psychological literature describing the new field of 'behaviour modification' techniques for the treatment and management of a wide range of conditions shown by adults and children. This chapter aims to outline the principles of this form of treatment, to describe its application to speech and language disorders with special reference to the condition of infantile autism, and to consider the evidence for the efficacy of these methods. The problems involved in evaluating the effectiveness of behaviour modification techniques in language disorders are no different in kind from those concerned in assessing any treatment (Ullman and Krasner 1965, Staats 1968, Bandura 1969, Yates 1970), and the principles outlined might well be applied to other forms of 'speech therapy'.

General Characteristics of Behaviour Modification

The guiding principle of behaviour modification procedures is that behaviour can be modified by its consequences. Behaviour followed by pleasant consequences will tend to increase in frequency, whereas behaviour which culminates in unpleasant consequences will tend to decrease (Ferster and Perrott 1968). Thus, the therapist undertakes a *functional analysis* of behaviour, leading to an identification of the 'sufficient and necessary conditions for a particular response to occur and persist' (Evans 1971). In practice, this involves systematically varying the environment and observing the effects on the child's behaviour, the aim being to specify the environmental conditions which affect the behaviour to be modified.

Having identified these conditions, these are deliberately varied to influence the behaviour in the appropriate direction. One of the most important characteristics of this approach is its reliance on the principle of 'contingent reinforcement'. In essence, this simply means that rewards or reinforcers are given systematically *only* when the child produces whatever behaviour it is the therapist wishes to encourage. Thus, the first point is to determine what does 'reward' the child, what is sufficiently important to him to make him 'work' to obtain it. For any individual child the particular reinforcer used will depend entirely on what the child will best respond to. His likes and dislikes determine what the therapist will use. Most normal children, and many handicapped children, respond best to social reinforcers such as praise and approval from an adult. Occasionally with poorly socialised children it may be necessary to use material rewards to provide motivation, but where tangible reinforcers are employed, care has to be taken to ensure that they are accompanied by social reinforcers so that these social cues may become more potent.

Of course, all teachers and all therapists utilise the principle of reinforcement as a matter of routine in their concern to encourage the child along the right lines. What is distinctive about behaviour modification procedures is their attention to detail, especially over timing, in order to maximise the child's motivation. The crucial feature of reinforcement is not what is given, but rather *when* it is given. It has been found that the accurate timing of rewards is crucial if success is to be achieved. Reward must *immediately* follow the desired behaviour and it must *only* follow that behaviour. At least in the initial stages, delayed or indiscriminate rewards do not obtain the same effects.

The second main characteristic of this approach is the analysis of the individual components of the behaviour which is sought. In order to develop complex behaviour, it is often necessary to break it down into its essential elements, which are then taught one at a time in easy stages. As a consequence of this functional analysis there is an emphasis on the 'shaping' of behaviour by dealing only with very small steps at a time.

A third major feature is the structuring of the environment to ensure that when the desired behaviour appears it is immediately reinforced. The degree of structure required is, in part, a function of the characteristics and problems of the individual child. Environmental structuring is necessary where, for example, the child is highly distractible or overactive. In such instances, a quiet bare treatment room may reduce the frequency of these behaviours and allow the target behaviours to become manifest. Similarly, if a child is found to be mute in the presence of strangers but not with his family, the environment may be structured in such a way that strangers gradually appear only in a situation where the child is talking with his mother (Reid *et al.* 1967). The imposition of structure is also a function of the therapist's need to evaluate the procedures used (see below).

These operant principles are particularly important in the early stages of treatment with severely disturbed, withdrawn autistic children and hence receive emphasis in the modification procedures outlined below. However, behaviour modification techniques utilise many other approaches which are also based on what is known about environmental influences on learning (Bandura 1969, Lovitt 1970). Bandura has emphasised that with socially responsive children it is often unnecessary to shape behaviour. The same effects can be achieved in a shorter time by instructing the child precisely in what is wanted of him, in showing him how to do what is required and by providing him with an appropriate behavioural or language model. Particular attention should always be paid to the use of imitation and modelling in the treatment of language disorders.

Reinforcement is probably not the most important factor in the normal child's acquisition of language (see chapter 5). However, we are concerned here with children who have *failed* to talk at the normal time and in this situation reinforcement principles are more important for several reasons. (a) The child's motivation may lag when he becomes aware that he is consistently failing to do what is expected of him. (b) The family may stop providing the appropriate language environment because it has not seemed to work with their child. (c) An abnormal lack of reinforcement in the environment may have been one factor in the speech delay. (d) The child's behaviour may be so abnormal or his social responsiveness so low that the ordinary social cues are ineffective and an *unusual* environment is required to produce the usual degree of response. (This applies particularly to autistic children.) (e) Some cases of speech delay are associated with *deviant* as well as delayed development (this also applies to autism), in which case again a special environment may be required to produce a normal language attainment. Finally, the efficacy of any form of speech therapy may be improved by the effect of discrimination attention and motivation, obtainable by reference to reinforcement principles.

Behaviour Modification and the Problems of Autistic Children

There are now many studies which have adopted behaviour modification approaches towards speech and language disorders and defects (Sloane and MacAulay 1968, Bricker and Bricker 1970). Stuttering (Goldiamond 1968, Beech and Fransella 1968), articulation difficulties (Mowrer *et al.* 1968, Marshall 1970), aphasia (Holland and Harris 1968), elective mutism (Straughan *et al.* 1965, Reid *et al.* 1967, Nolan and Pence 1970) are among the disorders which have been tackled. Because much has been written about establishing speech in autistic children we will use this literature to illustrate approaches to treatment founded on behavioural modification principles. A particular advantage to be gained in using this clinical group for illustrative purposes is that they present with diverse and severe forms of speech and language disorders. As a consequence, a variety of techniques has been developed to alleviate these problems, and readers will readily discern their applicability to other disorders.

Autistic children present major clinical problems in three areas (Rutter 1966*a* and *b*, 1968). Firstly, they are largely unsocialized and appear to be very withdrawn, *e.g.* young autistic children typically do not engage in eye-to-eye contact. From an early age they do not respond to the attention of their parents and, later, they do not join in the co-operative play of other children. Secondly, they show many bizarre behaviour patterns. Some people consider these to be secondary to the main, core handicap, but this does not make them any the less real. They are often very restless, and indulge in a variety of manneristic behaviours. Self-injury is not uncommon. All-in-all, autistic children show peculiar patterns of behaviour far outside the experience of most teachers and nurses, and can be extremely unresponsive to normal parental demands. In the third place, many autistic children have severe language problems. This is considered to be the major area of difficulty by some workers (Rutter 1968). In many cases, both speech and language are effectively absent. In other cases, children are echolalic. It has been shown that the presence of useful language before the age of 5 years is one of the best prognostic indicators(Rutter 1971). If one can establish speech in non-speaking autistic children after the age of five, the question is raised as to whether this also alters the ultimate prognosis.

Young autistic children are largely unresponsive to social rewards. Lovaas (1966) has argued that the autistic child's lack of socialization is the basis of all his behavioural deficits. Since speech and language form the main vehicle of social interaction, if speech could be established, the child should be more amenable to normal socialization influences. Thus Lovaas and his colleagues devised treatment programmes to establish useful speech in autistic children. (It has been strongly argued elsewhere (Rutter 1968) that the social withdrawal characteristic of younger autistic children is probably a phenomenon secondary to more central perceptual and cognitive deficits. Indeed, a strong case can be made for regarding early infantile autism as a severe cognitive disorder.) We need not however agree with Lovaas's reasoning to examine his techniques.

Planning Treatment

The first stage in planning a behaviour modification approach to language therapy with the autistic child is a detailed analysis of the child's language development, social responsiveness and behaviour. Before embarking on any form of treatment it is necessary to go far beyond the medical diagnosis of 'autism' to a systematic appraisal of the level of the child's understanding and production of language and of his assets and deficits in the cognitive and social skills required for the development of normal language competence. What is required to make this type of assessment is described in other chapters (see especially chapters 3, 6, 10 and 11).

However, the effects of this assessment on the planning of treatment need to be considered here. This can be done most easily by taking a few examples. If a young mute child is found to have a negligible understanding of spoken language, fails to use gestural communication, shows no imitative play, does not use toys appropriately and engages in no pretend or make-believe games it would seem that he is not yet at a stage when the production of language is possible. Speech training, using operant principles, might well achieve a small labelling vocabulary, but in the absence of language comprehension, it would be unlikely to produce a spoken language. In this case, treatment would probably focus on the development of pre-linguistic social skills and play behaviour. Operant techniques would be employed to develop social responsiveness, and systematic teaching would be used to aid the child's understanding of language and to facilitate the growth of imitative skills. Only after the child's comprehension was beginning to develop would *speech* training be used. A failure to take cognisance of the child's level of language comprehension may account for the poor results in some cases of operant speech training with autistic children (see below). Unfortunately it is not possible to determine whether this is so because of the linguistic naivety and lack of diagnostic detail in most of the published reports. Because of this lack, judgements of which therapeutic approach is most effective for children at each stage of language development are necessarily somewhat speculative. At present all that can be done is to decide on the basis of clinical experience and a knowledge of normal language development. Well planned evaluations of treatment are greatly needed to fill this hiatus in knowledge.

If a child remains without speech, has reasonable language comprehension but has grossly inco-ordinate tongue movements, there has to be a decision whether to concentrate on spoken language or gestural language. Many children with a language disorder show tongue inco-ordination and usually this proves no bar to speech. However, there are rare cases when the inco-ordination is so severe that fluent speech becomes unlikely. We had one case of an autistic child with this condition whose response to operant speech training was severely limited in spite of the boy's good social responsiveness and adequate language comprehension. In retrospect it seemed that a focus on developing gesture might have been more useful. A brief period of gestural training certainly produced more useful communications.

Where the child has an understanding of language at the 2 year level, but has only a few non-meaningful sounds in his repertoire, then a programme of operant speech training along the lines described by Lovaas (see below) might be appropriate. If the child's problem is one of echoing and lack of spontaneity in language production the techniques described by Risley and Wolf (1967) for encouraging flexible language usage should be considered. If the child is already speaking spontaneously in a social situation and is using phrases, methods employing imitation and modelling would probably be preferable to an operant approach. In short, which treatment programme is followed depends on what is found in the diagnostic assessment. In all cases, the therapist has to consider whether to try to take the child through the normal sequence of development of spoken language (in so far as we know it) or whether to use techniques which focus on one element (such as word production) which, initially, is modified in relative isolation from other aspects of language. In the present state of knowledge, there is no satisfactory answer to this question, but as a tentative guide it would seem that cases of deviant (as distinct from purely delayed) development would be more appropriate for the latter approach.

A further consideration is the extent to which treatment is focussed on the therapist-child interaction and the extent to which parents, teachers, and other key figures in his environment are employed as therapists. The principles of behaviour modification are easily taught to parents (Patterson and Gullion 1968, Schopler and Reichler 1971). They may easily be shown how to teach the child self-helping skills, how to deal with the child so as to eliminate temper tantrums and how to encourage peer-group interaction where appropriate, quite apart from encouraging language development. The child's home and wider environment provide the optimal setting for the growth of language whatever is done in a therapeutic session. Particularly where the child's language is deviant or severely delayed parents will need to be helped to know what to do to encourage language development. A good behaviour modification programme *always* needs to consider the child's environment as a whole and frequently the main emphasis will be placed on modifying the child's environment with the parents as co-therapists. It is essential to ensure an extension of the treatment programme outside the one-to-one therapy situation. However, for easier presentation the main description provided here concerns what may be done with the child.

Operant Speech Training with Autistic Children

The case we present here is of a mute autistic child with some understanding of language but with a profound lack of social responsiveness and the presence of deviant behaviour. This is the sort of challenging case which Lovaas and his colleagues have been working with over the past few years and in 1966 they presented the broad details of programmes for establishing speech in autistic children. Two main stages in the treatment programe were differentiated. In the first stage, previously mute children are taught to imitate the spoken utterances of the therapist, in the second stage they are taught to use these sounds meaningfully. Echolalic children, as Risley and Wolf (1967) showed, can be started at the second stage. As will be emphasised in a later section, the precise form of treatment is determined by the assets and deficits characterizing the individual child. What follows here is a brief general outline of Lovaas's techniques (Lovaas 1966).

Stage I

First the child must learn to sit with the therapist and attend to him. To achieve this, treatment is usually carried out in as bare a room as possible so that there is little to distract the child. Then the child is reinforced for sitting in the chair for progressively longer periods, starting with, say, 5 seconds. Wherever possible, the therapist should attempt to use normal social responses such as smiling, hugging, and praise as rewards for co-operation. However, by their very nature, many mute autistic children do not respond normally to such social reinforcers. Thus, reinforcement at this stage often consists of giving the child something tangible which he likes—such as a spoonful of ice-cream, or a flake of sugar-coated breakfast cereal.

Two points need to be emphasised about the giving of reinforcements: (a) they must be given immediately or 'contingently' (*i.e.* within a few seconds of the appearance of the *desired* behaviour); (b) at this early stage if it is necessary to use food as a reinforcer, it should be accompanied by obvious social behaviour on the part of the therapist saying 'well done' or 'good boy', and giving the child a hug or a pat. Thus, from a very early stage, material rewards are presented in the presence of social behaviour on the part of the therapist. The aim of this conjunction is to make the therapists' social behaviour rewarding in itself.

As might be expected, disruptive behaviours tend to occur, particularly in the early stages of treatment. Some techniques for modifying such behaviours are available. For example, if a child engages in self-destructive behaviour, the therapist removes all positive reinforcers for 5 to 15 seconds. He puts the sweets out of sight, and he looks away from the child during that period. This procedure is known as 'Time-out from positive reinforcement'. Lovaas reports that the systematic application of this procedure may result in the suppression of such interfering behaviours within one week. Next, speech training proper begins here, the child is reinforced every time he makes any noise. He is also rewarded for fixating on the therapist's face. When he is vocalizing at a rate of say one sound every 5 seconds, the therapist begins to bring the child's verbal behaviour under his verbal control. For example, the therapist may say 'ba-ba' once every 10 seconds. The child is then reinforced if he makes *any* sound within a few seconds. When the child is doing this reliably, the task is made more difficult, so that the child must match exactly the sound that the therapist produces. The therapist witholds the reward until the child approximates the sound that was produced. Closer and closer matching is required on each presentation before the reinforcement is forthcoming.

When this has been mastered, the whole procedure is re-cycled with a new, contrasting sound. The greater the difference between the sounds, the easier it is for the child to discriminate between them. Thus, if the child learned to copy 'ba-ba', he might then be taught 'ma-ma'. If he can still attach the correct sounds when the therapist presents them in mixed order, the therapist can then proceed to the next major stage.

209

Stage II

'The establishment of an appropriate context for speech' constitutes the second stage of Lovaas's approach. This stage is divided into three sections beginning with teaching the child to label common actions and objects, passing through the teaching of abstract terms such as pronouns and prepositions, and ending finally with techniques to encourage spontaneous conversational speech. This is the stage at which echolalic children can be started once the echoing has been brought under control. Other detailed techniques for modifying echolalia are also described by Risley and Wolf (1967).

In teaching labelling, for example, the therapist begins by holding up some fairly common object such as a doll. As soon as the child looks at it, the therapist says 'ba-ba' (prompt). Now, by this time, the child trained to imitate what the therapist says, should respond by saying 'ba-ba', and is immediately reinforced. The doll is then removed for a few seconds before the procedure is repeated.

Eventually the doll is shown again and the therapist does not say the whole label, but only the initial syllable. If the child still repeats the whole label, he receives the reinforcer. Gradually, the therapist fades the *prompts* which he gives until, eventually the child labels the doll correctly without any help. At this point, a new training stimulus is introduced, preferably one that is very different from the first. Only when the child shows that he can discriminate between the two stimuli, and can label them both correctly, can the therapist be sure that the labelling behaviour is firmly established. Once a few objects can be labelled, the emphasis of training in Lovaas's scheme shifts somewhat from the vocalization aspects to the cognitive or internal representation aspects. Thus, the child is taught to point to the correct objects on request. In this behaviour can be seen the beginnings of comprehension of speech.

An attempt is also made to teach the child to generalize certain labels. For example, he is shown a variety of dolls and pictures of dolls. The prompt, 'ba-ba', is used with each, and gradually faded as before. If the training has been successful, then any doll should elicit the spoken response, 'ba-ba'. The test that the child possesses a concept of doll comes when he correctly produces the label 'ba-ba' for a previously unseen doll. In this behaviour, too, can be seen the beginnings of concept formation.

Similar techniques of prompting and fading in highly structured situations are used to develop the other aspects of speech and language during the second stage.

Lovaas comments that: 'As in the case of all language training, it is crucial that the training be extended beyond the concrete training sessions into a more informal training within the child's day-to-day environment'. Lovaas's programme involves working with the child for 2 to 7 hours daily for several days per week. In our experience, noticeable gains can be achieved with two half-hour sessions per day, although the need to ensure continuity of treatment across the other 23 hours is as obvious as it is essential.

Lovaas's paper and that of Risley and Wolf (1967) describing very similar programmes for establishing functional speech in echolalic children are perhaps the most useful and influential papers so far published. They emphasize that '...the procedures as they are described here should not be taken as fixed and unchanging. The developing strength of behavioral technology lies in the continued refinement of its procedures'.

P   T

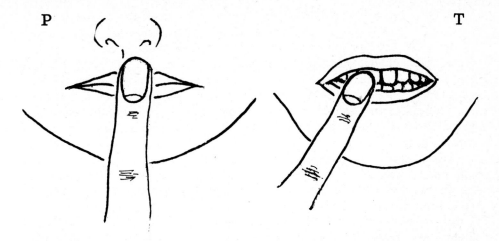

Fig. Adding visual and kinaesthetic cues to facilitate sound discrimination. *Left:* place the right index finger over mouth; produce 'p' through pursed lips, making a motion as if blowing the index finger away. *Right:* open mouth exposing teeth together making the 'T' sound. Tap teeth with the right index finger each time the 'T' sound is produced.
(Reproduced by kind permission of the Journal of Child Psychology and Psychiatry: see also Acknowledgements.)

Among the refinements introduced are those of Nelson and Evans (1968) who combined learning principles with traditional speech therapy techniques which employed additional visual and kinaesthetic cues to facilitate discriminations between sounds. Examples of these are illustrated in the Fig.

The Rôle of Imitation Training
The techniques used to build up a labelling vocabulary are, of necessity, time consuming, and require careful implementation. For more complex behaviours, successive approximation (or shaping) would be too slow, and as a result, a number of authors have devised techniques aimed at encouraging imitation (Metz 1965, Lovaas 1967, Bandura 1969, Bricker and Bricker 1970, Hartung 1970). Once a capacity to imitate has been developed in autistic children, this is then integrated into the speech and language training.

In normal children, it is obvious that much learning takes place by observing others and copying their actions (Bandura 1969). Sluckin (1970) has reported that infants at the age of 4 months will match some of the actions of other people, *e.g.* hand clapping. A major problem in dealing with autistic children is that they do not readily imitate the actions of others.

A method for the establishment of non-verbal imitation has been described by Lovaas *et al.* (1967). It involves what is called 'successive discriminations'. That is, the child is rewarded for closer and closer approximations to the behaviour of the therapist. What the therapist in effect does is train the child to copy his gestures. If, at a later stage, the child copies a novel pattern of behaviour, it is argued that the ability to imitate has been developed.

211

In the initial stage, the child is trained to play with simple toys such as banging a xylophone or placing pegs in a board. Later, more complex tasks are produced so that the child may be required to pick up the left-hand block when two blocks are placed in front of him, after watching the model pick up the left-hand block. When the child masters this set of tasks, he may then be required to match responses which select two or more attributes of an object such as picking up the card with the large triangle, then the card with the large red triangle, and so on. Some of the tasks require the child to copy sequences of movements without using objects, *e.g.* standing up, hand-clapping.

The variety of tasks used in the study reported by Lovaas *et al.* (1967) was varied from one occasion to the next to ensure that it was not simply a sequence being learned, but that the child was actually copying what the therapist was doing. The training techniques relied heavily on initial prompting with continuous food rewards for correct behaviour. As was the case with the establishment of verbal labelling, the prompts were gradually faded and the reinforcements gradually shifted to a partial reinforcement scheme, since it has been shown that behaviour which has been rewarded intermittently is more likely to persist.

Once the child learns to imitate these comparatively simple tasks, more complex skills are taught. In the process of building up these behaviour patterns, verbal labels are attached to the sequences so that eventually all that one may need to do is say to the child 'Hang up your coat' to elicit the appropriate behaviour.

The Behaviour Modification Strategy

An essential part of any behaviour modification strategy applied to children with speech and language problems is full assessment of the results. Briefly, four main stages in such an analysis can be identified.

(1) *The identification of target behaviours*

Those aspects of the behaviour of the child which need to be modified are selected and the goals of treatment are specified.

(2) *Baseline period*

The naturally occurring rate or duration of target behaviours is measured in the treatment setting.

(3) *Treatment*

Treatment is initiated using behaviour modification techniques. The child's responses to various procedures are monitored and the procedures are changed if they do not produce the desired effects.

(4) *Evaluation*

Short-term and long-term follow-up observations are initiated to evaluate the effects of treatment. Of course, if changes do occur this does not necessarily prove the treatment was responsible. Some techniques to test whether changes are causally related to therapy are described by Bandura (1969).

Outcome of Operant Training

Having described some of the behaviour modification techniques, we are now in a position to examine the outcome of operant training with autistic children.

The Table summarizes the results of many cases of operant speech and language training reported in the literature in recent years. Whilst we cannot pretend that these abstracts constitute a total coverage of the published literature, it is likely that the majority of studies involving autistic children have been incorporated. Wherever possible, an attempt has been made to present information under the following headings: author; sex and age of child; 'diagnosis'; initial speech/language characteristics; outcome of treatment and duration of treatment. Cases reported in more than one publication are listed only once.

TABLE
Outcome of operant training

Author	Sex	Age yrs/ mths	Diagnosis	Initial level	Outcome	Duration of treatment
Blake and Moss (1967)*	F	4.0	? (Mute)	No speech	2 words	—
Brawley et al. (1969)	M	7.0	Early infantile autism	Few words at 2 yrs	Simple naming, asks/answers questions, (appropriate speech remained at same level at 3 mth follow-up)	20 sessions
Chapel (1970)	M	4.0	Autism	Jargon and echolalia	Echoing, but some simple phrases used appropriately	—
Cook and Adams (1966)*	M	13.0	Retarded	No speech	Increase in sounds	12 hrs
	M	6.0	Retarded	No speech	Increase in syllables	20 sessions
	M	13.0	Retarded	3 words per day	76 words per session	—
Fygetakis and Grey (1969)	2M 1F	6.3	Aphasia	Disturbed grammatical functions	Novel sentences generated to rules	21 hrs
Hewett (1965)*	M	4.6	Autism	2 words	150 meaningful words	14 mths
Hingtgen and Trost (1964)	M	5.0	Autism-symbiotic	Few non-speech sounds, no communicating speech	Co-operative use of recognizable syllables generalised to adults	46
	M	5.6	Autism-symbiotic	Few non-speech sounds, no communicating speech	Co-operative use of recognizable syllables generalized to adults	30 minute sessions on average
	M	5.3	Autism	Few non-speech sounds, no communicating speech	Co-operative use of recognizable syllables generalised to adults	
	F	7.6	Autism	Few non-speech sounds, no communicating speech	No communicative vocalisations	

Outcome of operant training

Author	Sex	Age yrs/ mths	Diagnosis	Initial level	Outcome	Duration of treatment
Hingtgen et al. (1967)	M	6.6	Autism (no neurological damage)	Mute	18 word approximations (200 words at follow-up)	4-6 hrs
	F	5.5	Autism (no neurological damage)	Mute	17 sounds, 11 words (meaningful naming at 5 mth follow-up)	4-6 hrs
Hingtgen (1968)	M	5.11	Early childhood schizophrenia, possible brain damage	Mute	60 word approximations (raised to naming 50 objects after further 140 hrs)	48 hrs
	M	4.9	Early childhood schizophrenia, possible brain damage	Mute	25 word approximations, 10 labels (100 labels but no creative speech after further 140 hrs)	52 hrs
	M	4.1	Early childhood schizophrenia, possible brain damage	Mute	16 word approximations (no further progress after 600 hrs)	44 hrs
	M	4.0	Early childhood schizophrenia, possible brain damage	Mute	Imitates 9 sounds (no further progress after 600 hrs)	66 hrs
Jensen and Womack (1967)*	M	7.0	Autism	Single words	Word combinations with generalisations	—
Kerr et al. (1965)*	F	3.0	Retarded (Mute)	Grunts	Increased vocalization	—
Lovaas (1966)* Lovaas et al. (1967)	M	6.0	Schizophrenia	Occasional vowel sounds	Large imitative vocabulary	11 mths
	M	6.0	Schizophrenia	Occasional vowel sounds	Large imitative vocabulary	11 mths
	M	5.0	Schizophrenia	Mute	Extensive labelling	First 20 words in 38 days
	M	?	Schizophrenia	Echolalia	Spontaneous conversation	1 yr
	F	7.0	Schizophrenia	Echolalia	Used pronouns, prepositions and labelling, no spontaneous conversation	10 mths
	F	9.0	Schizophrenia	Echolalia	50 words, reduced echoing	2 mths
Ney (1967)	10M	?	Autism (6 of the 9 points)	No details	Improved more than matched group given play therapy	50 sessions
Nelson and Evans (1968)	M	6.0	Early childhood autism	20 'ideoglossic' utterances	200 words and phrases, some spontaneous speech	45 sessions over 6 mths

Outcome of operant training

Author	Sex	Age yrs/ mths	Diagnosis	Initial level	Outcome	Duration of treatment
Nelson and Evans (cont.)	M	6.0	Executive dysphasia, elective autism	6 dyslalic words (normal compre-hension)	20 words	29 sessions
	M	7.0	Expressive language disorder, brain damage? ESN	Echolalia	Labels, spontaneous speech	21 sessions
	M	5.0	Early childhood autism	Unintelligible sounds	Imitation only	26 sessions
Pelz (1969)	M	6.6	Autism	Few non-speech sounds	11 imitated sounds, 20 word approx-imations, 12 labels	139 hrs
Risley and Wolf (1967)*	M	7.0	Autism? Retarded?	Echolalia	Appropriate phrases	—
	M	8.0	Severely retarded	Echolalia	Labelling	—
	M	10.0	Autism	Echolalia	Labelling	—
	M	12.0	Autism	Echolalia	Labelling	—
Salzinger et al. (1965)*	M	3.6	Organic, IQ = 32	No words, no imitation	4-5 clear words	150 hrs
	M	3.10	Behaviour dis-order, normal IQ	Some words	Sentences	—
Schell et al. (1967)*	M	4.6	Autism	No speech	Few words, res-ponds to com-mands (labelling after further 8 mths)	45 sessions
Sloane et al. (1968)*	F	3.7	Retarded	No speech	40 words	8 mths
	M	4.7	Very retarded	10-15 single words	60 words, 60 phrases	7 mths
	M	7.5	Retarded, autism	24 'Tacts', 12 'Mands'	Increase from 100 to 600 response for 90 min session	—
	F	3.3	?	0-4 words	Regular naming	—
	F	4.8	Retarded	High verbal rate, poor articulation	Little change	1 mth
	F	4.0	Brain damage	No words	10 words	—
Straughan et al. (1965)	M	14.0	Retarded mute	Normal speech devel-opment but low rate of speaking	Frequency and sentence length increased	9 days
Weiss and Born (1967)*	M	7.6	?	Echolalia	Sentences, but he did not gen-eralise outside	9 mths
Wetzel et al. (1966)*	M	6.0	Autism	Echolalia	100 words, simple requests	20 sessions
Wolf et al. (1964)*	M	3.6	Schizophrenia	Echolalia	Normal 5yr level	2-3 yrs

*These 13 studies were summarized by Tilby (1968). We are grateful for the help of Mrs. P. Howlin in abstracting the other studies.

It can be seen that a wide variety of clinical problems have been treated with varying degrees of success. Even a cursory glance at the Table shows that the idealised behavioural modification model which we have presented above is, at best, approximated by only a few of the reported studies. Despite the obvious weaknesses in reporting, it can be seen that many dramatic advances are claimed.

For example, Lovaas (1967) has reported on 11 children who have taken part in his programme. All of them were severely delayed in speech development, and all got at least as far as the labelling stage. However, he noted huge individual differences in the rates of attaining imitative vocal behaviour. He comments that: 'When a child had some of this behavior at the onset of training, acquisition was rapid, and rather elaborate imitative behaviors were established within one or two weeks of training. In children who evinced no form of imitative behavior and consequently seemed more unresponsive to social stimuli, only extensive training efforts have brought about imitative speech'. In other words, echolalic children appear to respond much better to this treatment than mute children. In fact, '.... the variation extends from three or four trials upward to several thousand' and, as can be seen in the Table, some failures have been reported.

Some Methodological Criticisms

Many of the papers mentioned can be criticised on methodological grounds. Firstly, the descriptions of the children involved in the studies in terms of their physical, psychiatric, neurological and cognitive status, are generally absent or grossly inadequate. There are large individual differences in children's responses to treatment and, in order to advise rationally on which form of treatment is most likely to be beneficial to which sort of child, systematic and comprehensive clinical descriptions must be given. Secondly, whilst most authors have been careful to specify the details of their techniques, little attention has been paid to describing the pre- and post-treatment measures of speech and language attainment. Psychometric procedures are 'conspicuous by their absence' and the descriptions are generally too vague to be meaningful. Thirdly, almost all the studies reported to date have been individual case reports. Control groups will have to be used in future studies if for no other reason than that a significant number of mute autistic children do develop speech 'spontaneously' in middle childhood. In the Maudsley follow-up study (Rutter *et al.* 1967) of 32 children without speech at the age of 5 years, 7 subsequently developed speech; 2 of these at the late age of 11 years. In addition, control groups are necessary for comparing the relative efficacy of different forms of treatment when these alternatives have been sufficiently well-formulated. Finally, more attention needs to be paid to long-term follow-up to determine whether treatment induced changes persist.

Speech or Language Training?

One of the questions often raised about this type of treatment is, does operant training result in better speech, better language, or both? Critics claim that only speech is taught (Weiss and Born 1967), but in the absence of adequate data on treatment results and without a generally accepted definition of language, the issue must remain open. Fortunately, certain characteristics of language have been agreed by psychologists (Lenneberg 1967, Hockett 1970, Premack 1970) and these can be adapted

216

to permit measurement without the need for any global definition. For example, Brown and his colleagues (1969) have drawn attention to the 'pivot and open class' combination in early two word phrases. It would be useful to determine whether this type of sentence structure can be taught in a way which allows the child to generate new combinations.

It might also be questioned whether it should always be spoken words which are taught to children with speech delay. In some cases, gesture might prove a better way of initiating communication and preliminary techniques for teaching gesture are available (Levitt 1970).

Conclusions

Despite their limitations, the published studies indicate that the techniques described above are sufficiently valuable to warrant further examination. The volume of studies which has appeared recently in speech therapy journals is sufficient witness to the fact that behavioural approaches have a utility beyond psychology. Weiner (1969), for example, has cited 69 references linking speech therapy and behaviour modification practices. More recently, McReynolds (1970) has analysed some traditional speech therapy techniques in terms of the contingency reinforcement model. Hartung (1970) in the same journal, discusses practical ways of increasing imitation in mute autistic children, again within a behaviour modification framework. In Britain too, speech therapists are actively discussing the place of behaviour modification approaches in their discipline (Nelson and Evans 1968, Savage 1968).

Already, some workers in the field of speech pathology are conducting trials of traditional methods. Wilson (1966) undertook a controlled trial of the efficacy of speech therapy with mentally retarded children. Evaluating the effect of articulation therapy on sound error reduction over a three year period, he found no differences between the treatment and control groups. Other workers have been examining the problems of measurement in a speech therapy setting. Mowrer (1969) has discussed a novel method of recording the rate and accuracy of vocal responses during therapy sessions: 'The recording technique described may help provide a basic tool whereby empirical, normative data can be established, the process of correction studied, and the effectiveness of speech therapy procedures improved'.

Unequivocal conclusions are hard to come by in treatment research. We are fully aware that it is easier to formulate a theoretical ideal for treatment research than to achieve this in practice. Nevertheless, ongoing evaluation should form an integral part of any treatment procedure. It is only in so doing that premature and extravagant claims can be avoided. This is particularly important if we are to avoid creating an unwarranted optimism in already troubled parents.

Acknowledgements:
In collaboration with Drs. L. Hersov and M. Rutter, the authors are in receipt of a generous grant from the Department of Health and Social Security to evaluate the effects of behaviour modification techniques in the comprehensive treatment of autistic children. We would like to thank these colleagues, and Dr. S. Rachman, for their many helpful discussions and suggestions. We would also like to thank Drs. Nelson and Evans for giving us permission to use the Fig. in our chapter.

REFERENCES

Bandura, A. (1969) *Principles of Behavior Modification.* New York: Holt, Rinehart & Winston.

Beech, H. R., Fransella, F. (1968) *Research and Experiment in Stuttering.* Oxford; Pergamon.

Blake, P., Moss, T. (1967) 'The development of socialization skills in an electively mute child.' *Behav. Res. Ther.,* **5,** 349.

Brawley, E. R., Harris, F. R., Allen, K. E., Fleming, R. S., Peterson, R. F. (1969) 'Behavior modification of an autistic child.' *Behav. Sci.,* **14,** 87.

Bricker, W. A., Bricker, D. D. (1970) 'A program of language training for the severely language handicapped child.' *Except. Child.,* **37,** 101.

Brown, R., Cazden, C., Bellugi-Klima, U. (1969) 'The child's grammar from I to III.' *in* Hill, J. P. (Ed.) *Minnesota Symposia on Child Psychology,* Vol. 2. Minneapolis: University of Minnesota Press p. 28.

Chapel, J. L. (1970) 'Behavior modification techniques with children and adolescents.' *Canad. psychiat. Ass. J.,* **15,** 315.

Cook, C., Adams, H. E. (1966) 'Modification of verbal behavior in speech deficient children.' *Behav. Res. Ther.,* **4,** 625.

Evans, I. M. (1971) 'Theoretical and experimental aspects of the behaviour modification approach to autistic children.' *in* Rutter, M. (Ed.) *Infantile Autism: Concepts, Characteristics and Treatment.* London: Churchill Livingstone.

Ferster, C. E., De Meyer, M. K. (1961) 'The development of performances in autistic children in an automatically controlled environment.' *J. chron. Dis.,* **13,** 312.

—— —— (1962) 'A method for the experimental analysis of the behavior of autistic children.' *Amer. J. Ortho. psychiat.,* **32,** 89.

—— Perrott, M. C. (1968) *Behaviour Principles.* New York: Appleton-Century-Crofts.

Fygetakis, L., Grey, B. B. (1969) 'Programmed conditioning of linguistic competence.' *Behav. Res. Ther.,* **8,** 153.

Goldiamond, I. (1968) 'Stuttering and fluency as manipulatable operant response classes.' *in* Sloane, H. N., MacAulay, B. D. (Eds.) *Operant, Procedure in Remedial Speech and Language Training.* Boston: Houghton, Mifflin.

Hartung, J. R. (1970) 'A review of procedures to increase verbal imitation skills and functional speech in autistic children.' *J. speech. disord.,* **35,** 203.

Hewett, F. M. (1965) 'Teaching speech to an autistic child through operant conditioning.' *Amer. J. Orthopsychiat.,* **35,** 927.

Hingtgen, J. N. (1968) 'Differential effects on behaviour modification in four mute autistic boys.' *in* Churchill, D. W., Alpern, G. D., De Meyer, M. V. (Eds.) *Infantile Autism: Proceedings of the Indiana University Colloquium.* Indianapolis: University of Indiana Press.

—— Coulter, S. K., Churchill, D. W. (1967) 'Intensive reinforcement of imitative behavior in mute autistic children.' *Arch. gen. Psychiat.,* **17,** 36.

—— Trost, F. C. (1964) 'Shaping cooperative responses in early childhood schizophrenia. II. Reinforcement of mutual physical contact and vocal responses.' Paper presented at the Annual Meeting, American Psychological Association, September, 1964.

Hockett, C. F. (1960) 'The origin of speech.' *Sci.Amer.,* **203,** (3), 89.

Holland, A., Harris, A. (1968) 'Aphasia rehabilitation using programmed instruction: an intensive case history.' *in* Sloane, H. N., MacAulay, B. D. (Eds.) *Operant Procedure in Remedial Speech and Language Training.* Boston: Houghton, Mifflin.

Jensen, G. J., Womack, M. S. (1967) 'Operant conditioning techniques applied in the treatment of an autistic child.' *Amer. J. Orthopsychiat.,* **37,** 30.

Kerr, N., Meyerson, L., Michael, J. (1965) 'A procedure for shaping verbalizations in a mute child.' *in* Ullman, L. P., Krasner, L. (Eds.) *Case Studies in Behavior Modification.* New York: Holt, Rinehart & Winston.

Lenneberg, E. H. (1967) *Biological Foundations of Language.* New York: Wiley.

Levitt, L. M. (1970) *A Method of Communication for Non-speaking Severely Subnormal Children.* London: Spastics Society.

Lovaas, O. I. (1966) 'A programme for the establishment of speech in psychotic children.' *in* Wing, J. K. (Ed.) *Early Childhood Autism: Clinical, Educational and Social Aspects.* Oxford: Pergamon. p. 115.

—— (1967) 'A behaviour therapy approach to the treatment of childhood schizophrenia.' *in* Hill, J. P. (Ed.) *Minnesota Symposia on Child Psychology,* Vol. 1. Minneapolis: University of Minnesota Press. p. 108.

—— Freitas, L., Nelson, K., Whalen, C. (1967) 'The establishment of imitation and its use for the development of complex behaviour in schizophrenic children.' *Behav. Res. Ther.,* **5,** 171.

Lovitt, T. (1970) 'Behavior modification: the current scene.' *Except. Child.,* **37,** 85.

McReynolds, L. V. (1970) 'Contingencies and consequences in speech therapy.' *J. speech Disord.,* **35,** 12.

Marshall, R. C. (1970) 'The effects of response contingent punishment upon a defective articulation response.' *J. speech Disord.,* **35,** 236.

Metz, J. R. (1965) 'Conditioning generalized imitation in autistic children.' *J. exp. Child Psychol. Psychiat.*, **2**, 389.

Mowrer, D. E. (1969) 'Evaluating speech therapy through precision recording.' *J. speech. Disord.*, **34**, 239.

—— Baker, R. L., Schutz, R. E. (1968) 'Operant procedures in the control of speech articulation.' *in* Sloane, H. N., MacAulay, B. D. (Eds.) *Operant Procedure in Remedial Speech and Language Training.* Boston: Houghton, Mifflin.

Nelson, R. O., Evans, I. M. (1968) 'The combination of learning principles and speech therapy techniques in the treatment of non-communicating children.' *J. Child. Psychol. Psychiat.*, **9**, 111.

Ney, P. (1967) 'Operant conditioning of schizophrenic children.' *Canad. psychiat. Ass. J.*, **12**, 9.

Nolan, J. D., Pence, C. (1970) 'Operant conditioning principles in the treatment of a selectively mute child.' *J. consult. clin. Psychol.*, **35**, 265.

Patterson, G. R., Gullion, M. E. (1968) *Living with Children: New Methods for Parents and Teachers.* Champaign, Ill.: Research Press.

—— McNeal, S., Hawkins, N., Phelps, R. (1967) 'Re-programming the social environment.' *J.Child Psychol.Psychiat.*, **8**, 181.

Peltz, E. B. (1969) Infantile Autism: Operant Conditioning of a Single Case. University of Witwatersrand, B.A. Dissertation.

Premack, D. (1970) 'A functional analysis of language.' *J.exp.anal.Behav.*, **14**, 107.

Reid, J. B., Hawkins, N., Keutzer, C., McNeal, S. A., Phelps, R. E., Reid, K. M., Mees, H. L. (1967) 'A marathon behaviour modification of a selectively mute child.' *J. Child Psychol. Psychiat.*, **8**, 27.

Risley, T., Wolf, M. (1967) 'Establishing functional speech in echolalic children.' *Behav. Res. Ther.*, **5**, 73.

Rutter, M. (1966a) 'Behavioural and cognitive characteristics of a series of psychotic children.' *in* Wing, J. K. (Ed.) *Early Childhood Autism: Clinical, Educational and Social Aspects.* Oxford: Pergamon. p. 51.

—— (1966b) 'Prognosis: psychotic children in adolescence and early adult life.' *in* Wing, J. K. (Ed.) *Early Childhood Autism: Clinical, Educational and Social Aspects,* Oxford: Pergamon. p. 83.

—— (1968) 'Concepts of autism: a review of research.' *J. Child Psychol. Psychiat.*, **9**, 1.

—— (Ed.) (1971) *Infantile Autism: Concepts, Characteristics and Treatment.* London: Churchill Livingstone.

—— Greenfield, D., Lockyer, L. (1967) 'A five to fifteen year follow-up study of infantile psychosis. II. Social and behavioural outcome.' *Brit. J. Psychiat.*, **113**, 1183.

Salzinger, K., Feldman, R. S., Cowan, J. E., Salzinger, S. (1965) 'Operant conditioning of verbal behavior of two young speech deficient boys.' *in* Ullman, L. P., Krasner, L. (Eds.) *Case Studies in Behaviour Modification.* New York: Holt, Rinehart & Winston.

Savage, V. A. (1968) 'Childhood autism: a review of the literature with particular reference to the speech and language structure of the autistic child.' *Brit. J. Disord. Commun.*, **3**, 75.

Schell, R. E., Stark, J., Giddan, J. J. (1967) 'Development of language behavior in an autistic child.' *J. speech. Disord.*, **32**, 51.

Schopler, E., Reichler, R. J. (1969) 'Parents as therapists for their own autistic child.' Paper presented at the International Congress of Social Psychiatry, London, August, 1967.

Sloane, H. N., Johnston, M. K., Harris, F. R. (1968) 'Remedial procedures for teaching verbal behavior to speech deficient or defective young children.' *in* Sloane, H. N., MacAulay, B. D. (Eds.) *Operant Procedure in Remedial Speech and Language Training.* Boston: Houghton, Mifflin.

—— MacAulay, B. D. (Eds.) (1968) *Operant Procedure in Remedial Speech and Language Training.* Boston: Houghton, Mifflin.

Sluckin, W. (1970) *Early Learning in Man and Animal.* London: Allen & Unwin.

Staats, A. (1968) *Learning, Language and Cognition.* New York: Holt, Rinehart & Winston.

Straughan, J. H., Potter, W. K., Hamilton, S. H. (1965) 'The behavioural treatment of an elective mute.' *J. Child Psychol. Psychiat.*, **6**, 125.

Tilby, P. J. (1968) The Operant Approach to Remedial Speech and Language Training: A Critical Review. University of London, M.Sc. Thesis.

Ullman, L. P., Krasner, L. (Eds.) (1965) *Case Studies in Behavior Modification.* New York: Holt, Rinehart & Winston.

Weiner, A. E. (1969) 'Speech therapy and behavior modification: a conspectus.' *J. spec. Educ.*, **3**, 285.

Weiss, H. H., Born, B. (1967) 'Speech training or language acquisition? A distinction when speech training is taught by operant conditioning procedures.' *Amer. J. Orthopsychiat.*, **37**, 49.

Wetzel, J., Baker, J., Roney, M., Martin, M. (1966) 'Outpatient treatment of autistic behavior.' *Behav. Res. Ther.*, **4**, 169.

Wilson, F. B. (1966) 'Efficacy of speech therapy with educable mentally retarded children.' *J. speech Res.*, **9**, 423.

Wolf, M., Risley, T., Mees, H. (1964) 'Application of operant conditioning procedures to the behavior problems of an autistic child.' *Behav. Res. Ther.*, **1**, 305.

Yates, A. J. (1970) *Behavior Therapy.* New York: Wiley.

CHAPTER 18

The Management of the Hearing Impaired Child

J. A. M. MARTIN

The intimate relationship between hearing and speech is seen clearly in the young child who has difficulty in hearing. The hearing loss may be of such severity that he can never perceive speech at an adequate level of loudness and so fails to acquire language. At the other extreme, the loss may be of a degree and type that he learns his mother-tongue at the normal rate, but comprehension is unduly impaired by adverse factors such as noise, or the speech of unfamiliar adults. His speech may show defects of which he is unaware in the articulation of individual words and in the cadences and intonation patterns of the flow of speech, which he is unable to correct by ear alone. Hearing loss shows a wide variety of type and degree between these limits and is ordinarily measured by pure tone threshold audiometry. It is important to remember that there is no direct correlation between the picture of residual hearing so obtained and the child's facility in the comprehension and use of spoken language.

Management is dependent on very much more than the assessment in acoustical terms of hearing loss, and consequently makes great demands on those responsible for the care of these children in the formative pre-school years. Nevertheless, the time and effort spent during this period in the development of the child's language is of incalculable importance for so much of his cognitive, emotional and social maturation. In this chapter, the general principles of management will be discussed for the pre-school period, including the prescription and use of hearing aids, the development of language and school placement; and certain problems arising from the effect of a handicapped child on his parents. For details of management reference should be made to educational authorities such as Ewing and Ewing (1964) and Watson (1967).

The Child

Hearing Aids: Age of Child

The importance of early diagnosis needs to be emphasised continually, but let us assume the all too rare event of a four months old baby in whom the otologist has every reason to believe that there is a severe hearing loss. Does he prescribe a hearing aid? The child is deaf, babies under one year of age learn to use their hearing, the importance of early diagnosis has been stressed and a widely held view is that, unless there is immediate use of a hearing aid, the child will inevitably suffer. This line of reasoning may be acoustically correct but biologically harmful. Hearing aids are non-selective in their amplification, so that all sounds within the response range are brought to the subject's ear. The effect on the infant is twofold. There is a violent assault on his limited sensory world, confined initially as it is almost to the physical limits of his own body, internal sensation, mouth, hands, integument, soon associated with a progressive expansion of his world visually, and followed by an increasing awareness and expansion of the world of hearing. But a hearing aid cuts arcoss this orderly sensory

220

development necessary for the organisation of the world in which he begins to find himself. Sounds from near and far are fed into his ear and auditory space has no meaning. In addition to this he is exposed to the whole noisy world in which we live. Meaningful sounds, such as his mother's voice and the preparation of his feed, are submerged in the buzz and confusion of traffic, aeroplanes, and other noise long before he has learned to sort out and evaluate their significance. so that sounds cannot acquire any quality of meaning. Rather than prescribe an aid it is preferable to initiate auditory training by giving advice to the parents on how to talk to the infant, and how best to stimulate his interest in sound, preferably through regular visits from a peripatetic teacher of the deaf. The issue of a hearing aid may be deferred until the age of 9 to 12 months. The one year old is on the verge of walking and from this age on he will be intent on exploring the physical world through his own efforts. He is no longer a captive audience, obliged to sit on his mother's lap or restrained in pram or cot and so to hearing her voice nearby whenever she chooses. Instead he will be wandering away so that her speech and the sounds of her activity are progressively attenuated by the increasing distance, and soon submerged by the fascination of his new-found world.

Initial Prescription

It is advisable to avoid over-amplification and to resist the temptation to prescribe ultra-powerful hearing aids until one has had the opportunity to study the child's progress over many months. It is not possible always to rely on the parents' observations alone for details of progress, and discussion between clinician and teacher of the deaf is desirable and necessary. In this country, the government-issued Medresco OL56 has proved an excellent aid for initial prescription. Once the parents are confident in their handling of the aid and the child has accepted it, a second aid can be given so that both ears are receiving amplified sound from separate sources, though the parents should not be misled into thinking that two aids are twice as good as one. Where it is not economically feasible to use two aids, the output of the instrument can be taken to a receiver head in each ear by the so-called Y lead.

High Output Aids

An exception to the rule that two ears are better than one occurs in the severe forms of deafness in which there is little residual hearing, limited perhaps to 95/100dB in the low frequencies. A hearing loss of this magnitude almost always necessitates a powerful aid and modern instruments have a maximum output approaching 140dB. An aid of this type should be prescribed only after careful deliberation and when continuing assessment of the child's progress in the development of languages shows that he is doing badly. The maximum permitted noise level without time restriction in industry is 85dB for individuals with normal hearing. The effects of noise on the auditory pathways already damaged by *e.g.* rubella virus or bile pigments is not known, and the clinician needs to adopt an attitude of caution, conserving hearing rather than running the risk to the child of damaging it further. In such children binaural hearing is better omitted. Ballantyne (1970) has demonstrated the possibility of damage to hearing through this means, and one's own experience confirms it.

Once it is possible to gain a reasonably accurate picture of the hearing loss for each ear, and to determine the shape of the audiogram curve it may be necessary to modify the response characteristic of the aid. In the absence of detailed information the most suitable response is one of uniform, level gain across the speech range of frequencies within the limits of the instrument. A large minority of children have sensori-neural deafness of a type in which the low frequencies show no, or comparatively slight, loss whilst the frequencies above (and often including) 1000Hz are severely impaired. Uniform amplification in this type of deafness results in accentuating still further the loud low frequency sounds of speech and the mechanised world in which we live. A variety of aids include the facility of altering the response curve by reducing gain in the low frequencies. By a combination of different hearing aid settings and using receiver-heads of differing characteristics, a wide variety of overall response curves is possible. It should be emphasised that a pure tone threshold loss cannot be corrected so simply and it seems likely that we need other forms of testing hearing function before such accuracy of prescription is possible. Speech audiometry is limited in its application because the majority of children are too young and have limited vocabularies with highly personal content at the time when accurate prescription is first required. In the older child the results of speech audiometry may not be sufficiently precise to help evaluate the merits of alternative aids and settings except in relatively gross terms. Careful frequent observation of the pre-school child by teachers of the deaf experienced in this age group remains the best guide. The selection of an alternative instrument may therefore require several weeks of trial before a satisfactory opinion is reached.

Other facilities in hearing aids include some form of noise limitation, and induction coils. The former is useful in children in whom recruitment is demonstrable, or suspected through extreme intolerance of the aid particularly under noisy conditions, and where the pathology indicates (or cannot exclude) end-organ damage. It is possible to limit the high peaks of sudden noises by clipping or by compressing the dynamic range, with resultant increase in comfort to the child. Hearing aids with induction coils need to be prescribed when the child is due to go to a school or class in which the loop system is used. In this method, the teacher's voice is fed through a microphone and amplifier into a loop of wire arranged around or within the classroom and reconverted into sound waves through the coil in the child's own aid. The child is afforded a greater range of movement, though will not be able to monitor his own speech unless there is a setting on the aid allowing for this, which is not always present.

Many schools use group hearing aids. The classroom is equipped with a microphone and amplifier for the teacher and with specially fitted desks wired for headphones and a microphone for each child. In this way, high fidelity sound reaches the whole class of perhaps 4 or 6 children, each of whom can hear his own voice and the other childrens'. A similar arrangement can be used for one child and is then usually referred to as a 'speech trainer'. It is frequently recommended for the pre-school child and many mothers become adept in its use. There are certain disadvantages which tend to get overlooked. The situation is formal, requiring the co-operation of the child and his tolerance of the headphones, language may become artificial and an insistence on the child's output of spoken language can develop all too readily. Many teachers like to restrict its use in the home to various forms of games involving noise-making play material to stimulate interest in sound, and in telling simple stories with objects or pictures.

Ear Moulds

In order to conduct the sound efficiently from the receiver head of the hearing aid to the middle ear, it is necessary to have an ear mould. These should be made individually for each child and renewed as often as necessary. The difficulty of getting an accurate impression of the outer ear and meatus in a young struggling child means that several moulds may have to be made before a satisfactory fit is obtained. There are a variety of materials used in ear mould construction. One technique is to use a compound which serves both as impression material and final mould. This has obvious merits, particularly in the young child needing frequent changes of mould, but the material is more readily damaged, and the surface finish lacks the perfection of the more durable form. In this latter type, the impression is taken and a plaster of paris cast made, from which the final article is produced. Moulds need to be comfortable and firmly fitting with an adequate meatal prolongation, so that there is no leak of sound from within the external meatus back to the microphone of the aid causing a howl.

Development of Language

Once the hearing aid has been prescribed and fitted, the task of fostering the growth of languages is just beginning. No hearing aid can restore the hearing loss completely to normal and in the early stages, particularly in the severely deaf child who has not been diagnosed until two or three years old, it may be difficult to attract the child's attention to the world of sound. He may have become so competent in his visual assessment of the situation, and in communication of his needs by gesture and mime, that he relies on his eyes alone. It should not be assumed that a child, once given a hearing aid, will take the greatest pleasure in wearing it. It may on the contrary prove a long uphill task to gain his interest in music, nursery rhymes and speech.

The parents must bear the brunt of the training of their hearing-impaired child in the pre-school years and they need a great deal of detailed information and help to equip them for this task. It is not sufficient merely to tell them to talk to their child. Some parents need no instruction and have an intuitive grasp of the methods to adopt but they are in the minority and it is every parent's right to be taught the details of management. The principle is so simple that many, parents and teachers alike, are misled into believing that the practice is equally simple. To be told to 'talk meaningfully' requires a wealth of explanation and practical demonstration. Does it mean saying single words loudly and clearly over and over again, or is it immersing the child in a flood of words about what ever comes into the mother's mind? Some parents are taciturn by nature and if left to their own devices would say only a few brief words to the child in a day, others prattle incessantly and neither extreme is of any value. The child needs first to catch the cadences, the lilt and the pattern of the flow of speech so that it is necessary always to talk in short, clear, simple sentences.

Language is more than single words and the basic linguistic structures can only be built up if the child hears them in the speech which is used to him so that he learns not only intonation, stress and rhythm, but syntax as well. Stress has an important function in everyday speech and is an integral part of the language structure. It is characteristic of children with poor hearing that they develop an ungrammatical, telegraphic style partly because many of the particles, conjunctions and auxiliary verbs are unstressed and so poorly heard or omitted as unimportant.

Evaluation of the child's developing capacity in language should not rely purely upon the number of words which the child can say. One often gains the impression that this is the only criterion of success. It is harmful for the child and vitiates the approach of parents and teacher. The main concern must always be 'What does the child understand of what is said to him?'. Individual words have representational value for objects and activities and must be combined in the ways laid down by the syntax of the mother-tongue before language can be said to have developed. We are, after all, more than mobile vocabularies, and the collection of dictionary items is a vital but preliminary part in the learning of language. Excessive emphasis on output too early will short-cut the laborious elaboration of self-generated phrases and sentences with the result that 'word-items-in' will be replayed as 'word-items-out'. This can lead to the situation, so often witnessed, in which the child with a severe hearing loss on being told for instance to 'give it to Mummy' or 'sit down' will repeat the words after the speaker with no idea whatsoever that action is expected of him. Words have become things to repeat back, not sounds signals to initiate physical activity. The corollary of this failure to act on words is that words will not be used in the development of mental activity and cognitive skills. One can symphathise with the parents (and indeed the teachers) in their need to have tangible evidence of progress, but progress in the comprehension of what is said is an infinitely superior indicator when compared with the child's ability to say spontaneously or, worse still, simply repeat a few dozen words. The tragedy of the everlasting 'oralism' versus 'manualism' debate is that the insistence of either group of proponents on the output of spoken signs or the output of manual signs is diverting attention from where it should be directed, the reception and comprehension of language. And this redirection will itself fail unless language is considered as an integral part of human activity and behaviour as a whole. We are doing the deaf child a grave injustice if we continue to argue in such facile fashion that his problems can be resolved by training the mouth or the hands as a means of communication.

Schooling
Pre-school

Education in the more formal limited use of the word begins at 5 years and provision must be made for this group of handicapped children. Much can be done before this age to help the individual child; the vital rôle of the peripatetic teacher of the deaf in giving close personal assistance and advising constantly on management cannot be over-emphasised. The child with a hearing loss has peculiar problems of participation and involvement in the activities of ordinary children so that it is all-important to anticipate and over-come these difficulties as early as possible. If he has brothers and sisters who are older and younger, the problem is less than in the family setting where he is the only child or very much younger than the others. Young friends of his own age can be brought in and when the appropriate time comes he can spend a few hours a week in a nursery school. The difficulties he experiences in communicating verbally with the other children should not be underestimated, but the 2-and 3-year-olds can gain so much of the information required by situational clues that the individual's poverty of spoken language does not stand out so clearly. Fully aware of the needs of this age group, many principals of schools for the deaf have nursery classes attached to their schools where children can go from the age of $2\frac{1}{2}$ years onward. Special hearing units attached to ordinary infant schools are also opening nursery classes for their partial-hearing children. But if there is no provision locally in special schools and units, the nursery school, the day nursery or the well-managed play group can provide the right milieu for the young child. Communication is after all very much more than spoken language, and language itself is in part a highly social activity.

School Placement

There are a variety of ways in which the 5-year-old may be placed. He may go to an ordinary school, needing only the assistance of his hearing aid to enable him to compete on equal terms with the other children. It is always advisable for his progress to be checked by occasional visits from a peripatetic teacher of the deaf (Department of Education and Science 1969). He may go to a partial hearing unit (P.H.U.) which is a small class numbering not more than 8-10 children run by a teacher of the deaf, often with non-specialist assistants. Such units are attached to ordinary day schools and much will depend on the attitudes of the school principal and the unit teacher on how much integration into normal school activities there will be for the hearing-impaired (Department of Education and Science 1967). There are special schools reserved for the partially-hearing, and many long-established schools for the severely deaf. Such schools may be day or residential. Some schools cater for hearing-impaired children having other disabilities such as blindness or partial-sight, the educationally sub-normal and the maladjusted. The choice in practice is never so great as it may seem and many placements are an unsatisfactory compromise with the limited facilities available. One may have to recommend that a child whose parental care has been exemplary should go to a residential school for the deaf when he would ideally have been placed in a partial-hearing unit locally had there been one. A child with a profound loss and poor family background may have to be accommodated in a P.H.U., or even in a local infant school with occasional visits from a teacher of the deaf, rather than attend a deaf school on a boarding basis. Every decision on placement needs to be made in the knowledge of the facilities available, and the recommendation then discussed with the parents.

How does one come to a decision on optimum placement? The child's audiogram, a hearing test it must be remembered carried out using pure tones to determine a threshold measurement, can only give the crudest indication. There are too many children with apparently good residual hearing and a loss of no more than 70-80dB who have failed to develop language and who must have the special skills of a school

225

for the deaf. There are a variety of reasons for this. The diagnosis may not have been made until late; the parents may have been constantly on the move, or there was inadequate supervision by teachers because of staff shortages; the home circumstances may not be the most suitable for prolonged language stimulation, perhaps from overcrowding or isolation, both parents out at work all day, the limited use of language in the home. The child may have other handicaps such as defective vision, poor concentration and limited attention span, or a degree of mental retardation. It is often a number of factors working together that results in the child not being able to develop language as well as would have appeared likely at first acquaintance. Other children may have very severe losses, perhaps of the order of 95dB and still develop language at a near normal rate so that it becomes difficult to think of placing them in other than ordinary schools. Such children are often held up as the epitome of auditory training and the oral approach. Superlative results of this sort lead one to think that however intelligent the child and diligent the mother, there are other factors probably of an audiological and neurological nature which conspire to minimise the severity of the lesion. Less successful parents may be compared unfavourably. It is not necessarily their fault or indeed anyone's so much as the nature of the hearing disorder itself. We are very much in need of more sophisticated tests of hearing function to help us in the understanding of these apparent vagaries of linguistic development in the deaf child.

The most satisfactory evaluation of a child's language skills is made by those who see him most frequently. The parents can give invaluable information, but their estimate of a child's ability to understand is usually an over-estimate since they are describing situations which are well-worn, repetitive and in which much of the information is conveyed to the child quite unconsciously by movement and gesture. It is expecting too much of their objectivity to give a completely unbiased assessment of the child's comprehension of spoken language, and of his ability to produce intelligible words, phrases and sentences. The person whose observations in the question of school placement must most be relied upon is the peripatetic teacher of the deaf. He is in frequent, regular contact with the child, has been able to observe his increasing linguistic skills over months or years, has seen him at his best and his worst, and has come to know the family as a whole in a way no other member of the team responsible for the child's care can ever aspire to. His assessment of the child's abilities needs always to be sought when the question of which school, and what type of school, comes up for consideration.

The Parents

The child's mother and father play a vital rôle in fostering the growth of language and speech in their young hearing-impaired child. The clear recognition of this one fact played an important part in the development of the teaching of deaf children. Learning of language starts from soon after birth and any delay, such as the one under consideration in this chapter, arising from the inability to hear what is said to him and by him must inevitably impair the child's proficiency in this all important skill. No individual outside the family can hope to attain the intensity of 'teaching' which the parents can achieve. It is essential therefore, and economical, to give them all the help and guidance which they need. Before this can be done certain points need to be emphasised. The parents of a handicapped child have considerable problems of their own. Guilt, shame, despair may be the primary emotions attending the conveying of the diagnosis. Many mothers admit that it took them a great deal of effort and time before they were able to accept the true nature of the handicap, and that until they had done so progress was poor. Those responsible for diagnosis and management have a heavy burden of responsibility in ensuring that the nature of the deafness, and the implications this holds for alleviation and care, are fully understood. A child with a sensori-neural deafness is a child with a permanent handicap however well he learns to talk, and the parents have a constant need for detailed information and support, which is particularly acute in the first months and years after diagnosis.

They can be helped in two main ways. It is advisable whenever possible to put them in touch with other parents in a similar predicament and to arrange meetings both of an informative and social nature to enable them to talk out common problems. However understanding and experienced teachers and doctors may be, there is no answer to the admonition 'How do you know, you haven't got a deaf child'. And the same is true for the parents of a child with Down's syndrome, or a blind child, or an autistic or cerebral palsied child. The second way is to supply them with all the information they need to help in the intelligent management of their child. How to fit and adjust the hearing aid, how and when to use a speech trainer. How to talk meaningfully using all possible situations in the dining room, the bathroom and kitchen inside the house, and the fascinating activities going on in the outside world, children at play, shops, cars, trains, the crane on the building site, the men resurfacing the road. Detailed factual advice will enable them to come to terms with their child's disability by giving them the means to overcome or reduce it. Help is needed on such questions as discipline, and how to achieve the right balance of management within the family as a whole. The deaf child may be one child in a family of three or four and ill-considered advice may result in the alienation of all but one parent from him because of the excessive deference to his every need and wish. Those responsible for supervision of the care of a hearing impaired child need to consider him within the framework of the family as a whole lest a handicapped child begets a handicapped family.

REFERENCES

Ballantyne, J. (1970) 'Iatrogenic deafness.' *J. Laryng. Otol.*, **84**, 967.
Department of Education and Science (1967) *Education Survey, No. 1. Units for Partially Hearing Children.* London: H.M.S.O.
—— (1969) *Education Survey, No. 6. Peripatetic Teachers of the Deaf.* London: H.M.S.O.
Ewing, A. W. G., Ewing, E. C. (1964) *Teaching Deaf Children to Talk.* Manchester: University of Manchester Press.
Watson, T. J. (1967) *The Education of Hearing-handicapped Children.* London: University of London Press.

CHAPTER 19

A Diagnostic Aspect of Speech Therapy

M. K. F. HUTCHISON

Introduction

The ideas outlined in this paper are a product of several years of observation, diagnosis and therapy of pre-school children who have an auditory inattention problem combined with a marked language disability. A class of 4 such children was established in the Auditory Research Unit at Reading in 1969 (see chapter 20 for fuller details) and it has been possible to see that the features in therapy given in this chapter can be applied successfully to the group as well as to the individual situation.

At Reading, we have the opportunity of studying both normal and pathological language development during the joint paediatric and audiology clinic. Here, babies born within certain categories of risk are seen not only in a clinical situation but in a total situation, with guidance for the family and regular follow-up of the child until satisfactory progress has been made.

During the audiological examination, the babies' responses to a variety of auditory stimuli—presented at known intensities and frequency ranges—and their level of vocalisation are assessed and recorded in order to build-up a developmental profile in which the relationship between the two can be seen. The criteria we use for deciding whether or not a child's auditory behaviour and his vocal output are within normal limits are based on the research reported by Renfrew and Murphy (1964).

The following extracts have been taken from the records made of one infant's auditory behaviour and vocalisations. From these it will be seen that it was noted from the first that his vocalisation was significantly less mature than his auditory function.

$11\frac{1}{2}$ *weeks.* Initiation of generalised activity to moderately loud complex tone. No apparent startle.

7 *months.* Localised rattle. 30dB complex tones. Pure tones 500, 1000, 2000, 4000 at 30dB. Blowing bubbles, laughing, shouting. Inflected 'err', 'aha'—no other sounds.

Both rattles and pure tones were presented in free field. The intensities at the ear and testing conditions were based on earlier studies.

15 *months.* We are not happy about the quality of this child's vocalisations or response to sound. He appears to ignore voice and his own vocalisations are only at $4\frac{1}{2}$-5 month level. We should follow carefully.

16 *months.* Quick, accurate localisation to quiet rattle and pure tones. Response to voice unreliable.

17 *months.* Quick, accurate responses to pure tones, again at 40 dB. Head turn to voice. Mother feels he may know his name.

18 *months.* Response to auditory stimuli maintained—still no new vocalisation.

20 *months.* Responses again to pure tones and voice at 40dB, but less interested. No maturation of babble. No comprehension of language. Regular therapy commenced.

As just shown in these extracts, the audio-vocal function in the baby is regarded as of prime importance to language growth.

By the time an infant reaches the age of 9-12 months it is even more clear that the beginnings of language are present or absent. The following are examples of language behaviour usually present at this time: language here is divided into two forms of behaviour—(1) use of voice; and (2) development of comprehension.

Use of Voice

(1) The baby vocalises in response to familiar people; he may vocalise at sight of mother, father, siblings or relations and friends who see him frequently.
(2) He may call out to attract attention, usually of members of his family. (3) He may use utterances having a similar intonation pattern to that heard in an adult when 'commenting' on an event or idea. Claims that the infant has said something recognisable possibly come from the fact that at this age he is indeed acquiring the system of rise and fall pitch patterns he encounters in his language environment. (4) There may be an increase in the variety of consonant and vowel combinations within one utterance and often within one intonation pattern. (5) At 9 months the testing of audio-vocal function is increasingly important. One way of assessing this in a brief session is to attempt to change the infant's vocalisations; for example, by presenting him with a different pattern to the one he is making and hopefully to initiate a pattern of imitation to him.

Development of Comprehension

By 9-12 months, evidence of the beginnings of comprehension of spoken language assumes greatest importance to the tester. The baby can already understand changes in tones of voice, a stern tone, an angry tone, a pleased tone, and can probably discriminate his own name. He now demonstrates comprehension of a limited set of stereotyped and situation-framed phrases, such as 'wave bye-bye', 'clap hands', and may look for favourite toys when they are named, e.g. 'teddy' and 'panda'.

Certainly, over the next months, it is obvious that comprehension of the word is developing. By 18 months of age, the child discriminates a number of simple phrases and longer structures, e.g. 'Where's daddy?', 'Go, fetch Mummy's slippers', 'Bring me your cup from the kitchen', 'No, it's not yours', and reacts to them appropriately. He can use single words and two-word combinations spontaneously, and by the age of 2 his use of words may be anywhere along a continuum from a few words and phrases to long utterances of many words. The normal pattern of language development has been covered often before by psychologists and paediatricians and, more recently, linguists, and their accounts can be easily found in the literature.

In the next part of this paper I hope to relate maldevelopment to the parameters of normal development already mentioned. The appearance of a discrepancy between the level of auditory response and maturity of vocalisation has already been mentioned. This may become even more apparent as the child is reviewed regularly at the clinic.

Alerting Signals

The appearance of the following types of auditory and vocal behaviour in the first year of life are of concern to the clinician.

(*a*) Variable or inconsistent response to sounds.

(*b*) Response to sounds but failure to respond to voice.

(*c*) Deterioration of interest in sounds and apparent failure to learn from them or to give them domestic significance.

(*d*) Restricted vocalisation in both quantity and quality, or there may be a limited number of patterns of rise and fall in pitch; vowels and consonants may be present, but only a limited number.

(*e*) Failure to use sounds as a basis for his own language growth.

It is usually necessary to give the mother information about normal language acquisition (the broad sequences of development) and an explanation of the possible significance of her child's vocalisation pattern in relation to his future development of language.

As the baby gets older, any lack of progress will be more obviously seen, and direct therapy will be needed to maintain interest in sound and vocalisation. It is an even harder task to arouse such interest in a child of 3 or 4 who has not acquired it, or who, due to lack of help, has already lost it. It is obviously easier to *extend* an ability or activity possessed by the child than to develop new ones, especially if such lack of development has persisted for a considerable time.

In assessing the child's comprehension of language, it is necessary to remember that a child of normal intelligence and interest will show learning from situations that can be confused as comprehension of language. It is common for parents to say of their 15-to 18-month-old (as someone did recently): 'Oh, he understands everything I say; when the children come home from school he fetches their slippers for them, and when we are going out he goes and fetches his coat'. On closer enquiry, it appeared that this child did not respond to the word 'coat' as the word was not even used, and indeed he did not fetch or look towards his coat when named by his parent. Obviously these parents need to be told that comprehension of words means that the child responds by looking towards or fetching the desired article on verbal demands only; that he can discriminate it from other words, and, in the absence of any other cues, is able to select the correct object or action to match the spoken word. For the child with the type of disorder I am attempting to describe here, it can be demonstrated that increasing the quantity of language offered to him, or speaking louder to him, does not reliably improve his comprehension.

Environment

The first step in therapy is to regulate the child's language environment. Children who lack understanding frequently ignore what is said to them because to them speech is just meaningless noise. This needs to be corrected by ensuring that the language used in speaking to the child is within the limits of his understanding. In some instances, parents need to be shown what is meant by limiting language, *i.e.* restriction of the vocabulary used to the child, restrictions of the number of words per utterance addressed to him, and simplification of grammar.

The physical environment of the child needs to have similar control. Frequently, he may be easily distracted by visual patterns, by tactile sensation, by the least alteration in light intensity or change of furniture in a room, and until this behaviour is lessened, teaching him to attend to auditory stimuli is fruitless. During therapy sessions the physical environment can easily be made less distracting by keeping walls bare, cupboards closed, lights dimmed and only a small selection of materials for therapy to hand. Though it is more difficult in the home, parents should try to limit physical distractions.

I want now to outline the steps in diagnostic therapy that seem indicated in order to implement the hypothesis that the child will learn language if taught it specifically. Co-operation and a certain amount of attention are needed in the child for him to benefit from specific teaching. Both will develop under circumstances where language begins to have meaning and where they are, therefore, rewarded.

Communication

For the child and his parents there is the constant barrier of having no explicit system of communication, nothing beyond the crudities of voice tone (if the child is aware of voice), facial expression or perhaps gesture.

Parents frequently feel they should not use gesture: rather that they should force words from the child by not giving any clues other than verbal ones. Parents who first come for help when their toddler of 2 is not speaking, have very often been advised not to allow their child to use gesture. The assumption is made that he is too lazy to talk, and that by forbidding use of gesture he will be forced to talk. However, the expected change in language behaviour may not occur, as this advice may not be applicable.

Language

The parents of a non-comprehending child need careful and explicit guidance in their patterns of talking to their child. The following points need to be considered: (1) when to talk; (2) what words to use; (3) how many words to use in one utterance; (4) what voice level to use; (5) what distance to be from the child when talking; (6) what to do when the child is involved in other activities, *e.g.* it is necessary in some cases to make the child stop everything to attend; (7) how to deal with absence of response; (8) how much repetition to give; (9) what modality to use for communication, *i.e.* (a) visual and auditory patterns combined, (b) only auditory, and (c) when to use one modality and when to use both, or when to change to a new one, *e.g.* tactile.

With an older child, or even in the case of a child who has been followed through the joint clinic, investigations by other disciplines may need to be instigated (if not already begun): for example, surgery may be indicated to remedy a conductive overlay which will aggravate the child's ability to learn to attend auditorily.

The older child who has reached 3 to 4 years with no therapy, or what would appear to be inappropriate therapy, presents a similar picture to the younger child described earlier. The older child shows inattention to sound, yet is able to concentrate well on visual or manipulative tasks. Responses to auditory stimuli are inconsistent, as have been described in the younger child. Comprehension is grossly limited or absent. Vocalisation is musical, but limited in quantity and variety and no meaningful words are used, except perhaps some vocal patterns which are used predictably and therefore could be regarded as attempts to produce verbal communication.

Usually the case history, too, reflects some of the already mentioned symptoms suggesting a language disorder. For instance, there may be a history of very immature babble patterns, or a history of limited variation in phonemic combinations of vowel, consonant and pitch. The mother may describe her child as having been a 'quiet baby', or one who 'did not chat to himself much'. She may comment: 'He can hear if he wants to'. On testing, the child may respond to pure and complex tones and not to voice (as in the younger child), or he may respond to voice, including localisation. It is utterly bewildering to parents that the same child can actually respond to quieter sounds on one occasion and not respond to louder ones at other times.

In some instance, the child may be hyper-distractable and hyper-active and consequently may present problems in management and therapy. As with the younger child, this age group needs to be taught in a controlled environment.

Therapy

Initial therapy with these children is 'diagnostic' therapy. This term is used to describe a therapeutic programme in which success or failure in therapeutic progress assumes a diagnostic significance for the experienced therapist. As changes occur in the child's auditory awareness and understanding of language, the hypothesis from which the therapy is created is confirmed or otherwise.

The programme needs to be flexible so that it can be initiated at any age and at any stage of language uptake, and modified according to the parents' capabilities, the child's intellectual resources and the severity of the handicap. The parents of a young child who has been under regular review from a baby clinic are, hopefully, already greatly involved in the education of their child. The parents of an older child may need much explanation and encouragement to establish modes of communication before detailed language teaching can begin. For both groups of parents, it must be emphasised to them that they have a large part to play in language training, and such qualities as resource, flexibility, patience and confidence are called for.

Auditory Training

The dominant consideration is to teach the child that language used by the people around him is meaningful. It may be that the child has to learn that sound made by human voice is meaningful. The following is a suggested procedure for attempting to attach meaning to sound. The child is presented with a sound, visually and auditorily, and is asked to perform a relevant action. Then he is presented with the auditory stimulus alone. If the child can manage, then probably it is best to begin with a word, rather than a mechanical noise or a speech sound which is not so directly related to language. Progress in attaching meaning to a specified sound or word and an event may be slow, and possibly the auditory pathway will never be a reliable and consistent carrier of information.

Progress has been made when there is an increase in responsiveness to sound and there is some indication of awareness of the link between the visual lip pattern, the sound, and the required action performed by the child.

The next step comes in giving auditory and visual pattern of *two* words introduced separately (in conjunction with an action or an object or a picture), but which are visually/auditorily and semantically different from each other, *e.g.* car/baby, or mummy/car (but not mummy/daddy), or whatever two words fill these criteria and are relevant to the child's communication needs. It has been found that, if children are given two words of similar auditory or visual pattern, these two words will be confused, and at a later date it may be difficult to correct this confusion. It is essential that new words are not introduced until it can be seen that the child has retained previously taught words and can discriminate between them. It must surely be that kinesthetic feedback at this stage is as important as auditory and visual feedback, for it needs fine kinesthetic discrimination to distinguish between such words as 'bus', 'boat', 'boy', when such words are being produced as 'bu', 'boh', 'bo', by the child.

Once the child has learned some single words, the two-word combination can be introduced, using the language that he has learnt. From this point onwards, the therapist is constantly faced with the decision of what structures of language to teach and in what order.

The usual sequence in therapy is to begin by teaching the lip-pattern of a word, followed by teaching the auditory pattern of the word. It is possible to see that, once some words are familiar, the child can discriminate between them when only given the auditory pattern in conversational voice. The essence of therapy is to teach language, and, although more than one modality will be chosen via which the child will learn, it is utterly essential that the therapist knows how the child has comprehended— auditorily, visually, or auditorily and visually together. Surprisingly, frequently therapists do not know, and only when therapy sessions are tightly structured can the therapist be sure whether the child has comprehended a lip pattern or an auditory pattern.

As well as ensuring meaningful input of language, it is necessary to ensure that output is meaningful. The child ought to be encouraged to imitate, but this needs strict control so that he does not simply parrot words meaninglessly. He may make attempts to imitate, but these may be poor or stereotyped, *i.e.* the same sound for different words. This pattern of behaviour needs checking too. He needs to be taught to *use* the language he has. This means not just smiling encouragingly at any verbal attempts, but placing the child in situations where he wants to communicate and showing him that the language he has learnt is used for this function.

For a long time, this work may have little meaning for the child, yet his attention must be kept over a period of weeks and months. Frequently the child, especially the older child, can become bored with the repetition needed, and keeping his interest demands great resourcefulness on the part of the therapist and the parents.

REFERENCE

Renfrew, C., Murphy, K. (Eds.) (1964) *The Child who does not Talk*. Clinics in Developmental Medicine, No. 13. London: S.I.M.P. with Heinemann Medical.

CHAPTER 20

An Experimental Class for Language Disordered Children

MARGARET WHITE

In October 1969, concern over the lack of specific educational provision for the small, yet significant, population of young children with language disorders led to the setting up of an experimental class at the Royal Berkshire Hospital.* The aim was to establish a specialised environment in which teacher and speech therapist used their skills together to investigate methods of teaching these children. We present this report to indicate the way in which we have attempted to meet these children's needs. The report is necessarily anecdotal and experimental.

Four children were chosen to form the original class. These were selected in consultation with the organising teacher of the deaf and the therapist in the research unit responsible for therapy at that time.

Selection

Selection of the children was based on the following criteria:

(a) they were suffering from a severly impaired ability to develop spoken language;

(b) the basic cause of this disability did not seem to be related to peripheral auditory state, intellectual factors or severe emotional disorders;

(c) all children had been attending the Unit for investigations or therapy since infancy;

(d) each child had been meticulously investigated audiologically, paediatrically, psychiatrically, psychologically and otologically, and the usual pathological and virological tests had been completed;

(e) all of the children suffered from fluctuating conductive hearing losses which required careful and regular otological supervision.

The children now formed a relatively homogeneous group with ages ranging between 3-4 years. All were hyperdistractable, hyperactive, grossly visual and with severe impairment of attention span. All had created stress at home because of frustration and general lack of linguistic comprehension. Their auditory attention fluctuated markedly and minimal changes of auditory acuity had profound effects. Behaviour tended, therefore, to be variable and this, taken in relation to the factors mentioned above, led to obvious fears about psychiatric states.

---

*The Diagnosis and treatment of children with language disorders became a recognised and routine part of work of the Audiology Research Unit at the Royal Berkshire Hospital, Reading, about 8 years ago. The method of treatment and education outlined in the chapters by White and Hutchison was developed as a result of close daily work and discussion between the various disciplines involved. The two writers wish to emphasise that present treatment methods, although reflecting their own personal philosophy and daily patterns of therapy, are based on the work which has gone before.

The staff consists of a teacher of the deaf (myself), a senior research associate speech therapist/audiologist and a qualified nursery nurse working as an assistant. In addition to the several years experience of the education and therapy of such children that this staff supplies, we are able to call on the assistance of the Research Department of the hospital.

The initial aim of the class was to create a stable environment for these children and to contain them in a nursery situation from which they could be taken for very brief speech therapy sessions.

Sessions

Working together, teacher and nursery assistant aimed at giving the children the benefits of nursery education while controlling the linguistic environment. It was the teacher's job to establish a class programme flexible enough to absorb and complement the work of the speech therapist so that this was an integral part of the educational plan rather than a separate and therefore disrupting activity. The close working partnership between teacher, therapist and nursery assistant has been a very important factor in enabling us to assess and provide for the particular needs of these children through the class. Broadly speaking, there are three areas which we feel to be of major importance in helping the children and I will attempt to describe the specific function of the class in relation these areas. In addition to this, the teacher was to act as a liaison between the child at home and the child in the group.

1. The Need for Security

In terms of continuity of environmental stimulation the need for security is one of the basic and most important to be met by the class. Even now, if the children are taken from the room and play area to which they are accustomed, we see changes of ability to attend, fluctuation of auditory threshold and increased hyperactivity. To meet these needs we have designed both programme and environment for optimal predictability and try to ensure that the atmosphere is as serene as possible. The room we are working in as a base has been an advantage here. Space is limited. The children needed to have an area where they could play with reasonable freedom. At the same time there was need to have an area where visual distraction was cut to a minimum and individual work could be vigorously structured. This area has been created by fitting a folding partition into one corner which, when opened, creates a small rectangle where a table and two chairs will fit. The room is therefore divided into two sections, the individual teaching area formed by the screen and a free play area. In the free play area we have been careful to ensure that there is a high degree of consistency in the arrangement of furniture and also in the placement and selection of play materials.

To minimise distraction we began with no illustrations on the walls, at least until the children had become accustomed to the furniture and fittings. However, we have found that the children's ability to tolerate stimulation has increased. The first pictures to go up on the walls were enlarged photographs of each child with the appropriate name captioned below. Subsequent illustrations have had equal stress on clear visual reproduction and relevance to the child and are designed as an aid to communication, e.g., large pictures of simple domestic items through which the child might want to express his needs (milk, cup, toilet, coat).

The routine itself, of course, provides much of the framework for security. All our children rely on this heavily and we have found that in order to avoid stress this has had to be quite heavily structured. So when the children come in they know that after greeting they take off their coats, find their name-marked chair and sit down, before making their choice of play materials in the room.

After a period of free play each child has a session with the therapist or the teacher and when not receiving this individual attention he stays with the nursery assistant in the free play area. As part of the team she is aware both of the language level of each child and of his need for relaxation after a period of strenuous concentration. Though the nurse, teacher and therapist may appear to change rôles from time to time, consistency of approach to each child is essential. In this way one worker does not undermine the work of another and one of my own major responsibilities lies in the arrangement of educational processes which not only do not compete but which are mutually complementary.

2. *Specific Linguistic Needs*

Weekly case conferences are held during which the work of the previous week is reviewed and the programme for the coming week is agreed upon, often down to small details, particularly where new language or new concepts are planned. Plans have to be made to accommodate both the individual child and the group, bearing in mind the children's different language levels. This is an example (Sarah);

Work in free play area: emphasis this week on extending the use of structure, *person* wants *noun*, from individual situation into a group situation *e.g.* correct response required to the question, 'What does ———— want?'. Games involving this question-and-answer form. (N.B. structure has not yet been taught in combination with her own name or personal pronoun 'I'.)

Individual Work: Introduction of the under/on concept.
Two words to be taught singly until known, then in later weeks to be linked with nouns. New words such as these must be taught with face pattern until familiar, when she will be able to discriminate auditorily.

Auditory Training: 'Shopping Games'.
Asked to fetch two items of food when given only auditory pattern. She is finding this very difficult at the moment unless her vision is blocked while words are said.

Written Work: work on structure sentence, *e.g.* Sarah's *jumper is red*, aims at making her more aware of linking words and sentence rhythms.

Group Work: In addition to reinforcing each child's language in the group situation we have found it quite useful to concentrate on a single concept and/or word for a week or two at a time. This often provides a useful focal point for the creative work of the class and is another way of transferring language from the more specific individual session to use in the little 'group' community. For instance, during Easter week the word was 'egg' (so we boiled an egg, we painted an egg, we cut out egg shapes from polystyrene, and used all opportunities to reinforce the word).

Group auditory training is planned each week to increase the children's awareness and interest in sound. The range of sound to which the children can respond is extended by drawing their attention to the existence of different types of sound. Such concepts as loudness, pitch and rhythm are gradually being introduced. The children are also encouraged to discriminate familiar language, *e.g.* their own names.

The use of language and teaching methods in the class is carefully controlled. Only when a word is added to a child's vocabulary is it used in the class and later he is encouraged to use it spontaneously.

In our guidance to parents, research colleagues and visitors, we stress the necessity for a small quantity of meaningful words rather than a concentrated 'talk! talk! talk!' approach more common to classes for deaf children: silence is often more effective to highlight the meaning of a word or phrase with the children in our group.

Language Motivation

It is commonly believed that placement in a nursery school will provide language motivation. However, it is becoming increasingly clear with our children that only once the child begins to see the relevance of language in a structured situation does he begin to use it spontaneously. So often with these children, if language means anything at all, it is usually confusion, failure and stress. It is not enough to say that they cannot use language; they are often antipathetic to it and steps have to be taken to deal with such an attitude. We have found that greater encouragement is necessary for our particular group of children to begin to communicate with each other and the staff when within the group situation.

Group experience is of course important in our children. This is why we stress that a proportion of the morning be spent in group learning and social situations. The children still find it very difficult to *work* in a group with any degree of concentration, although, on a social level, awareness of each other and development of communication together has shown marked progress. Group games with any language content are very short so that concentration power and co-operation are not overtaxed.

Parental Support

One of the primary aims in establishing the class was to give the mother of each child some relief and there is no doubt that the strain has been reduced. Parental involvement has always been a characteristic of the work of the Audiology Unit. Part of my work in the afternoons is to visit each home at least once a week or more frequently, where it appears necessary. The parents are also encouraged to visit whenever they wish. In these ways they are kept actively involved in the language development of their child and they are encouraged to develop their own language skills with the child.

This, then, is an account of the lines along which we are developing in our experimental class at Reading. All four children are making progress, but I cannot stress too highly that the class is still very much at the beginning stage of one approach to the problem of giving these young children the combination of therapy, education and close clinical supervision which they require.

CHAPTER 21

Non-talkers: Therapy in the Pre-school Years

VALERIE SAVAGE

Introduction

With increasing emphasis on early diagnosis, one can hope and expect that the speech and language impaired child will present for treatment before school entry. Yet a dilemma presents in that principles of therapy have often been evolved from work with school-age children; and consequently have been largely 'corrective'. Especially in *speech* difficulties, this has meant that a school-age child, having reached some kind of articulatory plateau, can be treated and the effects of that treatment measured, using the child as his own baseline (Van Riper 1954). For this reason, many therapists have preferred to wait until articulatory habits were established before correcting, arguing that until then they were unable to distinguish the effects of therapy from normal maturation of the speech mechanism.

Measuring the effects of management is a problem in any developmental disorder, not least here because of the paucity of normative data. However, with children presenting in the speech clinic at an earlier age, it would seem reasonable to probe the nature of their difficulties afresh to determine whether there is a qualitative difference between the late talking 2-year-old and the 5-year-old with speech and language difficulties; and on these findings to evolve a dynamic therapy designed to meet the needs of a developing system.

Profiles for Therapy

There has always been a tendency in medicine, as frameworks for diagnosis have evolved, to pigeon-hole and classify disorders with ever more erudite terminology. Whilst this might be desirable for definable disease entities, it has never been entirely satisfactory for developmental disorders, which is perhaps reflected in the multitude of names in the literature used to describe non-talking children, *e.g.* congenital auditory imperception, developmental dysphasia, central word deafness. However, with the recent awakening of interest in the problems of language from so many and varied disciplines, it is becoming possible to see the problems of the language handicapped, not as a disease entity, but as a profile of ability and inability, the symptoms of which may be expressed as a language *score*. In viewing the scored comprehension and expressive abilities as the *result* of a perceptual-cognitive process, the underlying pathology starts to be probed and foci for therapy evolve. More important, as the problem is viewed less as an entity, the effects of treatment on one aspect of the problem can be measured, which in turn will modify both the profile and the measured symptoms.

After the most detailed and expert assessment highlighting the areas of greatest difficulty, the problem still remains for the therapist to determine the form therapy should take. Perhaps the most widely distributed advice to the mothers of young children is 'Talk to him'. Whilst there seems to be general agreement that this must be advantageous, there is little evidence to suggest exactly where this focuses the most help linguistically. It is here that the Reynell Developmental Language Scales are proving useful in measuring the area most affected by a given form of therapy, and thereby suggesting the form therapy might take in certain profiles of disability (Reynell 1969).

Language Stimulation

To return to the 'umbrella therapy' of language stimulation, we had observed for some time in clinical work that advice to parents on talking to small children might produce one of several effects: the child might improve dramatically both in his understanding of the spoken word and in speaking; he might improve in his understanding of speech; or he might not improve at all. So, in some children, inadequate language stimulation undoubtedly was a considerable factor influencing their development of spoken language, although this was by no means the whole answer. However, before trying to measure the effects of 'language stimulation', it is necessary to describe precisely what underlies the advice 'Talk to him, mother'.

The rationale behind this advice is that understanding of the spoken word precedes its expression developmentally, and therefore a child who hears little will say little. Yet bombarding a child with sound is not enough. If he is to make sense of his auditory environment, the sound—and especially speech sound—must be so structured that he can attach meaning to it. Therefore, the *way* in which he is spoken to is of paramount importance. To help a child to find speech meaningful, one can use the fact that he has already learned to make sense of his environment through his eyes. He knows what cups and spoons and clothes are for and he can demonstrate this. Therefore, the earliest, most meaningful language stimulation will be around the things he already knows and understands. Elephants and camels might be exotic, and even cows and sheep have a certain appeal, but for the child who might not see either from one month's end to the next except in picture books, these are not the most useful or meaningful things to talk about. Buses and cars and supermarkets and telephones and the whole paraphernalia of everyday living are the stuff language stimulation is made of. And not even 'Do you remember we saw a bus?', but rather 'Look, here's a bus'—right now in the immediate visual environment.

Not only must the language the child hears be relevant to his visual world, but also its presentation should be such that he derives the optimum information from it. Certainly the distance of the child from the speaker appears to be relevant and Dr. Sheridan (1964) talks about 'mother distance' as being the optimum listening distance. By this she means the distance of the child from his mother's voice when he is on her lap. Whatever the optimum, children do seem to be more aware of a normal conversational voice at a few feet than a sound of equal intensity across a room, and this is of relevance when talking to the slow talker. Also, the way information is presented can make a deal of difference. Children we have examined tend to develop understanding for simple phrases like 'Open the door', 'It's dinner time' and so on, before necessarily understanding the individual word meanings. They respond to the pattern of the utterance, initially within the visual and gestural context and later out of context, often before realising words have a use as 'labels'. Whilst it is important to duce information to its simplest for auditory processing, it does not follow that the one-word unit is necessarily the simplest. Therefore, when talking to children, one should give them a simple pattern from which to extract meaning rather than a bald word which differs only slightly accoustically from another, *e.g.* cat vs. cap; 'The *cat* wants his dinner.', 'Look, Johnny's putting his *cap* on'. Yet whilst talking in short sentences and simple phrases, it can happen that one's enthusiasm to 'stimulate' an endless stream of irrelevant chatter can act as a damper both to the child's listening and replying. Ultimately, it remains an art to determine the sensitive balance between talking to a child and listening for his replies.

No mention has been made of active attempts to get the child to repeat words, or to talk to order. It has been generally accepted that 'word-learning' *per se*, as undertaken by many parents, is usually a dismal failure. Children talk to express needs, ideas, and to comment on their environment, just as their parents have talked to them. Teaching words by rote is certainly not a part of the normal development of spoken language and, indeed, produces tremendous resistance in many children which can hinder the normal flow of spoken language.

Therapy for Language Stimulation

Whilst no detailed study of the effects of language stimulation has been undertaken, certain profiles begin to emerge which may, or may not, be substantiated by research using control groups.

Alex presented with no understanding of the spoken word and was quite speechless at chronological age (CA) 2 years 3 months. The first child in a wealthy family, he had suffered a succession of nannies together with a bi-lingual background. On measuring his non-verbal abilities, he scored in the superior range on the Merrill-Palmer scale. The Reynell profiles show a marked increase in his verbal comprehension over three months, accompanied by a comparable leap in his expressive language score. The only 'treatment' was advice and demonstrations to both mother and nanny on an appropriate level for talking to Alex (Figs. 1 and 2).

Peter, on presenting at CA 3 years 3 months with limited understanding of the spoken word and very little expressive language, was put on a similar regime. A child of average non-verbal abilities as measured on the Merrill-Palmer scales, he was the second boy in a family where the marriage suffered successive blows without ever completely breaking up. His scores over a six month period show a marked increase in verbal understanding, with expressive language barely holding the developmental curve (Figs. 1 and 2).

These two sets of scores are representative of the sort of results obtained on language stimulation therapy. It is probably fair to say this form of treatment is having a general effect on the child's understanding but that it does not necessarily affect the expressive language score.

Therapy for Expressive Difficulties

The problem then remains of influencing the child's spoken language. Will he in fact 'speak when he is ready', must he muddle along incompetently trying to get his needs met until such stage as he can tolerate correction, or is there some underlying

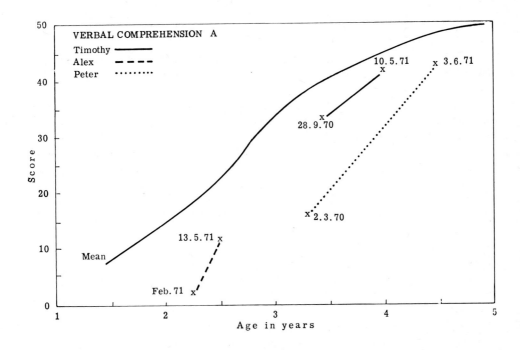

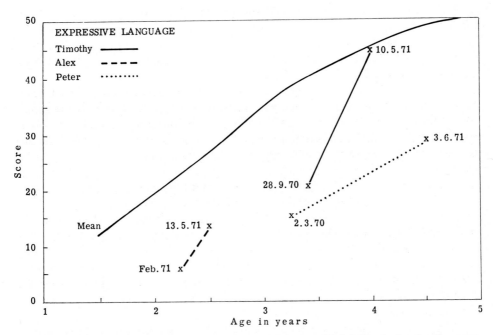

Figs. 1 and **2.** Simplified Reynell Developmental Language Scales (Boys), showing the scores of three speech retarded children before and after therapy. (The Reynell Scales are reproduced in this form by kind permission of the N.F.E.R. Publishing Company Ltd.)

241

pathology which can be probed and used as basis for therapy in the child with a discrepancy between understanding and verbal expression?

Some of the earliest workers (Stinchfield and Young 1938) recognised the importance of motor competence of the speech apparatus to the speech defective child. Unfortunately, the work was extended beyond the child with demonstrable motor incompetence to include stammerers and every manner of speech and language disorder. (In many ways it was not relevant, and, as results were disappointing, the techniques fell into disuse.)

In examining pre-school non-talking children, one of the most striking factors is the variability of the competence of their speech apparatus. Whilst some children can move their lips, tongues and palates efficiently and at will, a significant proportion show real difficulty both in motor and sensory awareness of the speech apparatus (Martin 1971). It seems likely in these children that their motor disabilities might be contributing to their poor speech and language output.

Studies are in hand by this author and others to probe this underlying motor incompetence and the effects of specific therapy upon it, but from data already available some information has begun to emerge. Before examining this, it is useful to consider exactly the form therapy can take in a child where an underlying motor incompetence has been detected from clinical examination and phonetic analysis of the child's utterances. At its simplest, a child can either be totally incompetent throughout the speech apparatus, or he can demonstrate inadequate control throughout, or he can have a more patchy profile—or an uneven spread of incompetence. It seems likely that the average adult and child speaker, although varying enormously from individual to individual, have a more or less even spread of competence across the speech apparatus. The first aim of 'motor' work, then, must be to give a child this even competence throughout, and then to progress to strengthening the apparatus as a co-ordinated whole.

This is being done in a group of late-talking children, using a series of games and exercises designed to strengthen each part of the speech apparatus in turn. The games are planned to be attractive to small children (lollipops and balloons and other enticements are used). It has been found that the most efficient way of getting exercises practised daily is to use the child's mother as therapist, and programme the work for her on a monthly basis.

The results of this study are not yet available, but the following profile of a child's progress gives some indication of the effects of this type of therapy.

Timothy presented at CA 3 years 5 months with a demonstrable motor incompetence of the speech apparatus. On testing, there was a marked discrepancy between his comprehension and expressive language. After 6 months of work, aimed at improving the control and efficiency of his speech apparatus, he has eliminated the gap, and, indeed, both fall within 1 SD of the mean. The interesting point here is that the therapy has not only affected his speech intelligibility (which was predictable) but also his total use of spoken language (Figs. 1 and 2).

The three main pre-requisites for successful management by using *solely* a programmed motor therapy are as follows:

(1) the child has an underlying motor pathology;

242

(2) he is young enough linguistically for this pathology to be largely uncontaminated by faulty learning patterns;

(3) there is someone available to work with him daily on the work programmed (*e.g.* his mother).

Conclusions

It is becoming possible, as various disciplines probe the problems of the late-talking child, to build up a more composite picture of underlying pathologies and their implications for therapy. As more refined tools for measuring disabilities become available, effects of therapy can be assessed more precisely and the therapy itself focussed on the cause of delay or disorder instead of modifying its symptoms.

This chapter describes two areas of difficulty which form a percentage of the problems encountered in the late-talking child. Management aimed at the underlying cause is outlined, and the effects measured using the Reynell Developmental Language scales.

REFERENCES

Martin, J. A. M. (1971) 'The otolaryngologist and the late talker.' *in Proceedings of the 11th World Congress of Rehabilitation of the International Society of Rehabilitation of the Disabled, Dublin, 1969.* Dublin: National Rehabilitation Board. p. 523.

Reynell , J. (1969) *Reynell Developmental Language Scales.* Slough, Bucks.: N.F.E.R.

Sheridan, M. D. (1964) 'Development of auditory attention and the use of language symbols.' *in* Renfew, C., Murphy, K. (Eds.) *The Child who does not Talk.* London: S.I.M.P. with Heinemann. p. 1.

Stinchfield, S. M., Young, E. H. (1938) *Children with Delayed or Defective Speech.* Stanford: Stanford University Press.

van Riper, C. (1954) *Speech Correction.* 3rd edn. New York: Prentice-Hall.

CHAPTER 22

Speech Therapy

CATHERINE E. RENFREW

A history of the treatment of speech disorders (Eldridge 1968) shows how, throughout the centuries, both medicine and education have been responsible for the development of the body of knowledge on which present theories of aetiology and therapy have been based. More recently, psychologists, linguists and biologists have contributed to this field.

In Britain, speech therapy had always been more closely linked with medicine, while in the U.S.A. affiliations with education, psychology and general speech have been much more common. When the professional body in Britain, the College of Speech Therapists, was founded in 1944, all members were registered medical auxiliaries. Fifteen years later, however, when more than three-quarters of the membership were working in education, they refused statutory registration among the professions associated with medicine. They have continued as a separate profession serving both medicine and education.

Training

The emphasis in the British speech therapist's training is nevertheless still on preparation for work in hospitals. The value of this practice is in the fact that students get experience more quickly with a great variety of more severely handicapping conditions in adults and children. National examinations are taken by all students except those in the University of Newcastle-upon-Tyne. The subjects examined are anatomy and physiology, phonetics and linguistics, psychology (including child development and psychopathology), speech pathology and therapeutics.

In the U.S.A., the training of the speech therapist can extend over a longer period than in the U.K. because students carry on their general education at the same time as their preparation for professional work. The professional body, the American Speech and Hearing Association, recommends that, for employment as speech therapists, candidates should have education up to the M.A. level, including the necessary study and examinations in speech pathology and audiology. The number of hours spent in theoretical preparation by students in both countries is very similar (Morley 1971), but the number of hours of clinical experience in the U.K. is very much higher. The other major difference is that the American speech therapist has spent more time in the study of hearing and its disorders than has the British student.

Scope of Work

Speech therapists are concerned with both adults and children who suffer from disorders of voice, articulation, language or fluency or any combination of these. They work mainly in hospitals and schools or school clinics.

In hospitals, patients are referred by doctors of the various specialities, *e.g.*

paediatrics, neurology, otolaryngology, geriatrics. In the education system, teachers are mainly responsible for referring children either by pointing out the child's speech defect to the medical officer or by informing him in a letter that speech therapy is requested so that if the child suffers from any medical condition that would contraindicate speech therapy, treatment would not be given.

In Britain, in contrast to the U.S.A. only a small proportion of the profession is engaged in teaching and a few individuals in full-time research.

Assessment

The title 'speech therapist' gives the wrong impression as to the nature and scope of the work done. Much of the speech therapist's time is spent in assessing and diagnosing and in a fair proportion of cases no therapy is given, perhaps because the individual referred is doing the best he can with the abilities he possesses, or perhaps because the assessment is only part of a larger scheme of assessment, *e.g.* pre- and post-surgery for cleft palate, Parkinson's disease or for a brain tumour.

Assessment, of course, is also necessary in all cases referred with a view to treatment. Few speech therapists receive guidance from a doctor who has studied speech disorders, although reports from a physician or surgeon as to the patient's medical condition and history are most helpful. Therefore, it is the duty of the speech therapist to identify which clinically significant features in a person's speech constitute the disturbance. She has to be sufficiently aware, for example, of the aberrations of the local accent to know whether vowel distortions, nasality and grammatical 'errors' are the accepted usual form of speech in the patient's environment before concluding they may be due to deafness, nasopharyngeal incompetence or expressive aphasia.

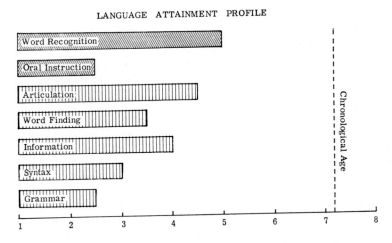

Fig. 1. Girl, 7 years 2 months, retarded in development of understanding and use of spoken language. Diagonal lines = receptive; vertical lines = expressive.

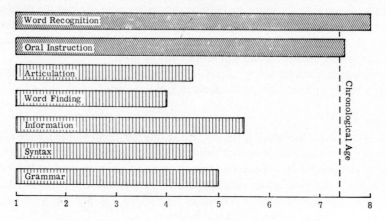

Fig. 2. Boy, 7 years 3 months, with articulation defect only.
Understanding and use of spoken language within normal.
Diagonal lines = receptive; vertical lines = expressive.

LANGUAGE ATTAINMENT PROFILE

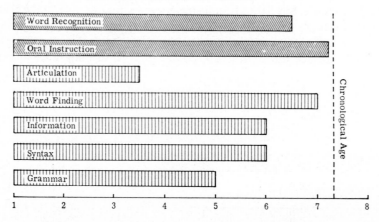

Fig. 3. Boy, 7 years 5 months, with normal understanding,
but retarded in all aspects of spoken language.

As spoken language is largely dependent on its reception and interpretation, the ability to respond appropriately by action or speech to words and commands, graded in difficulty related to age, is a vital part of the language examination. On the expressive side, we measure vocabulary, sentence length and structure, grammar, information and articulation. We obtain thereby a profile showing where weaknesses and strengths lie, *e.g.* see Figs. While making the assessment, it is important to design a situation whereby the therapist can listen to her patient in conversation in an off-guarded moment. In this way, it is possible to hear if speech deteriorates or improves, and in which respect, outside a 'formal' setting. Unusual stress or irregular rhythm may also contribute to the speech disorder, as is very obvious in cases of stammering, but these are not easily quantified and the speech therapist has to rely on descriptive terms which are not standard. In cases referred with voice disorders, special attention would be paid to the pitch used as well as possible range, the manner of breathing while talking, and so on.

It is particularly important when trying to assess a child's competence and performance that not only his age, but also the language used in the home environment, should be taken into account. Conversation with the mother can reveal something of her level of performance. Situations can be devised where one can listen-in while she makes explanations to the child. Bernstein (1968, 1971) in England and a host of writers in the U.S.A. have pointed out the wide variations in range, quality and frequency of the speech and language models to which children of different social classes are exposed, as well as the implications from the nature of the early teaching the child receives from his mother and other members of the family.

Speech Diagnosis
The diagnostic examination includes hearing, intelligence, social adjustment and motor development and should be carried out by audiometrician, psychologist and paediatrician. Often, however, these services are not readily available and the speech therapist has to make her own assessment of these factors and asks for a further examination only when some disability in these areas has been detected or is in doubt. The part of the examination always given by the speech therapist includes auditory discrimination and memory on the *receptive* side, the ability to imitate and the examination of the speech organs, at rest and in movement, on the *motor* side.

Much greater difficulty is experienced in deciding on causes and the appropriate measures to apply to those children whose ability to communicate is limited to vocal signs, manual and facial gesture, and others who do not communicate at all. Some of these children show good understanding of speech, but most of them respond poorly to spoken commands even when it is to their advantage to do so. For example, a child who ignores all instructions of a test and just plays with the material can give the impression that he doesn't understand speech until he is told to 'Put the sixpence in your pocket' or 'Eat the sweet that's in the red box', when he quickly complies. Some children, however, do not respond to such devices and react only to the emotional tones which accompany speech. While there is no doubt that these children have enormous problems of relationships and social adjustment associated with their inability to communicate in the way we expect, certainly their behaviour very often appears the logical result of language deprivation. In Rutter's (1970) article on the concepts of autism he says: 'Of all the hypotheses concerning the nature of autism, that which places the primary defect in terms of a language or coding problem appears most promising'.

In very young speechless children, one tries to find out how much and by what means they are making sense of their environment. This requires a considerable number of observation sessions. There are few generalisations to be made as each speechless child seems unclassifiable in terms of aetiology or behaviour.

A case-history is taken with special attention to speech and language development and the effect of the disability on a person's personality, social life, education and career. Reports from family doctors, health visitors and teachers are sought whenever relevant.

Adults and most children of five and upwards co-operate well in such assessment and diagnostic procedures. Younger children, however, are more likely to be distractible and negative at first and it requires time and skill to get their co-operation. One is wary of coming to a quick decision about the nature or extent of the problem until several periods of observation and trial treatment have added evidence justifying the original hypothesis.

In most cases, however, a speech diagnosis can be made at the first interview, *i.e.* we can usually decide that the patient is suffering from dysarthria or dysphasia; that a child's speech development is slow but of a normal pattern, or arrested in certain aspects only and so on. The speech therapist is not expected to specify which area of the CNS is damaged, but, for the purposes of treatment, assessment is usually much more useful than diagnosis.

Treatment

(In this section, description of treatment is restricted to children with retarded speech development only.)

There is a theory that there is no use in sending a child to a speech therapist until he has begun to talk. Nothing could be further from the truth. If a child has not started to talk (apart perhaps from 'Mummy' and 'Daddy') by 2 years of age, he should be examined by a speech therapist unless he is already found to be deaf or mentally defective. For those who are in doubt as to what can be done for such children, I recommend the article 'Speechless and Backward at Three' by Greene (1967). If a child has started talking ,but is still unintelligible at three, he should be seen by a speech therapist. A child who cannot be understood except by his family should certainly be seen before he goes to school. Most parents are desperately worried about their child's speech delay and are frustrated by their inability to communicate with him. Consequently, they are at the mercy of any one who, unencumbered by any knowledge of the subject, is happy to advise them how to deal with the child, often with unhappy results.

If a child with a speech disorder is not sent to the speech clinic prior to going to school, he is likely to be spotted once he gets there. Unless the child is suffering from a severe speech handicap, I am reluctant to treat him during his first six months of school life. As he is already making big adjustments socially, often these in themselves promote a spontaneous development in speech and language.

Treatment starts with giving the parents information concerning our assessment findings on the nature and cause (as far as we understand it) of the speech problem. In a few cases it is necessary only to demonstrate techniques that they might use at home. Suitable literature and sometimes material for practice can be handed out. There may be no need to see the child again, although a follow-up telephone call, letter, or visit will be necessary to ensure that the advice given has helped the child to make the expected progress and that parental anxiety has been reduced.

On the other hand, many children require regular visits to have skilled treatment by a speech therapist if they are going to make progress more quickly in all aspects of language development, *i.e.* including learning to read, count and measure, as well as learning to express themselves explicitly. The frequency of these visits is determined by the nature and complexity of the problem as well as by the child's age, intelligence and response to therapy and the amount of systematic co-operation from the mother. No rules can be laid down.

Some speech therapists are biased towards teaching, others to psychotherapy, still others to social work. We are trained to work through relationships and very few of us in Britain have experimented regularly with conditioning techniques and teaching machines such as are used in the U.S.A. We aim to develop in the child a desire to, and equip him with, the means of expressing himself and communicating with others by using language that makes his meaning clear. It is of primary importance that attending clinic is a happy experience for him. We gain our relationship with the young child mainly through co-operation in play, and in the older child through giving him the experience of success in learning while taking an interest in him personally, continually drawing him out, and letting him find the pleasure that can be enjoyed from verbal interchange.

Although the British speech therapist's background is mainly medical, her methods of treatment are largely educational (or re-educational) depending to a great extent on her application of phonetics and linguistics as well as her knowledge of psychology.

Articulation

Nearly all cases of slow speech development are sent to a speech therapist because their articulation defects draw attention to their condition. Most of these children are found to be retarded in one or more aspects of language development and this has to be treated concurrently with the articulation problem. Language therapy often continues after the articulation defects have cleared up.

The desire to communicate needs to be linked in the child's mind with the need to make one's meaning clear, and therefore attempts at improving the intelligibility of speech is tied up with the development of language.

The specific techniques we select are based on the findings at the diagnostic examination. Poor auditory discrimination in the presence of normal hearing results in the failure to appreciate the difference between sounds that have one or two features alike. This causes not only poor articulation but also some difficulty with understanding speech and developing a wide vocabulary. A poor auditory memory, whether for immediate repetition or the ability to store sounds in order, can also affect understanding of spoken commands, the development of complex sentences and the choosing of appropriate words.

If a child has a poor auditory discrimination we give him a carefully graded systematic programme of ear training to develop this function to the limits of its potential, at each stage linking *sound* differences to *meaning* differences, *e.g.* comparing *tar* with *car*, *foot* with *put*. Such a child usually increases his vocabulary markedly as a result, but sentence construction is likely to remain telegrammatic until he is taught to attend to the smaller words like *or*, *not*, *in*, *on*, *by*. He will come to a low ceiling beyond which he cannot progress in discriminating sounds, but he can usually make good use of visual cues. Little children are taught to watch the movements of other people's mouths and school-children learn to use the written letters as cues to the nature and order of sounds in a word. The written word, because of its relative permanence on the paper compared with the fleeting nature of spoken words in the ear, can be studied in detail, and the separation of one letter from another—like beads on a string—makes analysis easier. It is therefore vitally important that such a child learns to read well, *i.e.* with accuracy and understanding. He needs infinite practice in reading aloud to someone who will draw attention to his errors and also constantly test his understanding of unusual sentence constructions and the meaning of uncommon words. Then he has to learn how to formulate ideas himself, how to link ideas one to another in a logical sequence or in a time sequence. He should practice recounting events so that his need for self-expression is mediated by the necessity of communicating in a way that makes his meaning clear to others.

There is the large group of speech defective children who have little or no trouble in discriminating and remembering speech sounds but who are unable to produce these sounds at will. Sometimes they can produce the correct sound at the beginning of a word but not at the end of a word. Sometimes they can produce it adjacent to certain vowels or consonants but not adjacent to any others. The speech therapist studies the individual pattern of sound acquisition that the child is developing in each case and programmes her treatment accordingly. The type of movement or posture that is consistently causing the difficulty is identified, *e.g.* friction with the tongue tip. In most cases I find that the best exercise for speech is speech, so would advise practise with syllables, words and sentences using the various oral gymnastics required. One is merely trying to hasten the process which is normally made more gradually through the haphazard practice of everyday talking situations.

In some of these cases, each speech sound has to be taught separately by a form of motor-kinaesthetic training (Stinchfield and Young, 1938, Nelson and Evans 1968). This is often successful in producing good results in young children but is of doubtful value with most older children. Progress is particularly handicapped by the fact that the child seems unable to remember how to reproduce the sounds he has fortuitously made unless they are constantly reinforced by visual and tactile cues. Many of these children have an understanding of spoken language appropriate to their age but show a very retarded development in the ability to use even short sentences without wrongly-ordered words, and grammar which is bizarre rather than infantile. These aspects of language gradually, but very slowly, conform to normal usage at a simple level only, despite systematic and informed teaching.

Language
With the child whose language development is slow it is possible to gradually increase the child's need to use a wider vocabulary and complex *syntactical* constructions to convey his meaning more clearly. By providing practice on material and experiences appropriate to the child's language age and thereby establishing confidence in his ability to communicate and express himself. Pictures of everyday activities are used to help sentence structure, beginning with one person carrying out a single action

('the boy is running') and then by gradually up-grading the difficulty to more complicated pictures which have to be studied silently before a sentence can be formulated embodying the concurrent activities depicted. Rhymes are particularly useful because their rhythm aids the memory for words and those chosen should have simple sentences. Answering questions and conversing about the here-and-now is much easier, of course, to do satisfactorily than reply to 'What did you do last night?' or 'What will you do on Saturday?'. Even more difficult can be 'Tell me how you get dressed in the morning' or 'Tell me how you make a cup of tea'. On other occasions one lets the child ramble along in conversation to some extent if he needs practice in self-expression, but I find that most of them appreciate being questioned as to whom or to what they are referring and why one event should have followed another. Many opportunities for recapitulating stories are given, not only because it gives practice in ordering and linking sentences in a logical sequence, but also because this can help the therapist to pin-point unknown words or idiomatic phrases that are misunderstood.

In other cases, the development of language is not slow but bizarre. A school-age child may have a fair vocabulary but sentences are wrongly constructed and English grammatical rules have never been learned, *e.g.* 'I not went holiday long time yet; 'Me catched him ball; 'When us walk, fell I did'. Such children need a more structured approach to language use in which teacher, speech therapist and mother must work closely together to teach simple but correct sentence patterns. The teaching of reading and writing by the use of colours representing the different grammatical parts of speech is the best possible reinforcement of good sentence construction (Lea 1970).

Most children with defective speech and language have little verbal output. It is often difficult to determine whether they are unable or unwilling to communicate. Sometimes we know that their speech ability is sufficient for them to answer a question, but they will refuse to do so. O'Connor and Hermelin (1963) found their severely subnormal subjects avoided answering in words even when these were available to them unless the material reward made it worthwhile. Nevertheless, I have come to the conclusion that a child's lack of facility with speech is *usually* the main cause for his consistent reluctance to use it, except in cases of elective mutism. I would put the emphasis on trying first to improve the speech skill, although I am only too happy to alternate my periods of treatment with those of a psycho-therapist or to work concurrently with a social worker who is helping the mother.

Results

The use of attainment tests at intervals is the best way we know of objectively measuring progress, although so often we see progress subjectively in the blossoming of the child's personality as he gains confidence in his ability to communicate with those around him. Verbal aggression has to be tolerated for a period from the previously withdrawn child, just as verbosity and constant questioning has to be coped with in the child who has just 'found his tongue'.

There are certain types of difficulty with articulation and language that clear up quite quickly with speech therapy and there are others that persist—though in a less severe form—into adult life. There are children who will never be able to make effective use of speech as a means of communication. It is important that the speech therapist recognises each of those conditions as quickly as possible so that a short course of intensive treatment can be given in certain cases; blocks of treatment alternate with breaks for consolidation for others who will progress slowly and by fits and starts; and, for those who will never learn to speak, assistance with developing a non-verbal means of communication.

The outcome of treatment is fairly easy to forecast in most cases when one takes into account the nature and severity of the child's speech problem, his intelligence and his willingness or drive to communicate. Another guide towards success is the attitude of the family; whether it is one of sensible encouragement or of over-indulgence or of constant nagging. Often the part of treatment that is working for the child's benefit has nothing to do with *his* attending the speech clinic but rather the change of attitude gradually achieved through many conversations with the mother. Very few evaluative studies of speech therapy have been carried out and statements about results at the moment are based on clinical experience rather than controlled studies.

In my experience, from $5\frac{1}{2}$-7 is the age when quickest improvement is achieved (although I would never suggest that one should wait till a child is this age before starting treatment). Unless the speech difficulty is severe, children of average intelligence usually make a good response to speech therapy with a once-weekly attendance for three months and, after a break, one month's further attendance. It is important to ensure in these cases that the child has made a good start in reading before he is finally discharged.

It is not possible to predict when children *severely* handicapped in speech will make strides forward in progress. I have worked with children, barely intelligible at the age of 10 or 12, who have suddenly made a spurt in speech development and within six months have become not only intelligible but able to form fairly long and sometimes complex sentences. Their progress in reading and writing did not, however, match that in spoken language and they remained barely literate into adult life.

Pierre Janet has said: 'Happy is the physician to whom the patient comes when he's about to recover'. Many of our apparent successes fall into this category and may well mislead us into thinking that the specific techniques used were responsible.

REFERENCES

Bernstein, B. (1968) *Everyday Problems of the Child with Learning Difficulties.* New York: John Day.
—— (1971) *Class Codes and Control.* London: Routledge & Kegan Paul.
Eldridge, M. (1968) *A History of the Treatment of Speech Disorders.* Edinburgh: E. & S. Livingstone.
Green, M. C. L. (1967) 'Speechless and backward at three.' *Brit. J. Dis. Commun.,* **4,** 134.
Lea, J. (1970) *The Colour Pattern Scheme.* Hurst Green, Oxted, Surrey: Moor House School.
Morley, M. E. (1971) *Reciprocal Recognition of Qualifications.* United States and United Kingdom Colleges of Speech Therapy, Bulletin No. 225. London: College of Speech Therapists.
Nelson, R. O., Evans, I. M. (1968) 'The combination of learning principles and speech therapy techniques in the treatment of non-communicating children.' *J. Child Psychol. Psychiat.,* **9,** 111
O'Connor, N., Hermelin, B. (1963) *Speech and Thought in Severe Subnormality.* Oxford: Pergamon.
Rutter, M. (1970) 'Autism: concepts and consequences.' *Spec. Educ.,* **59,** (2), 20.
Stinchfield, S. M., Young, E. H. (1938) *Children with Delayed Speech or Defective Speech.* Stanford: Stanford University Press.

CHAPTER 23

Services for Children with Delayed Speech

ESTHER SIMPSON

The value of expert services depends on how effectively they are applied to those who need them. Children with delayed speech are not themselves going to make contact with specialists about their problems. In many instances, parents may fail to recognise their child's problems or may not appreciate the need for educational and medical facilities. It is the task of those who work with children in need of help, together with administrators, to see that existing services are effectively applied.

In different countries, different systems exist for the delivery of services. None is entirely adequate in quantity or quality, but the relative merits and demerits of the various approaches are largely unknown. The measurement of the effectiveness of any particular service is a difficult task and has rarely been undertaken. Nevertheless, it is essential that such measurement should be carried out if we are to make rational decisions on how services are to develop. In this chapter, some of the main considerations will be discussed and the currently existing services in the United Kingdom will be outlined.

Screening

The first issue is whether it can be assumed that all disorders will become manifest in such a way that all parents will know when to bring their children for assessment, or whether special steps must be taken to ensure that some form of screening is applied to the general population to pick out those children in need of help. Specific investigations to answer this question have not been carried out with respect to speech delay, but it is evident from clinical experience that many children are diagnosed too late if it is left to parents to bring children to medical services when they are worried. Parents cannot know all the indications for concern and some form of screening is required.

How such screening should be carried out remains a matter for debate. Of all the remediable conditions likely to be missed, deafness is the most important, and it is generally agreed that screening tests of hearing in infancy are of paramount importance. Because tests are of imperfect reliability, and because children change, it is necessary that those tests be repeated when the children are older. This is particularly the case when other handicaps (such as mental retardation) have made testing more difficult. At present, the situation with respect to screening for hearing defects is less than satisfactory. An enquiry in 1969 (D.H.S.S. 1970) showed that 97 local authorities out of 160 attempted to screen the *whole* child population between the ages of 6 and 12 months, but that only 45 of these were satisfied they actually did so. One hundred and thirty-eight authorities had some type of scheme for screening hearing between these ages, but 42 screened only special groups, *e.g.* children thought to be at 'risk', or those attending clinics. Several studies have shown that this method misses many children with handicaps, and 'at risk' registers are not a reliable means of picking out handicapped children (Rogers 1967, Alberman and Goldstein 1970, Knox and Mahon 1970). Arrangements for screening hearing obviously vary from area to area and it is clear from what has been said already that the situation remains inadequate. Nevertheless, in recent years there has been an increasing awareness of the importance of this sort of service, with an upgrading in the quality of what is provided, as well as a realisation that establishing that a child can hear pure tones is only a beginning. It is still necessary to assess *how* a child is able to use what he hears in order to develop spoken language.

The National Health Service in the U.K. provides direct access to a general practitioner (G.P.), or family doctor, for *all* children, and also to the preventive services of the local authority child health (or welfare) centres. Through the G.P., children may be referred to a complete range of specialist hospital services. When the freely available G.P. service was introduced in 1948, it was thought by some that the number of children attending health or welfare centres would fall, but in fact this did not happen. From 1951 to 1968, the number of children attending these centres rose from 1,370,000 to 1,980,000. However, as the Sheldon Committee reported (Central Health Services Council 1967), the proportion of children attending falls rapidly with increasing age. Most infants attend, but between 2 and 5 years of age only some 20 per cent do so. This fall-off need not happen when much better coverage is provided by some local authorities, but special efforts are needed to ensure regular attendance. An alternative approach is for the G.P. systematically to see all children in his practice at specified ages. This is done by a few family doctors with a special interest in preventive paediatrics but it is very much an exception to the usual procedure. It is evident that at the present time large sections of the population are not being covered by any type of screening procedure and this must be remedied. To effect this requires an appreciation by all those concerned that screening is necessary, and a concerted effort to provide what is required.

Who should carry out *what* sort of screening at *which* ages remains a matter for controversy and further evidence is required on the cost benefits involved. A Spastics Society Working Party (Egan *et al.* 1969) has suggested one possible scheme. This may be more than can be achieved immediately, but a simple assessment of developmental milestones for *all* children on several occasions during the pre-school years is well within the capacity of all local authorities. For this to be effective, however, would require that whoever carried out the screening should have the necessary skills and should be aware of the criteria determining the need for a fuller assessment. In the past, family doctors, health clinic doctors, and indeed hospital specialists, have had little training in developmental assessment. This is gradually being rectified by the provision of post-graduate courses and by changes in medical school training. These improvements in medical education are an essential part of any programme to provide better screening and assessment services for speech retarded children.

Assessment

Once a child has been identified as possibly having a problem with speech development, he needs full and expert assessment. As described in previous chapters, there are many causes of speech delay and many accompanying handicaps. This means

254

that, according to the presenting symptoms, children may be referred to paediatric, psychiatric, audiological or neurological clinics. Specialists in each of these disciplines need to be able to undertake a broad-based assessment of the kind outlined in chapters 3, 6, 7, and 14. As a minimum, assessment should include an evaluation of neurological and general medical function, response to sounds, intellectual level, and overall psychological development, as well as speech and language competence.

Psychological assessment of young children is very important and is available at psychiatric and some paediatric clinics. However, as the Summerfield Report pointed out, there is not at present a clearly defined source in community services from which psychological help and advice can be obtained for children below school-age (Department of Education and Science 1968). Furthermore, not all psychologists have the skills and experience necessary for a detailed assessment of the very young child and for giving firm advice about the management of the problems of children with speech and language delay. Nevertheless, the necessary skills and experience will not be obtained unless psychologists are asked, on a much larger scale than has been the case to date, for an opinion on these children.

Where should the assessment be carried out? There are two main considerations in this connection, which have somewhat contradictory implications. First, assessment must be an ongoing affair having close links with the provision of services. A once-and-for-all assessment, however expert, is not enough because children change and their needs differ as they grow older. Secondly, some children will need specialised diagnostic facilities and evaluation by experts with specialised knowledge which may only be obtainable in large hospital centres with a particular interest in developmental problems. The first is most easily provided in local clinics with close ties with educational and social, as well as medical services, whereas the second may require a regional centre serving a large population. The pros and cons of the latter have been debated on various occasions (Whitmore 1969). Different areas probably require different patterns of services, but in all cases some local provision will be needed as well as more specialised centres to which difficult problems can be referred.

Management and Treatment

The care of children with speech delay requires a multi-faceted approach including: (a) the specific treatment of medical disorders (such as deafness); (b) the prevention of secondary handicaps; (c) advice and counselling of parents; (d) speech and language therapy; (e) nursery school provision; and (f) remedial education. In some cases, other facilities, such as social assistance or genetic counselling, will be needed.

Some of these facilities are described in earlier chapters. The evidence concerning the effects of language delay on psychological development (see chapter 15) emphasises the importance of providing the child and his family with advice and counselling so that secondary handicaps may be avoided. Parents need practical suggestions on what they should and should not do in order to give their child the best opportunity for normal development. Speech therapists, among others, have an important part to play in this respect, as well as in direct therapy with the child. At one time speech therapy was mainly pre-occupied with the correction of speech defects, but there is

255

now a much greater awareness of the importance of *language*, and well-trained speech therapists may guide parents on how to help their child's language development. Some aspects of speech therapists' work have been described in chapters 6, 9, 21, and 22. In the U.K., although some work in paediatric or psychiatric clinics, most speech therapists are employed by the local authority, so that their main link is with community, rather than with hospital, services. The need for close liaison between speech therapists and medical specialists has been emphasised in chapter 6.

Because this book has been primarily written for doctors, less attention has been given to the provision of education for children with speech delay. This in no way reflects its importance. Both in the pre-school years and after 5 years of age, educational measures have a *crucial* rôle. If these are to be effectively applied, doctors must be aware of the needs and what is available.

All local education authorities have powers to provide for the special needs of handicapped children from the age of 2 onwards. This provision may take the form of play-groups, nursery schools, special classes, units and schools, and authorities carry out their duties in different ways and to different degrees. Before any special arrangements can be provided, the local authority must be made aware of the need for them, and this emphasises an important responsibility of those who carry out the initial medical and psychological assessment of children with speech delay. There is a definite onus on those who see children with possible learning difficulties to communicate with the local education authority giving details about the children involved and advice concerning the kind of special educational setting most likely to help the individual child.

Nursery schools and play groups may be helpful for some children with speech delay, but the benefit varies greatly with the type of provision and the type of child, so that pre-school educational services need very careful planning. The experience of teachers in dealing with speech retarded children is one factor and the more severely affected children often do better in nursery groups specifically catering for handicapped children. The amount of supervision and attention is important and the content of activities is also relevant. Nursery schools must make deliberate efforts to provide *specific* training appropriate to the child's handicaps.

Speech delay is often followed by difficulties in learning to read (see chapter 15) and for this reason alone (as well as the need to take account of the child's communication difficulties in devising teaching methods), special attention must be paid to the type of schooling provided. Some children with language difficulties will cope perfectly adequately in ordinary schools with additional specialist help (such as from speech therapists). Others will require full-time or part-time attendance at special classes, and some will be properly placed in special schools. Educational provision for children with hearing impairment, cerebral palsy or mental retardation is the most developed, and special training is available for teachers wishing to teach children with these handicaps. The provision for children with other handicaps is less satisfactory, although in recent years there have been important developments in the establishment of special classes and special schools for children with speech delay and autistic children. The extent of these developments varies greatly among local authorities and provision is still inadequate in many areas.

The hard-and-fast categories of handicap laid down by the Department of Education and Science in *Handicapped Pupils and Special Schools Regulations, 1959*, may sometimes impede the placement of children with language disorders who often have other problems as well. As diagnosis, both medical and educational, has improved, there has come a greater awareness of how seldom a child has a single handicap and how infrequently he can be placed unreservedly in a single recognised category of handicap. Instead of this categorisation, perhaps in future it will be possible to provide schools which offer a particular kind of education rather than a place for a child with a particular kind of handicap. This would make placement easier and would allow more ready modification and greater flexibility in the educational environment. Such a change, however, would depend, even more than present arrangements, on detailed guidance from doctors and psychologists about the sort of educational milieu required for the individual child and about the educational implications of the medical and psychological findings.

In providing services for speech retarded children, co-operation and communication between all concerned is vital. Education authorities see assessment units mainly as sources of advice about the educational placement of handicapped children. Paediatricians view diagnosis principally in terms of children's medical needs. However, there is a very encouraging tendency for paediatricians to include response to education as an important factor in the overall evaluation of young children. The aim of services must be to provide earlier, and more skilful, recognition of children with delayed or deviant development of speech and language, and, having recognised them, to provide an individual programme of education designed to minimise the child's disability and to enable the child to make the best possible use of his assets.

REFERENCES

Alberman, E. D., Goldstein, H. (1970) The 'At Risk' Register: a statistical evaluation.' *Brit J. prev. soc. Med.*, **24**, 129.

Central Health Services Council. (1967) Child Welfare Centres. Report of the Sub-committee 1967. London: H.M.S.O.

Department of Education and Science. (1968) Psychologists in Education Services: the Report of a Working Party appointed by the Secretary of State for Education and Science. London: H.M.S.O.

D.H.S.S. (1970) On the State of the Public Health. The Annual Report of the Chief Medical Officer of the Department of Health and Social Security for the Year 1969. London: H.M.S.O.

Egan, D., Illingworth, R. S., MacKeith, R. C. (1969) *Developmental Screening 0-5 Years*. Clinics in Developmental Medicine, No. 30. London: S.I.M.P. with Heinemann.

Knox, E. G., Mahon, D. F. (1970) Evaluation of 'infant at risk' registers.' *Arch. Dis. Childh.*, **45**, 634-639.

Rogers, M. G. H. (1967) 'The "at risk" register. *Med. Offr.*, **118**, p. 253.

Whitmore, K. (1969) 'An assessment service for handicapped children.' *Med. Offr.*, **122**, p. 263.

APPENDIX I: Tests Used Routinely in the Speech Clinic

A Picture Screening Test of Hearing. (Reed 1960). Age Range 2-4 years. This test is in book form. Each page has four pictures representing words with acoustically similar names, which have to be identified on request. The intensity of the tester's voice is constant at a specific level relevant to the child's threshold for speech. The number of items confused are recorded and may be analysed acoustically. No lip-reading is allowed.

The Kendal Toy Vocabulary Test. Age range 2-4 years. There are ten small objects (toys) to be identified on request. In each series the 'key' objects have names which are acoustically similar to others presented at the same time. These objects are placed in front of the child in such positions that there is an equal chance of any being selected. The number of errors are noted together with the level of loudness of the speaker's voice, which must be constant throughout the test, and may be analysed acoustically. No lip-reading is allowed.

The Manchester Picture Vocabulary Test. Age range 4-7 years. There are six lists of 20 monosyllabic words. The vocabulary range is simple and an attempt has been made, within the length of the lists, to secure homogeneity and equality of difficulty. The words were chosen to give as wide a selection as possible of the phonemes in Standard English. The words are depicted on three sets of 20 cards each. On each card are six pictures, one of which illustrates the stimulus word. A varying number of the other five words contain the same vowels or the same consonants. The child is asked to point to the stimulus word on request. The errors are noted and the percentage correctly selected is recorded together with the intensity of the speaker's voice as it reaches the ear.

The Manchester Junior Word Lists. Age range 7-10 years. There are eight lists of 25 words containing vocabulary based on that of children entering school. Each list is presented at a specific intensity and each word is repeated by the child. The number of errors are noted and the percentage correct at a specific level of loudness is also noted. This test is not suitable for a child with an articulation defect.

A Test of Understanding the Spoken Word (Richards 1967) (Speech Audiometry). This test was intended for speech defective children and requires no speech from the child. It consists of 20 oral instructions requiring the child to carry out actions with the test equipment of dolls' furniture. During the development of the test, about 50 normal children were tested in each of the four main groups with median ages of $3\frac{1}{2}$, 4, $4\frac{1}{2}$ and 5 years, and the mean scores noted. The standard deviation shown by each age group was approximately 3.7. The scores are calculated from the number of commands the child carries out correctly.

Kuhlmann-Anderson Test (*Modified*). Age range 1.4-4.4 years. Simple commands and gesture are used at the start of this test, then identification by pointing. Subsequent commands involve activity, then simple questions are asked requiring some verbal response. At the end of the test the child is asked to identify pictures according to what is happening and then according to the relationship of the objects. The number of correct responses are scored and then those partially correct are also scored. The total score is interpreted in terms of age levels and the test is used to arrive at the level of comprehension the child is showing relative to the norm. (Obtainable from N.F.E.R., Windsor, Berks.)

The English Picture Vocabulary Test (Brimer and Dunn 1963). Age range 3-5 years, 5-9 years and 7-12 years. (This is the English adaptation of the Peabody Test.) It is designed to test comprehension in terms of recognition of specific items of vocabulary in picture form. It is in book form. There are four black and white pictures per page. The stimulus picture has to be identified on request. The vocabulary becomes progressively more advanced. The total number of correct responses are scored and the level of comprehension calculated from normative data supplied.

An English Language Scale (Watts 1964). Age range 4-10 years. This is a picture description test designed to measure the progress of young children in mastering the basic varieties of the English sentence. It tests the ability to frame a fresh sentence on a given pattern. Each page has six black and white pictures. The tester describes the first two twice according to specific instructions. The child's description of the other four pictures is noted in full and scored according to instructions for structure of sentences and content. The level of language used is calculated from normative data supplied.

The Edinburgh Articulation Test (Anthony *et al.* 1971). Age range 3-6 years. Forty-one coloured pictures in book form have to be named or repeated. These present a balanced and comprehensive selection of consonants and consonant clusters occurring in English at various positions in the word structure in monosyllabic, disyllabic and a few polysyllabic words. It is concerned with consonants since it is considered that vowel systems are established in children's speech at an early age. It does not test articulation in continuous speech. The pictures are presented one at a time and the response of

259

the child is noted A raw score of consonants correctly pronounced when naming pictures is calculated and converted into a standard score. An 'articulatory age' can be determined from the normative data supplied. From phonetic representations of the consonants actually produced by the child, the degree of immaturity of articulatory forms can be worked out using the qualitative data supplied, and deviant patterns of articulation can be readily identified.

For full references to the tests see chapter 6.

*See chapter 7, page 85.

For the Reynell Developmental Language Scales (1969) and the Renfrew Word Finding Vocabulary Scale (1964) see chapter 9.

APPENDIX II: Case Histories

CASE 1. An Adolescent Boy Suffering from Stammering

The mother, who was Norwegian in origin, had three pregnancies. The first resulted in the birth of the patient, the second in a miscarriage, and the third in the birth of a boy who is healthy, intelligent and successful educationally and socially.

The mother's uncle on her father's side had had a stammer. Her husband had suffered recurrent severe episodes of depression for seventeen years and had been retired from the Overseas Civil Service. His disorder had caused a great upset in his parents lives and had resulted in a great deal of domestic stress. During her first pregnancy with T., the mother was admitted to hospital at about four months gestation for a period of three weeks. There she felt tired and ill. The labour occurred at term and lasted about six hours. Delivery was in hospital and the child weighed 3.2 kg. He seemed healthy, though he was unable to breast feed and bottle feeding had to be instituted, after which he thrived. His early milestones of motor, linguistic, adaptive and social behaviour were within normal limits. He was walking without support quite steadily at the age of fourteen months and could feed himself by the age of fifteen months. No clumsiness in handling objects was ever observed. He could dress himself before the age of six except for small buttons and laces which he managed before the age of seven. He was toilet trained night and day shortly after the age of four.

He went to the local primary school and managed to retain his place in an A stream with some difficulty. He stayed there until the age of 10½ when the family returned home on account of the father's illness. He then went to a primary school in the North of Scotland but failed an intelligence test to assess his suitability for senior secondary education. He was only admitted after his parents had appealed to the Director of Education when the boy was 12½ years old. He has held his place in the senior secondary school, however, and is in the middle of his class, though he is about one year older than most of the children in it. No behaviour difficulties were reported. At home he was intensely jealous of his more gifted younger brother who did rather better at school, and he made no effort to conceal his feelings. His reaction to the situation was to concern himself in his own persuits in an independent way, making model aeroplanes with petrol engines and radio control which actually flew. He has always been liable to become anxious in stressful situations such as examination and complains of 'feeling a lump in my chest'. He perspires excessively when he is anxious. During the episode of his father's depression which necessitated the family coming home to Scotland, he was very concerned and his concern was increased when his classmates told him that his father had been admitted 'to the loony bin'. His general health had been good though he had suffered from measles and chickenpox. He had been vaccinated and immunised against diphtheria, tetanus, whooping-cough and poliomyelitis without adverse reactions.

He said his first intelligible words, other than 'ma' and 'da', at the age of about a year but was not an 'early talker'. He had phrases before the age of two years and at the age of two was talking in sentences quite clearly. At the age of four and a half, a few months after the birth of his brother, he began to hesitate when talking and had 'difficulty in getting his words out'. This difficulty was most prominent in single words, especially those at the beginning of phrases or sentences, but he would 'force them out' even though he would become red or blue in the face in the process of doing so. In the course of time he had learnt a great many 'tricks' to avoid words on which he thought he would stammer. His mother observed that he would begin sentences with 'And' or 'Is it possible', or if asked a question would say 'Now wait', in order, as he said, to give him time to organise his answer. His mother did not think that his speech difficulties had altered in any way until the family had come back to Scotland, since when they had lead to increasing difficulty. The boy had trouble not only in initiating sentences and phrases but also in the middle of sentences so that there might be arrest of speech, repetition of individual syllables or single words or even a number of words.

He had become increasingly aware of his speech difficulties and had been teased about them to some extent by other pupils at school. He had observed to his mother: 'Sometimes I wonder what life is going to be like with this'. He tended to avoid talking as much as possible and many of his pursuits had become increasingly solitary as his speech difficulties worsened.

The severity of his stammer and hesitations varied considerably in different situations. No stammer occurred when he was relaxed and model-making with close friends but if, for example, he was asked to read aloud in school, his stammering became severe. Between the ages of 12 and 14 he had received quite prolonged speech therapy locally, but though the speech therapist felt that he had derived benefit from treatment, neither the boy nor the mother felt his speech had improved. In desperation, Mrs. T. asked to be referred to the Speech Clinic in the Royal Hospital for Sick Children.

On examination, no physical abnormalities were found and his hearing appeared to be acute. He showed a marked speech dysrhythmia, however, which involved hesitations, repetition of syllables. words and word-groups, and he had a large repertoire of 'tricks' by which he tried to overcome his difficulties. In particular, he tried to avoid words beginning with 'h', 'b'. 'l' and 's' on which he knew he was likely to stammer. Stammering and hesitation was apparent when he was in conversation and also when he was reading aloud.

The speech therapist who saw him in the clinic assessed his speech and hearing and submitted the following report.

'This boy has a severe secondary stammer. He shows initial blocking of consonants and re-petition of initial syllables of words. He starts phrases with 'and' or 'um' and is generally unable to initiate speech without these aids. He uses circumlocution to avoid feared words and replaces difficult words by those he finds easier to produce. He has a marked facial grimace when speaking.

Breathing. He has a poor breathing pattern. Inspiration is shallow and he expires most of the air on the first word then completes the phrase rapidly.

Speed of utterance is excessive. 186 words were recorded in one minute. His speech accelerated rapidly in conversation and he showed a strong tendency to 'clutter'.

Voice has recently 'broken' and is extremely variable in pitch. *Comprehension*. He achieved a comprehension level of 16.5 years on the Peabody Picture Vocabulary Test.

Expressive language was comparatively retarded and he achieved a 12 year level on both the Watts Ideational Addition Test and the Watts Sentence Completion Test. These tests were selected in this case as they did not involve much use of continuous speech which might be distorted on account of his stammer.

Auditory discrimination was exceptionally poor and the errors produced indicated that it was defective at a 5 year level on the Wepman Test of Auditory Discrimination. This test requires the subject to judge whether pairs of words spoken are the same or different.

Hearing. This was excellent on formal audiometric testing and no problems had occurred previously.'

Since he was interested in aeroplanes of the Second World War, he was asked to write a composi-tion about this subject and he wrote an excited description of the development of fighter command be-tween 1931 and 1940 which was accurate and included extracts from Sir Winston Churchill's speeches which were also accurately remembered, but his writing was poor and clumsy and he made a large number of grammatical mistakes, tending to omit verbs, prepositions and articles, and using incorrect tenses. These mistakes became more frequent as he warmed to his theme. He drew quite skilfully.

It was felt that the boy, who was very aware of his severe hesitations and stammer and was in-creasingly embarrassed by them, should receive intensive speech therapy and this was arranged as an inpatient in view of the fact that he lived so far away from Edinburgh. He was admitted to hospital a few days after he had been seen in the outpatient clinic. The speech therapist was treating a group of children of similar age suffering from speech dysrhythmia. He stayed in the hospital convalescent ward and received daily therapy in this group.

Therapy

Intensive speech therapy was given for three weeks during which time he received therapy daily in a group situation with two other adolescent boys. A modified course in 'syllable-timed speech, was provided after the pattern evolved by Andrews and Harris (1964).

The problem was tackled in three ways. First, the spontaneous use of syllable-timed speech in all conversational situations was established. The boys were instructed in the use of this new speech pattern, their rhythmic skills were developed, and they were instructed in the techniques of correct breathing patterns and general relaxation.

The next stage of therapy aimed at improving their general confidence in the use of syllable-timed speech in conversation outside the clinic. General discussion and counselling preceded this stage of therapy. Independence of action and thought was encouraged in routine situations in the hospital and outside: they asked questions from strangers, planned outings, answered the phone and took messages. General linguistic skills were improved by formal language work, reading and discussion: they wrote a play for public performance to staff and parents. Manipulative and artistic skills were encouraged by letting them make equipment and decorations for use in the department.

The parents were helped by advice on ways to encourage their child at home. They attended as a group for discussion of mutual problems under the guidance of the therapist. The actual process of syllable-timed speech and the mechanism by which it helps the stammerer was discussed together with the aims and expectations of the course.

Response to Therapy

This was excellent. At the end of the course he was able to control his speech in all conversational situations encountered routinely. He mastered the techniques of syllable-timed speech immediately and his general confidence increased daily. Confidence in his ability to use syllable-timed speech in conversation with strangers followed.

His parents were pleased with his progress and co-operated fully with all stages of treatment. He was, however, garrulous by nature and showed minimal awareness of any errors he made in speech and the possibility of relapse was great. When he attended for review six months after the course of therapy his speech was normal and he was discharged from the Speech Clinic.

CASE 2.   A Boy with Post-traumatic Dysarthria due to Bulbar Palsy

There was no family history of speech problems. Labour was at term and the baby weighed 3.4 kg. At the age of three years and eight months he was knocked down by a car, was immediately unconscious and suffered a fractured skull. He remained unconscious for three-and-a-half weeks, during which time neurosurgical explorations showed no evidence of intra-cerebral or meningeal haemorrhage. There was some brain swelling at the time of the first exploration. Because of a markedly abnormal electroencephalogram showing bursts of epileptic activity, sodium hydantoate was prescribed. He was admitted to a convalescent home eight weeks after the accident. He showed limited comprehension and had only a few, unintelligible words. There was a marked inco-ordination when he tried to handle objects or to walk and involuntary movements were present in the lips, tongue, palate and in all four limbs. Eight months after his accident he could walk reasonably steadily but he was apathetic and had considerable drooling from the mouth. He became more active and developed restless and destructive behaviour. Sodium hydantoate continued to be administered. By the age of four years and nine months he could obey simple commands but his speech was limited and difficult to understand. Two years after the accident he was discharged home and referred to the Speech Clinic because his speech was poor and partly on account of his over-activity.

On examination he was seen to drool continuously from the mouth. There was marked dysarthria with slow speech, omission or substitution of consonants and vowel sounds and much intelligibility. There was paresis of the tongue, more marked on the right side. His movements were rather clumsy. He was found to be deaf bilaterally and was thought to have a sensori-neural deafness with a conductive overlap. It was considered that the boy showed evidence of bulbar paresis with dysarthria and a hyperkinetic behaviour disorder which had not responded to treatment with sodium hydantoate.

He was referred to the Royal Hospital for Sick Children, Edinburgh. Here, his severe dysphonia indicated unilateral paresis of the vocal cords and subsequent laryngoscopy revealed swelling of the left false cord and scarring of the related tissues. It was thought that the left cord was paralysed. Sodium hydantoate was replaced by sulphiame (100 mg three times per day) and there was a mild but definite improvement in his over-activity. His electroencephalogram continued to show generalised bursts of epileptic activity more evident in the left hemisphere than the right.

He received a course of intensive speech therapy twice daily for eight weeks and co-operated well in these sessions. Response to therapy was satisfactory as shown by his improvement in test scores and increased use of speech in the play group. Imitation of speech sounds was sufficiently poor for dyspraxia to be suspected. It was recommended that he should have a full audiological investigation by a medical and educational team and that he should receive remedial teaching and speech therapy after discharge.

CASE 3.   A Boy with Dysarthria Associated with Nuclear Agenesis (Moebius' Syndrome)

The family history was unremarkable. The mother was rh negative and because of this was admitted to hospital at an estimated 38 weeks gestation where delivery was by forceps. The baby weighed 2.1 kg.

He sat without support shortly before the age of one year, crawled at about 16 months but did not walk until the age of 20 months. Although he could not speak at the time of referral, his parents were convinced that he could hear and comprehend what was said to him. The only physical abnormality his parents noted was that he had an alternating convergent strabismus. They also noted that his face was rather expressionless.

On examination he was observed to play with toys in an aimless way and his concentration was limited. He was hyperdistractible. There was continuous mouth breathing without drooling saliva. Swallowing was somewhat laboured and associated with tongue protrusion.

The medical opinion was that B. showed generalised retardation of all aspects of behaviour development: in addition there was evidence of nuclear agenesis affecting the third, sixth, seventh, ninth, tenth and twelfth cranial nerves. The neurological findings were confirmed. It proved impossible to obtain any reliable assessment of his intelligence.

At the age of five, arrangements were made for him to attend the Speech Therapy Department twice weekly. Therapy aimed at encouraging direct imitation of speech sounds in a play situation, increasing vocabulary and training him to listen. This proved unsuccessful in an individual situation but he did well in a nursery group. Therapy was then given in the presence of a child with similar problems. There was immediate improvement in co-operation and although articulation was very immature he was soon volunteering single words in response to pictures.

262

At the age of six he was given the Peabody Picture Vocabulary Test which showed that he was understanding speech at a 3.7 year level. General language stimulation was given with particular attention to discrimination of nouns, *e.g.* the names of animals, and adjectives like 'big' and 'little'. He could soon use two-word phrases spontaneously and these were expanded into three-word phrases. He developed an increasing interest in written material. His speech was hyper-nasal and dysarthric. Specific articulation therapy was then added to language therapy. All successful attempts at articulation of plosives were reinforced by smiles, verbal praise and 'stars' in his speech book. The results were good and his confidence increased. Interest in the written presentation of speech work continued and he soon began to copy letters and words. He is now able to communicate intelligibly by speech, his reading and writing skills are developing, and he is benefitting from an increased ability to communicate in all fields.

CASE 4. A Boy with Slow Speech Development associated with Mental Retardation

The boy was born at term and weighed 3.1 kg. There were no complications. His eldest sister had spastic cerebral palsy with mental retardation. There was no other family history of abnormality. Motor development was normal but speech development was slow; much of what he said was unintelligible. He was operated on for strabismus on two occasions between the ages of two-and-a-half and three years. At the age of four-and-a-half he was referred to the Speech Clinic with retarded speech.

On examination no neurological abnormalities were found apart from a persisting mild bilateral strabismus associated with hypometropia. The medical opinion was that the boy was not deaf or psychotic but that he was somewhat mentally retarded and had a disproportionately severe developmental speech disorder. He was referred for psychometric assessment. Examination of his chromosomes showed a normal pattern and examination of his blood and urine by amino acid chromatography and a Guthrie test showed no abnormality. At the speech therapy dept. which he attended once weekly for six weeks, he was generally silent during the sessions unless stimulated to produce words. It was reported that he did not speak at school but that he 'chattered away' at home. A fluctuating dysphonia was noted. His hearing was tested and was normal but his auditory discrimination was poor.

He went to primary school at the age of five years and eight months. He made little progress in reading but had some grasp of numbers.

He was seen by the medical team in the Speech Clinic at six monthly intervals and speech therapy was carried out weekly. When he was eight-and-a-half years old a full reassessment was made. At this time involuntary movements of the lips, tongue and palate and of the outstretched hands were noted. It was suspected that he was suffering from 'rheumatic chorea' though there was no evidence of carditis.

He was seen again three months later and his choreoid movements had virtually disappeared. It was considered that a period of intensive speech therapy as an inpatient would be worthwhile, and he was admitted to a convalescent unit.

CASE 5. A Boy with Specific Retardation of Speech Development (Specific Speech Development Syndrome)

There was no family history of slow speech development known to the parents. Birth was at term by breech extraction and there was prolapse of the cord for several minutes before birth. Birth weight was 3.3 kg. The boy was cyanosed and required intermittent positive pressure ventilation. As a precaution he was placed in an incubator for 24 hours. His speech development was slow and his articulation was defective. His mother thought that his hearing was intact and that he 'understood everything that was said to him'. He was referred to the Speech Clinic at four years and five months of age.

On examination, no neurological or physical abnormalities were found. His hearing seemed acute. His speech showed substitutions of 't' for 'k', 'd' for 'g', 's' for 'v', 'sh' for 'f' and 'ta' for 'ti'. Occasionally he could not pronounce 'th' and had difficulty with consonant clusters especially at the end of words. Auditory discrimination was normal. On the Peabody Picture Vocabulary Test his comprehension was at a 4 year level, but his expressive language scores were at a 3½ year level for both information and grammar on the Action Picture Test. On the Edinburgh Articulation Test his articulation was very immature, below a 3 year level. He showed retarded speech development without any associated mental retardation, mental defect or psychiatric disorder. His IQ was assessed as 118 on the Stanford-Binet L-M Scale. It was considered that progress would be made without the help of speech therapy and that the child should be reviewed after six months.

After six months, his mother reported that his speech was much improved and was intelligible to other members of the family and to neighbours. He was attending a local nursery school. A second neurological examination found no abnormalities. His comprehension had improved to a 4 year level and his expressive language levels for information and grammar were at a 4.5 year level. His articulation was almost mature and measured at 3.5 years on the Edinburgh Articulation Test. As he was soon to enter school, it was decided that the best course would be to refer the boy to the local school speech therapist to be observed periodically and treated if teachers or other pupils found him significantly difficult to understand.

263

CASE 6. A Boy Suffering from the Effects of High Tone Hearing Loss with a Choreoid Syndrome Secondary to Kernicterus

There was no known family history of hearing loss or speech difficulties. The mother had a high antibody titre and an intra-uterine transfusion was carried out at an estimated 24 weeks gestation. At an estimated 28 weeks gestation, labour occurred spontaneously and the child was delivered by assisted breech. He weighed 1.59 kg. He was apnoeic, oedematous, and jaundiced. His blood group was A-rhesus-positive and the Coomb's test was positive. Resuscitation was carried out by tracheal intubation and intermittent positive pressure respiration. An immediate exchange transfusion was given through the umbilical cord. Two further transfusions were given on the second and third days after birth. He was tube fed and suffered five apnoeic attacks associated with cyanosis during the first week of life. He was in an incubator for approximately six weeks and was discharged at the age of 12 weeks weighing 2.72 kg.

His early motor milestones were within normal limits. At about one year of age his mother became worried by his lack of response to sounds. At between one year and eighteen months of age he was seen by a local E.N.T. surgeon who diagnosed serious hearing impairment. Subsequently he was seen by a teacher of the deaf and an audiologist who prescribed a Medrasco hearing aid. The child responded immediately. He began to babble 'furiously'. Tonsillectomy and adenoidectomy were performed after a series of tonsillitis and enlargment of neck glands with fever attacks. At the age of two-and-a-half he was still without any words. He received private speech therapy and developed some words of speech. He became more sociable and seemed to understand more of what was said to him as long as whoever was speaking faced him. At the age of three years and two months he was seen at the Speech Clinic.

The history was noted. During examination he responded to loud sounds, showed no gross abnormalities of adaptive behaviour and tried to be social within the limits of his language. He could understand simple commands if he was facing the person giving them. He uttered many single words, some of which were intelligible to everyone present. He showed impairment of upward gaze and some involuntary movements of the lips, tongue and palate especially when he was under emotional stress. Slight involuntary choreoid and athetoid movements were present in the right hand. Muscle tone was slightly reduced, and biceps, triceps, supinator, knee and ankle jerks were sluggish, more so on the right than the left. As far as could be tested there was no defect in other systems. It was thought that the boy had severe hearing impairment, probably as a result of severe rhesus incompatability. He had an above average intelligence.

A high tone hearing aid was prescribed and the child immediately improved. Auditory training and speech therapy continued. Therapy aimed at improving auditory attention by the use of the hearing aid and lip-reading and by increased use of auditory training techniques at home and in the nursery school. Parental sympathy and interest in the child's problem was encouraged by involving the mother in the clinical training sessions. The boy received specific language therapy in formal structured play situations using toys to correspond to real life activities. His response to therapy was excellent. His mother became increasingly interested and proficient in the techniques of auditory training and showed amazing insight into his problems. The boy improved dramatically.

Therapy continues on a weekly basis. The boy's speech is readily intelligible to all.

Subject Index

A

Adenoids: 19.
Approach to the child: 173.
Articulation: 7, 42, 70, 152, 204, 249.
——, defects, prevalence of: 48.
Assessment, clinical: 33 *et seq.*, 68 *et seq.*, 254.
——, psychological: 106 *et seq.*, 255.
At risk concept: 83.
Attention: 37, 95 *et seq.*
Audiometry: 79, 85 *et seq.*, 222, 259.
——, EEG: see EEG audiometry.
Audio-visual integration test: 124.
Auditory discrimination: 2, 29, 95 *et seq.*, 249.
Auditory Discrimination Test: 116, 124.
Autism: 26, 36, 38, 43, 45, 93, 130, 150 *et seq.*, 206 *et seq.*, 247.
——, prevalence of: 50.
Autism, and thinking: 178.

B

Babble: 4, 39, 53, 148, 151, 169.
Behaviour modification techniques: 117, 156, 204 *et seq.*
——, evaluation of results: 212 *et seq.*
Bilingualism: 59.
Binet test: 122, 137.
Blocking, speech: 16.
Brain development: 1, 102.
Brain injury: 1, 187.
Brain, unilateral lesions of: 2.
British Intelligence Scales: 106.
Brooklands experiment: 142.

C

Cerebral palsy: 21, 93, 96, 182.
——, prevalence of: 50.
Child-minding arrangements: 149.
Chimpanzees, language in: 9.
Classification of speech and language disorders: 13 *et seq.*
Cleft palate: 18.
Clutter: 15.
'Codeme': 192.
Code, symbolic: 33, 96, 180, 189 *et seq.*
Codes of communication: 189 *et seq.*

Codes, restricted and elaborated: 27, 61, 144.
Columbia Mental Maturity Scale: 122.
Comprehension, assessment of: 36 *et seq.*, 72, 109 *et seq.*
Concepts, learning of: 4. 177.
Cognition: see intelligence.
Communication: 33, 43, 191 *et seq.*, 231.
Cries, types of: 2, 168.

D

Deaf environment: 59, 102.
Deafness: see hearing loss.
——, psychogenic: 89.
Decision to respond to sounds: 90.
Deep structure: 9.
Definitions of speech and language: 33, 189.
Denver Developmental Screening Test: 116, 121.
Deprivation: see environmental influences.
Development of brain: see brain development.
Development of speech and language: 1 *et seq.*, 191 *et seq.*, 223.
Developmental diagnosis: 69 *et seq.*, 116, 169.
Developmental speech disorder syndrome: 27 *et seq.*, 36, 38, 39, 40, 78, 179, 263.
——, prevalence of: 49.
Deviant speech or language: 28, 40, 41, 55, 63, 148, 161 *et seq.*
Diagnosis: 30, 33 *et seq.*, 79, 172, 173, 195, 247.
Disproportion of jaw or palate: 19 *et seq.*
Down's syndrome: 2, 17, 73, 138, 142, 143, 148.
Dysarthria: 17 *et seq.*, 43, 262.
Dysphasia, acquired: 25.
Dysphonia: 14, 44, 73.
Dysrhythmia, speech: 15 *et seq.*, 44, 73.

E

Echoing: 7, 42, 151, 208.
Edinburgh Articulation Test: 78, 259.
EEG audiometry: 79, 92.
Emotional development: 100, 181 *et seq.*
Environment, meaning of: 52, 63.
——, structuring of: 205, 230, 235.
Environmental influences: 10, 39, 52 *et seq.*, 101, 142.
English Picture Vocabulary Test: 140, 259.
Expansions: 55.

F

Family doctor: 254.
Family history of speech disturbances: 15, 28.
Family influences: 24, 57, 171.
Family size: 14, 57.
Feedback: 95 *et seq.*
Frostig Developmental Perception Test: 106, 121, 124.
Fry list: 85.
Functional analysis: 204.

G

Genetic factors: 15, 57, 59, 60, 83, 86, 153.
Gesell schedules: 69, 121.
Gesture: 4, 40, 178, 194, 231.
'Go' game: 85.
Grammar: see syntax.
Grammatical rules: see rules of grammar.
Griffiths Scale: 121.
Gunzburg charts: 116.

H

Hare-lip: 18.
Head circumference: 73.
Hearing aids: 220 *et seq.*
Hearing, assessment of: 37, 76, 84 *et seq.*
Hearing behaviour: 83 *et seq.*
Hearing loss: 21, 24, 36, 39, 40, 70, 73, 80, 83 *et seq.*, 181, 184.
——, and thinking: 177.
Hearing loss, high tone: 43, 73, 88, 264.
——, prevalence of: 49.
Heller's syndrome: 156.
Hester Adrian Research Centre charts: 116.
Hobsbaum test: 111.
Houston Test of Language Development: 116.
Hyporhinophonia: 19, 21.

I

Identification of sounds: 90.
Illinois Test of Psycholinguistic Abilities: 58, 107, 111 *et seq.*, 121, 137, 143.
Imitation: 35, 53, 180, 196, 207.
Imitation training: 211.
Inner language: see language, inner.
Institutional influences: 27, 56 *et seq.*, 92, 149.
Intellectual development: 44, 120 *et seq.*, 136 *et seq.*
Intelligence, assessment of: 44, 106, 120 *et seq.*

K

Kendall Toy Vocabulary Test: 85, 259.
Kibbutzim: 56.

Knobloch Developmental Scales: 121.
Kuhlmann-Anderson Test: 259.

L

Labelling: 4, 210.
Language acquisition device: 103, 144.
Language, comprehension: 3, 4, 7, 28, 36 *et seq.*, 72, 79, 107 *et seq.*, 149, 180, 182, 229, 247.
Language delay, effects on development: 176 *et seq.*
Language environment, clarity of: 57.
Language, inner: 6, 35, 178, 193, 195, 196.
Language production: 40 *et seq.*, 78 *et seq.*, 111 *et seq.*
Language tests: 80, 106 *et seq.*, 251.
Language training: 208, 238, 250.
Laryngoscopy: 14.
Laterality, testing: 75.
Leiter International Performance Scale: 122.
Listening: 37, 95.
Localisation of sound: 3, 48, 91.

M

Manchester Picture Vocabulary Test: 259.
Manchester Word Lists: 85, 259.
'Memord': 192.
Mental retardation: see retardation, mental.
Merrill-Palmer Scale: 122, 137.
Michigan Picture Language Inventory: 115.
Mime: see gesture.
Models of language development: 103.
Moebius' syndrome: 23, 76, 262.
Motivation: 90, 99, 125, 237.
Motor impersistence test: 124.
Movements, involuntary: 76.
Mutism, elective: 26, 36, 38, 43, 45, 156 *et seq.*, 206.

N

Neoligisms: 42.
Neonatal period: 2, 168.
Neurological disorder: 21, 43, 142, 147, 153, 182, 185 (see also cerebral palsy).
Neurological examination: 75.
Nodules, vocal cord: 14.
Nursery schools: see pre-school programmes.

O

Open class words: see pivot.
Operant techniques: see behaviour modification.
Oseretsky test of motor co-ordination: 124.
Otitis media: 18, 88.